DOG BREEDING
A complete reference book

Dr KGM de Cramer

Reference book on dog breeding for beginners and seasoned breeders

Author
Kurt G.M. De Cramer, BVSc, MMedVet (Gyn), PhD
Small Animal Reproductive specialist
Veterinary Surgeon in private practice
Rant en Dal Animal Hospital
Mogale City
Gauteng
South Africa

Co-Author (Genetics chapter 16)
Dr Sooryakanth Sasidharan BVSc, MSc, PhD, MRCVS
Veterinary Surgeon with special interest in genetics
United Kingdom

This book is dedicated to all breeders who are as passionate about their hobby as I am about my profession

DOG BREEDING
A complete reference book

Dr KGM de Cramer

Disclaimer
The information in this book is the opinion of the respective authors and is based on experience gained in private practice, in academic hospitals, during research projects and through the study of relevant literature. The authors do not accept responsibility for any loss or damages due to the misinterpretation of information provided in this book. Please do not use this book as a self-help manual; always consult your veterinary surgeon regarding any health issue which may affect your dog. The fact that many treatments are described in this book should not be misconstrued as instructions for breeders to self-treatment. Descriptions of treatments in this book are included for the mere purpose of detailing the various options breeders have regarding numerous conditions and for them making informed decisions which they could explore and discuss with their veterinary surgeons. The authors have made every attempt to ensure that the information contained in this book, is current and sourced from prominent publications, up-to-date papers, reviews and books.

© Copyright 2019
All rights reserved.
No part of this publication may be duplicated in any form what so ever without written permission from the copyright holders.

Published by

KeJaFa
KNOWLEDGE WORKS

35 Piet Retief Avenue
Noordheuwel,
Krugersdorp, 1739
South Africa

www.kejafa.co.za
kejafa@mweb.co.za

Dog Breeding
A Complete Reference Book

First published 2018
First print 2018
Second print 2019

ISBN: 978-0-9947174-4-3

Proofreading by Eileen de Bruyn
Layout by Christina van Straaten
Cover photo by Freddie Marriage
Printed and bound by Ingram Spark, England

ABOUT THE BOOK

DOG BREEDING: A complete reference book is virtually an identical remake of the book previously published in 2014 as "Breeding is a Bitch". The tittle and cover was changed to more attractively portray the subject of dog breeding for a global market. Although this book is primarily written for dog breeders, it will also be of value to anyone who works with dogs on a daily basis, i.e. dog trainers and personnel working in: canine protection and security services, service dogs for the military, police canine units, animal shelters and dog boarding kennels, as it also deals with conditions unique to larger dog colonies. Veterinary students and veterinary surgeons who have a special interest in dog breeding may all benefit from the wealth of knowledge compiled in this handy reference book. Likewise, veterinary specialists in theriogenology (animal reproduction) may also benefit from the in-depth discussions pertaining to unusual cases.

Whether you are a beginner or an experienced breeder, DOG BREEDING: A complete reference book will help you identify, correct or prevent many problems which you are sure to encounter. Its comprehensive nature classes it as a complete reference book on dog breeding.

Its main focus is reproduction in both the male and female and the subjects it covers are extensive. It entails detailed discussions of; the heat cycle, determining optimal breeding time, management of studs, puberty, breeding soundness in the stud and bitch, genital diseases, pregnancy, lactation, whelping, dystocia, caesarean section, artificial reproductive techniques, fertility problems, reproductive efficiency, neonatal disease and puppy survival. It also covers the ethical aspects of dog breeding, how most breeders start off, nutrition, routine preventative health measures, parasite control and various matters and conditions relating to the keeping of dogs and large dog colonies. In addition it comprehensively covers practical basic and advanced genetics for dog breeders.

DOG BREEDING: A complete reference book, will enable beginners to start off on a less rocky path as it deals with problems which even the most experienced dog breeders find challenging.

The book comprehensively covers:
- Animal husbandry, nutrition and how to start off as dog breeder
- Breeding management and modern artificial reproductive techniques
- Genital diseases, pregnancy, whelping, lactation, caesarean section, fertility problems, reproductive efficiency, neonatal disease and puppy survival
- Routine preventative health measures, parasite control and various matters and conditions relating to the keeping of dogs and large dog colonies
- Basic and advanced genetics for dog breeders

PREFACE

For centuries dogs have been bred and selected at whim by their human custodians. This has led to a fascinating diversity not equalled by any other species, domesticated or wild. This is an evolving process with new breeds continuously emerging. At the same time, numerous diseases and genetic conditions have emerged and are still emerging.

Significant progress has been made in veterinary science regarding diagnostics, treatment and nutrition. Recent advances in DNA biotechnology is attracting increasing attention and has led to more accurate diagnosis. The identification of genetic markers enables the accurate identification of carriers of genetic conditions. Sustained research in this field is sure to make an increasing number of tests available as a selection tool for breeders.

The world is becoming increasingly smaller with few places exempt from global influence. Given the continued movement of domestic animals and wildlife from one continent to the next, through continuous exportation and importation, it is very likely that diseases and genetically linked afflictions which are encountered elsewhere in the world will emerge in local dog populations. With particular reference to genetic diversity, this global trade is sure to bring both the good and the bad. On the other hand, locally isolated breeds may lack this diversity and therefore become increasingly inbred. Assisted reproductive techniques such as artificial insemination of imported frozen semen can help in this regard.

CONTENTS

ABOUT THE BOOK i

PREFACE ii

Definitions, Terminology and Synonyms used in text xiii

Abbreviations used in text xvii

INTRODUCTION 1

1. **HISTORY AND EVOLUTION OF DOGS** 3

2. **ETHICS OF DOG BREEDING** 5

3. **BEGINNING AND EVOLVING AS A BREEDER** 9
   3.1. Choosing a breed 9
   3.2. Purchasing stock 11
   3.2.1. Purchasing foundation stock 11
   3.2.2. Purchasing puppies 11
   3.2.3. Purchasing adult brood bitches 11
   3.2.4. Purchasing an adult stud dog 12
   3.3. Pre-purchase veterinary examinations and certification 13
   3.4. Number of dogs kept 14
   3.5. Animal hoarders 15
   3.6. Breed rescue organizations 16
   3.7. Closed kennel concept 16
   3.8. What to do with non-productive stock? 17
   3.9. Showing dogs 18

4. **NUTRITION** 21
   4.1. History of commercial pet foods 21
   4.2. Homemade diets 22
   4.3. The key nutrients in dog food 24
   4.3.1. Fats 24
   4.3.2. Carbohydrates 24
   4.3.3. Proteins 25
   4.4. Choosing the right diet for your dogs 27
   4.5. Food for the different life stages and life styles 29
   4.6. Feeding for pregnancy and lactation 30
   4.7. How much and how often to feed my dog 32
   4.7.1. Volume 32
   4.7.2. How often to feed 32
   4.8. Obesity 33

4.9.	Underweight dogs	34
4.10.	Feeding of bones	34
4.11.	Dental care and diet	35
4.12.	Pica	36
4.13.	Coprophagia	37
4.14.	Appetite stimulants	37
4.15.	Supplementing commercial diets	37
4.15.1.	Calcium supplementation	38
4.15.2.	Vitamin D	39
4.15.3.	Vitamin C	39
4.15.4.	Vitamin B complex	40
4.15.5.	Folic acid supplementation and pregnancy	41
4.15.6.	Vitamin A	41
4.15.7.	Vitamin E	42
4.15.8.	Glutamine	42
4.15.9.	Prebiotic and probiotics	42
4.15.10.	Kelp and algae	42
4.15.11.	Table scraps	42
4.15.12.	Treats	43
4.16.	Nutraceuticals	43
4.16.1.	Glucosamine and chondroitin	43
4.16.2.	Antioxidants	43
4.16.3.	Omega-3 and-6 fatty acids	43
4.17.	Ergogenic aids (performance enhancing substances)	44
4.18.	Substances which are potentially toxic to dogs	44
4.18.1.	Poisonous flora (plants, mushrooms and algae)	44
4.18.2.	Pesticides	45
4.18.3.	Prescription and over-the-counter drugs	46
4.18.4.	Commercial dog foods	47
4.18.5.	Common house-hold hazards	47
4.19.	Water	47
5.	**REPRODUCTION IN THE BITCH**	**49**
5.1.	Puberty in bitches and age of first breeding	49
5.2.	Delayed puberty	50
5.3.	The oestrous cycle (reproductive cycle or heat cycle) of the bitch	50
5.3.1.	The stages of the oestrous cycle of the bitch	52
5.4.	Aberrant heat cycles in the bitch	55
5.4.1.	Split heat	55
5.4.2.	Silent heat	56
5.4.3.	Persistent heat	56
5.5.	Bitches which do not cycle at all (anoestrus)	56
5.6.	Short intervals between heat cycles (short interoestrus intervals)	56
5.7.	Dormitory effect	56
5.8.	Excessive vaginal haemorrhage during heat	57
5.9.	Vaginal fold prolapse (vaginal hyperplasia)	57

5.10.	Vestibulo-vaginal strictures	58
5.11.	The genital lock	59
5.12.	Vaginitis	62
5.12.1.	Vaginitis during oestrus	62
5.12.2.	Dioestrus vaginitis	62
5.12.3.	Skin fold vaginitis	63
5.12.4.	Puppy vaginitis	63
5.13.	Cystic endometrial hyperplasia	63
5.14.	Ovarian cysts	64
5.15.	Para-uterine cysts	64
5.16.	Pyometra	65
5.17.	Monitoring of the oestrous cycle and determining optimal breeding time	66
5.17.1.	Methods used by breeders to determine optimal breeding time	67
5.17.2.	Methods used by veterinary surgeons and breeders to determine optimal breeding time	69
5.18.	Breeding protocols for optimum fertility	71
5.18.1.	Natural mating with unlimited access to a stud dog; without heat timing	71
5.18.2.	Natural mating using one stud dog on two bitches, alternating matings, without heat timing	71
5.18.3.	Natural mating with limited access to a stud dog (2-3 matings)	72
5.18.4.	Natural mating with access limited to a single mating	72
5.18.5.	Breeding using compromised semen	72
5.19.	Examination for breeding soundness	73
5.19.1.	Pre-breeding bacterial cultures	73
5.19.2.	White cell count	74
5.19.3.	Ultrasonography of uterus and ovaries	74
5.19.4.	Thyroid function	74
5.19.5.	Brucellosis	74
5.20.	Oestrus induction and oestrus synchronization	74
5.21.	Superovulation of the bitch	75
5.22.	Fertility drugs	75
6.	**PREGNANCY**	**77**
6.1.	Prevention of pregnancy	77
6.1.1.	The pharmacological control of the heat cycle	77
6.1.2.	Surgical control of reproduction in bitches	77
6.2.	Fertilization	79
6.3.	Early development in the womb	80
6.4.	Sex ratios	81
6.5.	Diagnosis of pregnancy	82
6.6.	Phantom pregnancy (pseudopregnancy)	85
6.7.	Parentage testing	85
6.8.	Gestation length	86
6.9.	Prediction of whelping date	86
6.9.1.	Whelping date relative to breeding dates	86
6.9.2.	Whelping date relative to decline in rectal temperature before labour	87
6.9.3.	Whelping date relative to behavioural signs of impending labour	87

6.9.4.	Whelping date relative to veterinary observations made during heat	88
6.10.	Complications of pregnancy	88
6.10.1.	Loss of pregnancy	88
6.10.2.	Vaginal discharges during pregnancy	88
6.10.3.	Torsion of the uterus	89
6.10.4.	Pregnancy associated oedema (swelling) of hind legs and surrounding areas	89
6.10.5.	Retained placentas (afterbirths)	90
6.10.6.	Retained foetus	90
6.10.7.	Uterine infections after whelping	90
6.10.8.	Post-whelping "blues"	91
6.10.9.	Continued haemorrhaging after whelping	91
6.10.10.	Uterine rupture	91
6.10.11.	Uterine or vaginal prolapse	92
6.10.12.	Post whelp hair loss	92
6.11.	Safety of drugs during pregnancy	92
6.12.	Pregnancy termination	93
6.13.	Labour induction in the bitch	93
7.	**MAMMARY GLANDS AND LACTATION**	**95**
7.1.	Uptake of colostrum by puppies	95
7.2.	Lactation and agalactia (poor or no milk production)	97
7.3.	Galactostasis	98
7.4.	Mastitis	98
7.5.	Milk fever (eclampsia)	99
8.	**WHELPING**	**101**
8.1.	Signs of impending labour	101
8.1.1.	First stage	101
8.1.2.	Second stage	103
8.2.	Management of the whelping bitch	105
8.2.1.	The whelping quarters	106
8.2.2.	Observation of the whelping process	108
8.3.	Dystocia (difficulty in labour) in the bitch	112
8.3.1.	Deciding when to intervene	113
8.3.2.	Medical management of dystocia	115
8.3.3.	Oxytocin and its role in dystocia	115
8.3.4.	Calcium gluconate	116
8.3.5.	Glucose	116
8.3.6.	Traction on foetuses	116
9.	**CAESAREAN SECTION IN THE BITCH**	**117**
9.1.	Indications for caesarean sections	117
9.1.1.	Dystocia as indication for caesarean section	118
9.1.2.	Singleton pregnancies	119
9.1.3.	Prolonged pregnancy	120
9.2.	Complications of caesarean sections	120

9.3.	Post-operative care	122
9.4.	Resuscitative aids in neonates following caesarean section	123
9.5.	Concepts which require explanation relevant to size of puppies	123
9.5.1.	Synchrony of ovulation	123
9.5.2.	Prematurity	124
9.5.3.	Dysmaturity	124
9.5.4.	Superfoetation (pregnancy with foetuses of different age)	125
9.5.5.	Runts	125
9.5.6.	Twinning	126
9.5.7.	Sharing of placentas	126
10.	**REPRODUCTION IN THE MALE**	**129**
10.1.	Puberty in males and age of first breeding	129
10.2.	Spermatogenesis	129
10.3.	Vasectomization	130
10.4.	Castration (neutering)	131
10.5.	Breeding soundness examination of the stud	132
10.6.	Semen collection	132
10.7.	Semen quality	133
10.8.	Poor semen quality	134
10.9.	Treatment of poor semen parameters	135
10.10.	Daily sperm output (DSO)	135
10.11.	Superfecundation (multiple sires of one litter) achieved by multiple sire matings	136
10.11.1.	Using two or more sires with poor semen parameters on one bitch	137
10.11.2.	Using compromised semen or stud of poor fertility in combination with a semen of optimal quality	137
10.11.3.	Concerns of breeding authorities regarding multiple sire breeding	138
10.12.	Prostatic disease	138
10.12.1.	Benign prostatic hypertrophy	138
10.12.2.	Prostatitis	139
10.12.3.	Prostatic and paraprostatic cysts and prostatic abscesses	139
10.12.4.	Prostatic cancer	139
10.13.	Testicular conditions	140
10.13.1.	Cryptorchidism (undescended testis)	140
10.13.2.	Testicular torsion	142
10.13.3.	Testicular infection (orchitis) and epididymitis	142
10.13.4.	Testicular trauma	143
10.13.5.	Testicular neoplasia (cancer or tumours)	143
10.13.6.	Testicular hypoplasia	144
10.13.7.	Testicular degeneration	144
10.13.8.	Inguinoscrotal hernia	144
10.13.9.	Hemiorchidectomy (removal of one testis)	145
10.14.	Penis and prepuce conditions	145
10.14.1.	Phimosis	145
10.14.2.	Paraphimosis	146
10.14.3.	Balanosposthitis	146

10.14.4.	Priapism	147
10.14.5.	Persistent frenulum	147
10.14.6.	Urethral prolapse	147
10.14.7.	Transmissible venereal tumour (TVT)	148
10.15.	Libido	149

11. ARTIFICIAL REPRODUCTIVE TECHNIQUES 151

11.1.	Artificial insemination using fresh semen	151
11.1.1.	Intravaginal use of fresh semen	151
11.1.2.	Intra uterine use of fresh semen	153
11.2.	Artificial insemination using chilled semen	153
11.3.	Artificial insemination using frozen semen	153
11.3.1.	Reasons for semen freezing	154
11.3.2.	Age of stud at freezing	154
11.3.3.	Freezability of dog semen	154
11.3.4.	Number of ejaculates which need to be frozen	155
11.3.5.	Number of inseminations	155
11.3.6.	The insemination method and site	155
11.3.7.	The number of straws or pellets required (insemination dose or "breeding unit")	157
11.3.8.	Import and export of semen	157
11.3.9.	Thawing (defrosting) of the semen	157
11.3.10.	Semen banking	158
11.3.11.	The ideal recipient of the frozen semen	158
11.3.12.	Deliberate superfecundation following artificial insemination	158
11.3.13.	The insemination centre	158
11.4.	Advanced artificial reproductive techniques	159
11.4.1.	Embryo transfer	159
11.4.2.	Freezing canine ovaries	159
11.4.3.	Cloning	159
11.4.4.	Chimeras	160

12. FECUNDITY (REPRODUCTIVE EFFICIENCY) IN DOG BREEDING 161

12.1.	Canine herpesvirus	162
12.1.1.	Fate of foetuses from bitches exposed whilst pregnant (prenatal exposure)	162
12.1.2.	Fate of puppies exposed from birth to 4 weeks (post natal exposure)	163
12.1.3.	Fate of dogs older than 4 weeks	164
12.1.4.	Control of canine herpesvirus	164
12.1.5.	Practical significance of herpesvirus to breeders	164
12.2.	Minute virus of canines	165
12.3.	Canine brucellosis	165
12.4.	Bacterial infections	166
12.5.	Obesity of bitches	167
12.6.	Selection for fecundity	167

13. THE NORMAL NEONATE 169

13.1.	Birth to weaning	169

13.2.	Dewclaw removal	170
13.3.	Tail docking	171
13.4.	Rearing orphan puppies	172
13.4.1.	Foster mothers for orphan puppies	175
13.4.2.	Milk replacers during the first 3 weeks	177
13.4.3.	Creep feeding	179
13.5.	Weaning puppies	180
13.6.	Selling puppies	181
13.6.1.	Disputes regarding puppy sales	181
13.6.2.	Dispute regarding puppy falling ill post sale	181
13.6.3.	Dispute regarding defects that become evident post sale	182
13.6.4.	Dispute regarding suitability for breeding post sale	182
13.6.5.	Outcome of these disputes	182
13.6.6.	Solutions to these disputes	182
14.	**NEONATAL DISEASE**	**185**
14.1.	Therapeutic principles in puppies	186
14.2.	Neonatal disease and conditions in puppies from birth to 3 weeks of age	186
14.2.1.	Low birth-mass puppies	187
14.2.2.	Weak puppies	187
14.2.3.	Neonatal septicaemia	189
14.2.4.	Colic puppies	190
14.2.5.	Toxic milk syndrome	191
14.2.6.	Congenital abnormalities	191
14.2.7.	Fading puppy syndrome	197
14.3.	Neonatal disease and conditions in puppies from 3 weeks of age till weaning	198
14.3.1.	Neonatal opthalmia (opthalmitis neonatorum)	198
14.3.2.	Puppy strangles (juvenile cellulitis, juvenile pyoderma, submandibular abscesses)	198
14.3.3.	White scours	198
14.3.4.	Infectious juvenile pneumonia	199
14.3.5.	Hypoglycaemia in toy breeds	199
14.4.	Neonatal disease and conditions in puppies from weaning onwards	199
14.4.1.	Concept of erosive and multifactorial disease	200
14.4.2.	Impact of crowding on disease	200
14.4.3.	Non-specific diarrhoea at weaning age	201
14.4.4.	Canine parvovirus	201
14.4.5.	Nosocomial (hospital-acquired) disease	205
14.4.6.	Canine coccidiosis	205
14.4.7.	Giardiasis	206
14.4.8.	Ringworm (dermatophytosis)	206
14.4.9.	Encephalitozoon	207
15.	**ROUTINE PREVENTATIVE HEALTH MEASURES**	**209**
15.1.	Choosing a veterinary practice	209
15.2.	Control of diseases preventable by vaccination	210
15.3.	Should breeders annually vaccinate all their dogs?	212

15.4.	Strategic vaccination	212
15.5.	Vaccinating breeding bitches	213
15.6.	What about rabies vaccination?	213
15.7.	Import and export regulations	213
15.8.	Routine veterinary check of puppies prior to sale	213
16.	**GENETICS FOR DOG BREEDERS**	**215**
16.1.	Foreword on genetics	215
16.2.	Introductory terminology	216
16.2.1.	Congenital	216
16.2.2.	Heritable (hereditary, inherited)	216
16.2.3.	Genetics	216
16.2.4.	Genetic disorder	216
16.2.5.	Genomics	216
16.2.6.	Genotype (what the animal has within its genes)	216
16.2.7.	Genes, alleles and locus	216
16.2.8.	Chromosomes	217
16.2.9.	Genetic testing	217
16.2.10.	Homozygous and heterozygous	218
16.2.11.	Dominance, co-dominance and penetrance	218
16.2.12.	Developmental anomaly (defect)	218
16.2.13.	Heritability and heritability coefficient	219
16.2.14.	Mutation	219
16.3.	Hybridisation	219
16.4.	Mixed breeds	220
16.5.	Designer dogs	221
16.6.	Polygenic inheritance and complex conditions	221
16.7.	Genetics of dog breeds	222
16.8.	Genetic theory & testing: a status check for the dog breeder	222
16.9.	Genetic testing: practical considerations for the dog breeder	223
16.9.1.	Testing for coat colour traits	225
16.9.2.	Testing for coat colour, length and type	225
16.10.	Breeding strategies for the management of genetic disorders	226
16.11.	Selection in practice	226
16.11.1.	Science or art	226
16.11.2.	Inbreeding as genetic "tool"	227
16.11.3.	Measurement of intensity of inbreeding	228
16.11.4.	Outbreeding (outcrossing)	229
16.12.	DNA profiling services	229
16.13.	Parentage testing services	229
16.14.	Breed identification services	230
16.14.1.	Identification of purebred dogs	230
16.14.2.	Identification of mixed breed dogs	230
16.15.	List of currently identifiable breeds (2013)	230
16.16.	Genetic testing and dog breeding the way forward	231
16.17.	Concept of genetic registries	235

16.18.	DNA tests possible and offered by various laboratories worldwide	235
16.19.	Genetic counselling	242
16.19.1.	Breeding recommendations for dogs carrying known recessive genes for which there is a test available	242
16.19.2.	Breeding recommendations for dogs carrying known dominant genes	242
16.19.3.	In the above cases, what does the breeder do with affected dogs?	243
16.19.4.	Breeding recommendations for conditions for which there are no tests for carriers	243
16.19.5.	How much of the defect could have been influenced by the environment and how do they know its presence is not purely a fluke (an unpredictably expressed trait)?	243
16.19.6.	How can one determine if the defect is not purely environmental?	243
16.19.7.	What role does the environment play in complex conditions?	243
16.19.8.	Is it possible to determine if a genetic condition is 'caused' by the sire or dam only?	244
16.19.9.	How do we manage sex-linked genes?	244
16.19.10.	If the inheritability of the trait (excepting a very serious defect) is very low, may we risk breeding with these dogs?	244
16.19.11.	What does the breeder do if the defect is not very detrimental to the breed and they have other issues of greater importance in the breed which requires stringent selection	245
16.20.	Breeding recommendations summary	245
17.	**INTERNAL PARASITES (ENDOPARASITES) OF DOGS**	**247**
17.1.	Verminosis (worm infestation)	247
17.2.	Roundworms (*Toxacara canis* and other *Toxacara spp*)	247
17.3.	Hookworms (*Ancylostoma spp*)	248
17.4.	Common flea associated tapeworm (*Dipylidium caninum*)	248
17.5.	Whipworm (*Trichuris vulpis*)	249
17.6.	Other tape worms (*Taenia spp, Echinococcus spp*)	249
17.7.	Treatment and control of worms in dogs	249
17.7.1.	Deworming program for dogs by ordinary pet owners	249
17.7.2.	Deworming program for dogs in breeding kennels	250
17.7.3.	Unsuccessful control of worms	250
17.7.4.	Strategic deworming versus routine deworming	251
17.8.	Heartworm (*Dirofilaria immitis*)	251
17.9.	Spirocerca lupi	251
18.	**EXTERNAL (ECTOPARASITES) OF DOGS**	**255**
18.1.1.	Ticks	255
18.1.2.	Skin mites and ear mites	256
18.1.3.	Demodectic mange (*Demodex canis* associated mange)	256
18.1.4.	Fleas	257
18.1.5.	Flies and maggots	257
19.	**MATTERS AND CONDITIONS RELATING TO DOGS KEPT IN BREEDING KENNELS**	**259**
19.1.	Kennel management	259
19.1.1.	Hygiene and sanitation	259
19.1.2.	Keeping breeding dogs and other animals on the same premises	260

19.1.3.	Health and safety issues regarding kennel staff	260
19.1.4.	Positive identification of dogs	261
19.2.	Self-treatment by breeders	261
19.3.	Alternative healing methods	261
19.4.	Performance enhancing drugs	262
19.4.1.	Corticosteroids	262
19.4.2.	Non-steroidal anti-inflammatory agents	262
19.4.3.	Behavioural modification using drugs	262
19.4.4.	Anabolic steroid abuse in dogs	262
19.5.	Behavioural aspects in dogs	263
19.5.1.	Socialization, critical factors for socialising of companion dogs	263
19.5.2.	Puppy temperament assessments	266
19.5.3.	Stress and associated conditions	267
19.5.4.	Aggression in dogs	269
19.6.	Common conditions in dog breeding kennels	269
19.6.1.	Respiratory infections (kennel cough)	269
19.6.2.	Musculoskeletal disorders	270
19.6.3.	Pressure point hygroma	276
19.6.4.	Miscellaneous conditions	276
19.7.	Sudden death	280
19.7.1.	Gastric dilatation and volvulus (stomach torsion)	280
19.7.2.	Heart conditions	281
19.7.3.	Heat exhaustion (hyperthermia)	282
19.7.4.	Restricted airway syndrome	282
19.7.5.	Bee sting attack	283
19.7.6.	Strokes	284
19.7.7.	Snake bite	284
19.7.8.	Canine red gut (*clostridial enterotoxaemia*) (mainly of interest to veterinary surgeons)	285
19.7.9.	*Spirocerca lupi*	288
19.8.	Zoonoses	288
19.8.1.	Rabies	288
19.8.2.	Bacterial infections	288
19.8.3.	Endo and ectoparasites	289
19.8.4.	Protozoal infections	290

ACKNOWLEDGEMENTS 293

ABOUT THE AUTHORS 294

KEYWORD INDEX 296

REFERENCES 301

Definitions, Terminology and Synonyms used in text

Where synonyms apply, preferred terms are used in this book. Terms and terminology specific to genetics are discussed in the chapter dealing with genetics.

Abortion Expulsion of non-viable foetuses from dam

Acidosis Abnormal increase in blood acidity

Ad lib (ad libitum feeding) The practice of leaving out as much food as the dog wants, all the time, also known as free access feeding

Aetiology Cause

Agalactia Poor or no milk production

Alopecia Hair loss

Anecdotal Hearsay or lacking scientific proof

Auscultation Listening with stethoscope

Azoospermia Total absence of sperm in the ejaculate

Bilateral On both sides

Birth interval See interpup interval

Birthing See parturition

Brachycephaly Short snouted and broad faced

Breeding May refer to natural mating, artificial insemination using fresh, frozen or chilled semen

Caesarean section Surgical procedure to remove offspring from a pregnant animal or woman

Carcinogen Agent which may cause cancer

Castration Neutering, removal of testicles

Coitus Synonymous with act of mating, breeding, copulation or sexual intercourse

Colostrum The first milk present in the mammary glands following delivery of the puppies

Coprophagia Act of eating faeces

Cornuectomy Refers to only removal of one uterine horn without its associated ovary

Cryptorchidism Failure of one or both testes to descend into the scrotum at the time normal for the species of interest

Dam Mother of offspring in dogs

Delivery Freeing of foetus from mother

Dioestrus Phase of the oestrous cycle of the bitch that follows oestrus and is dominated by progesterone from corpora lutea

Dormitory effect The effect that one oestrous bitch have on other bitches in synchronizing their cycles, is termed the dormitory effect.

Due date Date that dam is expected to give birth

Dysmaturity Apparent prematurity of one or more puppies in presence of normal full term puppies in the same litter

Dystocia Difficulty in giving birth, whelping or labour

Ecbolic Drug that enhances contractility of the uterus during parturition

Eclampsia Synonymous to milk fever, puerperal tetany or hypocalcaemia

Elective caesarean section Refers to a caesarean section that is performed on a pregnant woman/animal on the basis of an obstetrical or medical indication or at the request from the owner

Definitions, Terminology and Synonyms used in text

Emergency caesarean section Caesarean section performed during labour (intra-partum) by necessity
Endometrium Wall of the uterus
Entropion Curling-in of eyelids
Fecundity The potential reproductive capacity of an individual dog (dog or bitch) or dog population whereas fertility is the natural capacity to reproduce
Fertilization rate The ratio between the number of fertilised oocytes and the number of ovulated oocytes.
Full term Refers to pregnancy has gone its full tem and that partus is now imminent
Genital lock Synonymous with copulatory lock or tie (genital tie) in the domestic dog and basically entails the stud and the bitch getting stuck at mating
Gestation length Time that is required for foetus to fully develop from conception or other constant (key event or "chronological landmark"), until birth of offspring
Gestation Synonym for pregnancy
Hemi-ovarectomy Surgical removal of ovary on the one side (unilateral)
Hemi-ovariohystorectomy Surgical removal of ovary and its associated uterine horn
Heterologous From another species
Homozygotic twinning Twin offspring formed from the splitting of an embryo
Hyperfoetation Refers to an excessively large litter for a specific breed or species and usually results from superovulation and or assisted reproductive techniques
Hyperplasia Enlargement of organ as result of increase in number of cells
Hypertrophy Enlargement of organ as result of increase in size of cells in the organ
Hypoglycaemia Low blood glucose
Hypoplasia The failure of an organ or body part to grow or develop fully
Hysterectomy Surgical removal of uterus without removal of ovaries
Idiopathic Of unknown origin
Idiosyncratic Unusual but characteristic yet unexplained
Immunoglobulins Antibodies
In vitro In the laboratory
Infertility Total inability to produce offspring
Interoestrous interval Interval between two consecutive oestrus cycles
Inter-pup interval Interval between puppies
Labour induction See partus induction
Labour See parturition
Lactation Milk production
Lactogenic Via milk
Libido Sex drive
Maiden Bitch See Nulliparous
Melaena Blood in stool
Metastasis Spreading to other parts of the body
Monoestrous Meaning exhibiting one or two oestrous (heat) cycles per year irrespective of whether the bitch falls pregnant or not
Monorchidism Implies that one testicle did not develop at all
Multiparous An animal is multiparous if it has produced offspring on more than one occasion
Myiasis Maggot infestation
Myometrium Uterine muscles
Neoplasia Cancer

Definitions, Terminology and Synonyms used in text

Nosocomial Hospital acquired

Nulliparous An animal is nulliparous if it has never produced offspring

Obstetrics Science of delivering offspring from its dam

Oedema Swelling

Oestrus Synonymous with the words, "in heat" and "in season", refer to the bitch exhibiting typical external visible signs of heat. What the breeder, thus, commonly refers to as "in heat" or "in season", should be construed by scientists as a combination of two phases of oestrous known as pro-oestrus and oestrus combined

Oestrus induction Induction of a new oestrus cycle

Ovariectomy Surgical removal of ovaries

Ovariohysterectomy Surgical removal of both uterus and ovaries

Ovulate Process of releasing egg/s from ovary

Parity Refers to number of times the mother has given birth to offspring

Parturient Patient in parturition or labour

Parturition date The date of normal anticipated parturition

Parturition management Refers to the management of the pregnant bitch from the time of admission until her discharge with the litter delivered. Management of parturition may include partus observation, various diagnostic procedures and

Parturition number See parity

Parturition Is the expulsion of the foetus (and its membranes) from the uterus via the maternal birth canal also termed; birthing, whelping, labour or partus

Partus See parturition

Patella Kneecap

Pathogens Infectious agents that may harm the host

Perineum Region of the abdomen surrounding the urogenital and anal openings

Placentas Afterbirths

Poliovular species Species that normally have several offspring in one litter

Polygynous species (from the word polygamy) Species in which males have multiple partners

Polyoestrous Numerous oestrous cycles during the same season

Polytocous An animal is polytocous if it produces a litter consisting of more than one offspring as a rule

Pregnancy termination Refers to terminating the pregnancy at any stage prior to full term

Pregnancy See gestation

Prematurity Refers to the immaturity of offspring born prior to full term and thus development. These puppies are identified by sparse hair covering, are usually weak and have difficulty breathing

Prepartal Before parturition

Pre-term Refers to a time before full term

Primigravida bitches Maiden bitches

Primiparous Refers to a first time pregnancy

Pseudopregnancy Synonymous with pseudocyesis, false pregnancy or phantom pregnancy and refers to a state following heat where a bitch appears to be pregnant whilst in fact she is not

Rumen Large stomach of ruminants where plant material ferments

Runts Runts are small looking puppies that seem to be weaker, grow slower, mature slower and are usually in poor body condition

Safe window for intervention Refers to the time frame in which one may perform a caesarean section without adversely affecting outcome

Definitions, Terminology and Synonyms used in text

Septicaemia Blood poisoning
Singleton Pregnancy with only one foetus
Spermatogenesis Process of sperm production
Stenosis Constriction of usually a circular structure
Suboestrus Silent heat
Super-fecundation Occurs when two or more eggs that were ovulated during a single cycle of a bitch are fertilized by spermatozoa from different males
Superfoetation Occurs when a pregnant female, already carrying one or more live foetuses, is bred again at a second oestrous cycle and a second conception occurs
Superovulation Ovulation of a larger than normal number of ova
Symbiosis Mutually beneficial
Term See full term
Transponder Microchip
Twinning Homozygous twins (identical twins) are twin offspring formed from the splitting of an embryo
Uterine inertia Synonymous with uterine fatigue) and it is the inability to expel a foetus from the uterus when no obstruction exists
Uterotomy Refers to the surgical procedure to open one or both uterine horns usually to selectively remove one or more foetuses prematurely
Vas deferens Tubular system that transports the sperm from the testis to the ejaculatory apparatus
Venereal By sexual contact
Verminosis Worm infestation
Vulva Vagina lips
Whelping rate The ratio between the number of bitches bred and the number of bitches that whelped
Whelping Species specific term for parturition or giving birth in the dog
Zoonosis (zoonoses = plural) Is a disease that can be transmitted from animal species to humans

Abbreviations used in text

/kg	per kilogram
®	Registered trade mark
°C	Degrees Celsius
A.I.	Artificial Insemination
ALP	Alkaline Phosphatase
BARF	Bones and Raw Food Diet or Biologically Appropriate Raw Food
BPH	Benign Prostatic Hypertrophy
BSE	Breeding Soundness Examination
BV	Biological Value
BW	Bodyweight
CEH	Cystic Endometrial Hyperplasia
CLIA	Chemiluminescent Immune-assay
CPV	Canine Parvovirus
CS	Caesarean Section or Caesarean Sections
d	Day or days
D1	Day one of cytological dioestrus
DEXA	Dual-energy X-ray absorptiometry
DHA	Docohexaenoic acid
DNA	Deoxyribonucleic acid
DSO	Daily sperm output
ED	Elbow dysplasia
ELISA	Enzyme-linked immunosorbent assay
et al.	And others
FEDIAF	Guide for the manufacture of safe pet food
GDV	Gastric dilatation and volvulus
GNRH	Gonadotrophin releasing hormone
HD	Hip dysplasia
HIV	Human immunodeficiency virus
HOD	Hypertrophic osteodystrophy
IU	International units
LH	Luteinising hormone
MDA	Maternally derived antibodies
MDR1	Multiple drug resistance gene 1
NSAID	Non steroidal anti-inflammatory drugs
OCD	Obsessive-compulsive disorder
PPS	Painful progressive swelling
PTA	Puppy temperament assessment
RIA	Radioimmunoassay
RDA	Recommended daily allowance
TCI	Trans cervical insemination
TVT	Transmissible venereal tumour

Introduction

The psychological value of having a hobby is well researched and recognized. A hobby makes you a more interesting person and it gives you something fascinating to talk about. It alleviates boredom and provides the opportunity to meet people who have similar interests. It not only keeps you mentally alert because you constantly learn new things, but it has the added advantage in that it keeps you physically active. The happier people amongst us are those who are passionate about a hobby. It may be biking, hiking, painting, gardening or one of many other activities. If you have chosen dog breeding as a hobby; this book is for you. It will help you irrespective of whether you are a beginner or a seasoned breeder. Whatever your reason and motivation for becoming a dog breeder, there are certain fundamentals which must be considered. First and foremost, you should have an innate love for animals and in particular a love for dogs. Secondly, you should analyse your motives as they should be pure. Also consider what impact the added responsibilities will have on your lifestyle. Factors such as time constraints, space requirements, the regional restrictions on the number of dogs which may be kept, nuisance factors such as noise and smell, financial considerations and neighbour tolerance, should also be taken into account.

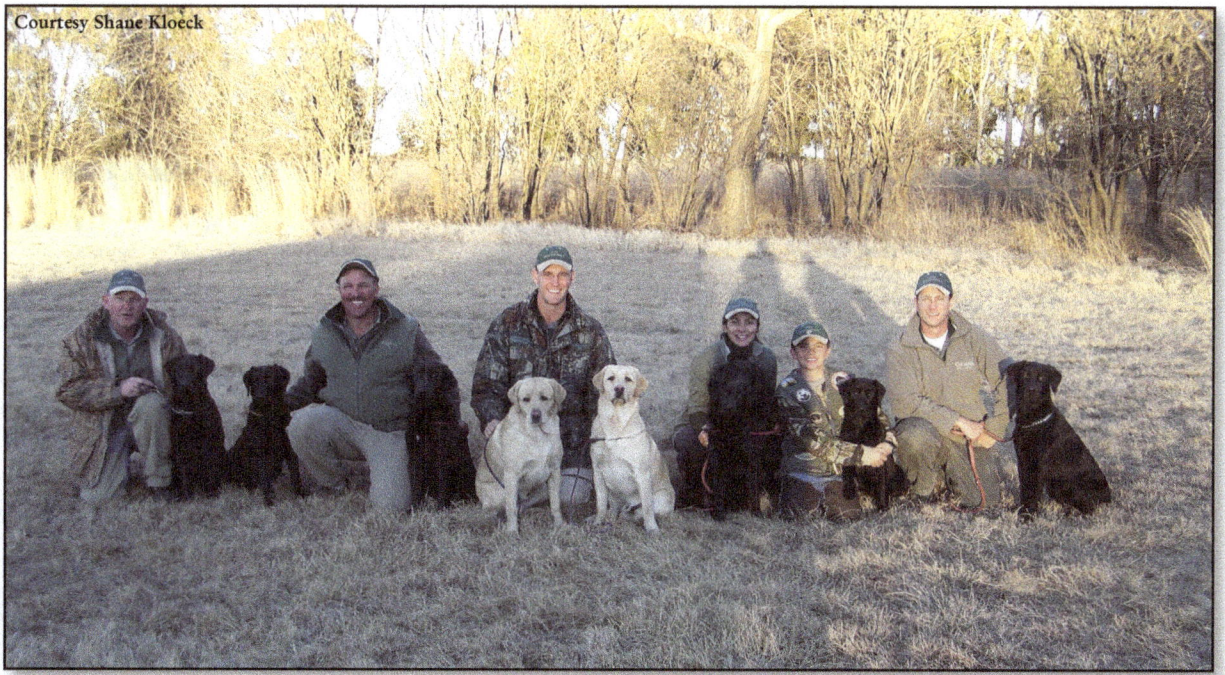

Family and friends enjoying both their hobby and dogs whilst bonding with their kids

Most people start by buying a purebred bitch and then allow it to have a litter. This novel experience, perhaps traumatic if something goes wrong, in all probability determines whether a person will become a breeder or not. For the others, the wonder of reproduction, or the fascination of the resulting litter, or a passion for the breed, or all three, inspires them to become dog breeders. Many breeders eventually enter the competitive arena in a quest for perfection and accolade.

Typically most hobbyist breeders have around 3-6 breeding bitches and may or may not become actively involved in showing or dog sport activities. It is in the interest of the breed that a breeder does enter the competitive arena, as this is where success or failure is measured. To breed purely for

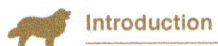
Introduction

the fun of it, without measuring your success against a breed standard and also other dogs of the same breed, is not conducive to the improvement of the breed. Hobbyist breeders by far make up the bulk of dog breeders and undoubtedly make the greatest contribution to the annual number of purebred puppies registered worldwide. It is for this reason that all aspects of a dog breeding endeavour should be of the highest standard.

Some breeders might progress to large-scale dog breeding or commercial breeding. These breeders are involved with the commercial production of dogs for the security industry, the armed forces, guide dog associations or the pet trade. These breeding enterprises (if ably assisted by experienced veterinary surgeons) are in many instances at the forefront of technology regarding animal husbandry, disease control and assisted reproductive techniques. Large-scale or commercial breeders, by virtue of the large number of dogs which they keep, face a greater risk of outbreaks of serious diseases. The latter is particularly true if financial constraints prohibit the introduction of routine health controls and interventions.

Irrespective of the scale which you wish to breed at, this book is designed to help you. It will hopefully increase the sweet and decrease the sour associated with dog breeding, as ultimately dog breeding should remain fun.

I sincerely hope that this book will encourage and inspire both newcomers and experienced breeders to excel at a challenging yet fascinating and amazing hobby. In conclusion, prospective breeders as well as experienced breeders and others involved in the dog breeding fraternity, including veterinary surgeons, may all benefit from the wealth of knowledge compiled in this handy reference book.

Chapter 1

History and Evolution of Dogs

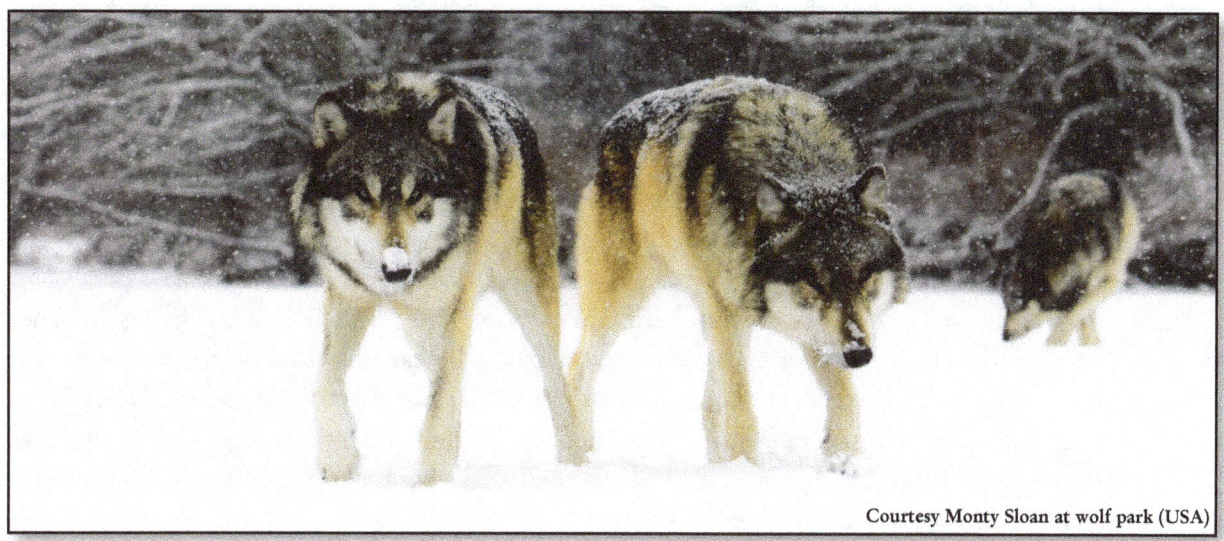

Wolves (Canis Lupus) in natural habitat. They are the only proven ancestors of the domestic dog. The other dog-like animals featured below did not contribute to the domestic dog. Of these, only the Golden jackal and Ethiopian wolf is known to hybridise successfully with the domestic dog

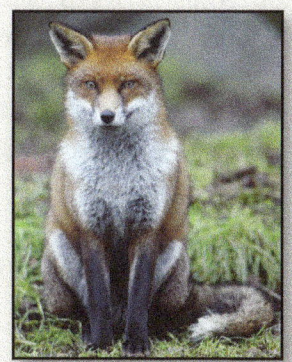

Red fox (Vulpes vulpes)

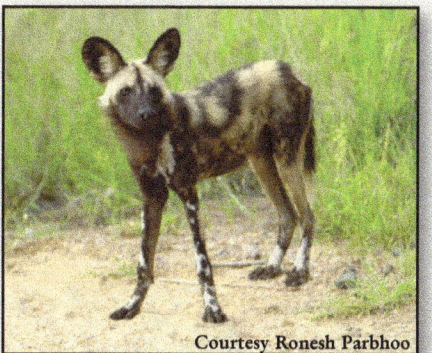

African Wild Dog (Lycaon pictus) also aptly named African painted dog

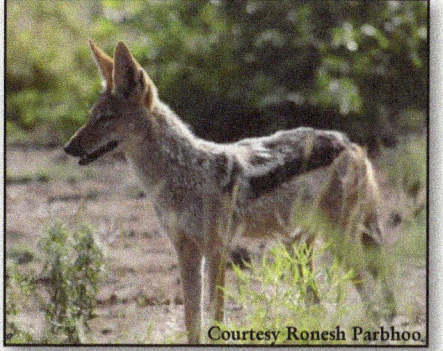

Black-backed jackal (Canis mesomelas)

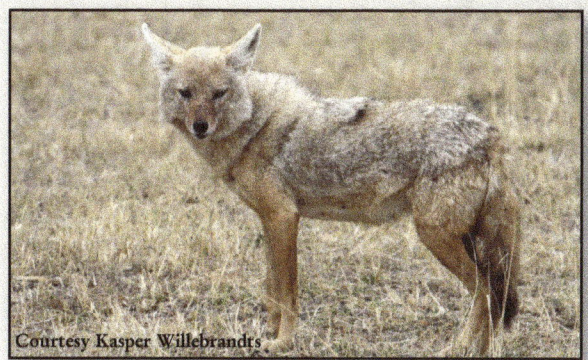

Golden jackal (Canis aureus) is found in Africa and Asia

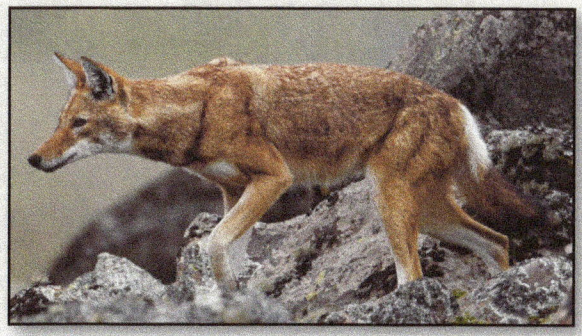

Ethiopian wolf (Canis simensis) (This is the most endangered canid on earth)

Chapter 1 History and Evolution of Dogs

The scientific family Canidae includes domestic dogs and dog-like animals such as wolves, wild dogs, foxes, coyotes and jackals. The general consensus is that dogs directly descended from *Canis lupus* (Wolf) ancestors. Archaeological evidence suggests that domestic dogs appear to have been domesticated around 10,000 - 15,000 years ago. However, some biologists question this belief which sparked a debate over the history and evolution of the domestic dog which continues to this day. Exactly how the initial population of wolves became domesticated remains unclear but is presumed to be wolves living in near proximity to hunter-gatherers who then developed a symbiotic (mutually beneficial) co-existence. It is speculated that this co-existence led to tamed wolves which enabled early man to start the process of selective breeding. This selective breeding was probably limited to characteristics such as aggression and loyalty, followed later by functional traits which were of value to their human owners. The selection process is also most likely to have occurred on many different geographic areas more or less at the same time.

Dogs are genetically very similar to wolves, sharing in excess of 98% of their DNA. The resemblance between the German Shepherd Dog and a wolf is obvious, whereas this similarity is not that clear when other breeds are compared to the ancestral wolf. The fact is; less than two per cent of DNA in the domestic dog *Canis familiaris* separates it from its ancestor, the wolf. However, considering the large number of genes in question, two percent is still a lot of genes, hence the large genetic diversity in dog breeds, which in turn suggests a diverse ancestral pool.

Within a breed, genetic uniformity exists only for genes affecting morphological, conformational and behavioural traits. Remarkable differences in size, conformation, behavioural traits, coat type, coat length and coat colour exist between the different breeds. The domestic dog is the most morphologically diverse mammalian species. Following the initial selection, which was for functional traits useful to man, a shift occurred towards selection for conformation and or performance in dog sport competitions. In some breeds, selection for both traits took place in the same line and in others the same breed has two distinct looking "lines" namely a working dog "line" and a show dog "line".

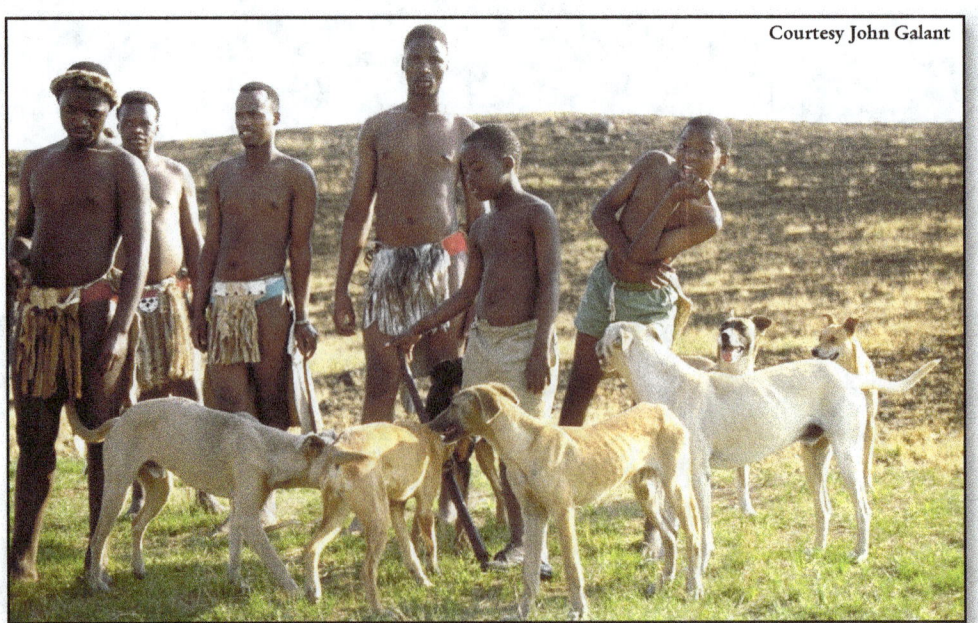

Young boys with their hunting dogs on the African savannah. In some parts of the world, hunting for "bush meat" provides a significant part of local population's protein diet. Interestingly, these dogs all look very similar irrespective of location on the African continent.

Chapter 2

Ethics of Dog Breeding

There has been an up swell of negative sentiment in recent times directed towards purebred dog breeding and per implication dog breeders. Unfortunately the fire of negative sentiment is stoked by anti-breeding activists who have no interest in examining the bigger picture or who are unwilling to consider the merits of any opinion which is in conflict with their own radical beliefs. Matters relating to animal welfare are notoriously emotive. The dynamism with which activists defend their views should not be underestimated and neither should the support which they have, from a sizeable portion of the public or even legislators, be taken lightly. It is therefore incumbent upon the proponents of dog breeding that they take note of the negative aspects associated with breeding and seek to address them.

Personally, I find the thought of hunting reprehensible despite the fact that I do eat meat. I do however fully understand that a well-controlled hunting industry makes a significant contribution to the conservation of animals and responsible land use. The "inconvenient truth" in both the developed and underdeveloped worlds is that, if there is no financial interest in nature, there will be no incentive to preserve it. Likewise, without dog breeders, there can be no purebred dogs.

One of the main arguments by anti-breeding activists is that the breeding of purebred dogs for the pet trade is wrong in the face of all the homeless pets which are destroyed at animal shelters and pounds. They make the point that breeding contributes to pet overpopulation. However, evidence shows that irresponsible pet ownership and failure to sterilise female pets are the main contributors to the disturbingly high number of abandoned and homeless pets which have to be euthanized. Those who are willing to pay a premium price for a purebred dog contribute little to the unfortunate animal shelter statistics. The genetic purity of breed also has little to do with it. In most countries, mixed breeds far outnumber purebred dogs in dog shelters. It is no coincidence that many stray dogs, unsterilized bitches and pet abandonments occur in regions where socio-economic hardship and poor education is rife. Cultural perceptions also play a role.

Another argument is that breeding inevitably leads to the kennelling of dogs. For some, the mere thought of confining "man's best friend" to a kennel, is perceived to be cruel. Most animal lovers will concur that the solitary confinement of animals without providing an enriched environment, human contact, interaction and exercise is not only sad, but also wrong. Responsible breeders are those who practise and encourage responsible and humane animal confinement.

Ethical objections are made against breed standards that encourage the selection for a "desired look", that unfortunately contributes to a higher incidence of certain defects in that breed. For instance, breeding for short snouts and broad faces (brachycephaly) can increase the incidence of restricted respiratory airways whereas breeding for a "wrinkly look" can increase the incidence of entropion (curling-in of eyelids). Much discussion and a lot of soul-searching has to take place and if changes to a breed standard will bring about healthier dogs, the changes have to be made, as it is the ethical thing to do.

Chapter 2 Ethics of Dog Breeding

The main players in this field are the many breeder associations, clubs and dog registering authorities all over the world. They are the custodians of the breeds and have the responsibility to dictate or strongly influence the direction of genetic selection within a breed. However, dog breeders are their members and ultimately fund the machinery of their breed's governing organization. I hope that responsible breeders all over the world will take appropriate action to effect the much needed changes to breed standards which negatively affect the health of a breed. This does not mean that selection for breed specific traits or even "oddities" is wrong, but the custodians of the breed standards have a responsibility to ensure that these specific standards do not negatively affect their breed's health.

Some animal activists claim that certain breed standards blatantly promote selection for anatomical and conformational defects. These accusations must be considered and if there is merit in them, action must be taken to change the standard. Hats off to the brave few who attempt to improve breed standards amidst fierce opposition from those who wish to uphold "old school thoughts". It is my wish that this book will inspire more breeders to courageously support those individual breeders who have suggested drastic changes to breed standards which negatively affect the health and wellbeing of the breeds concerned.

The vast number of genes and polygenetic nature regulating certain undesired traits are an impediment to progress. Biotechnology has a lot to offer in the quest to eradicate these traits and promises to make a huge contribution in times to come. These technologies (genetic testing), when they become available, will enable the breeder to prospectively eliminate negative traits as opposed to retrospective selection and elimination based on the manifestation of defects in the offspring (progeny testing), when essentially the "damage" is already done.

Ethical objections are sometimes made against the intended use of the dog. For instance, dogs bred for security purposes attract criticism because of the way which these dogs are kennelled, trained, handled; their working conditions and the dangers they may be exposed to. Clearly, few will object if a herding dog is employed to do the work it is bred for, or if the sport dog competes in a working trial. This is so because it is apparent to everybody that these dogs love doing their "job". In contrast, negative perceptions exist about the "job" of the security dog, perhaps fuelled by the aggression training that security dogs undergo. There are those who find the sport of greyhound racing objectionable whereas others view it as a perfectly humane sport which the owners and their dogs equally enjoy. Some argue that this sport draws individuals who value profit above the welfare

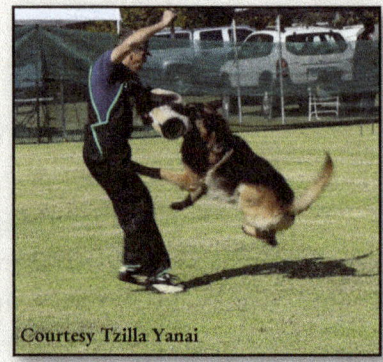
Security dog training in progress

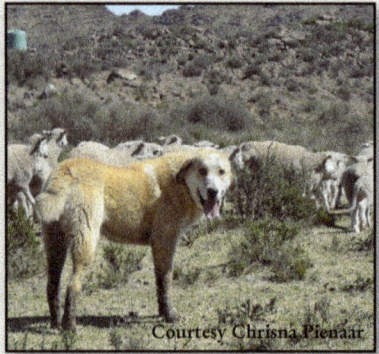
Central Asian Ovtcharka guarding flock from predators

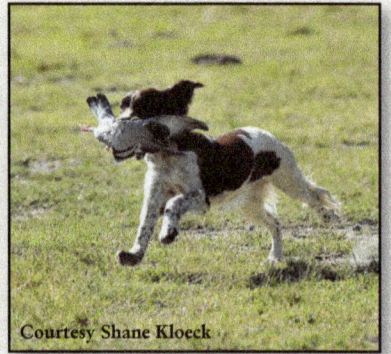
Gundog returning its catch

of their dogs. Others argue that a well-controlled dog racing industry is no different from any of the other dog sport and that it should not be singled out.

Criticism is sometimes directed at those who breed dogs on a large scale. This is particularly true if it is evident that these breeders either do not have the resources or the will to properly care for their animals. Conditions at these kennels are then usually characterised by poor disease control and hygiene, inadequate housing and poor nutrition. Many worry about the fate of dogs which have reached the end of their reproductive or working careers and what will happen to them if they become a burden to the breeder. Many fear that these animals are simply euthanized. This is a real problem and breeders have a responsibly towards these animals. Appropriate re-homing is one option but it is not always easy to find the right home for an ageing dog. However, notwithstanding the difficulties, the welfare of the dog must always be uppermost in the breeders mind. The bottom line is this; dog breeders must manage their dog breeding concern in such a way that enough resources are available to take appropriate care of whatever number of dogs they keep.

Whether antagonists like it or not, dog breeding is here to stay. To those captivated by it, comes the responsibility to improve the breed, to observe good animal husbandry, to take good care of their animals and finally to ensure that their puppies go to owners who will do the same. This book advocates responsible breeding practices. Responsible breeding involves the utmost devotion to the breeding of healthy puppies. It involves meeting and exceeding the minimum requirements regarding the elimination of genetic faults. Responsible dog breeders are those that make the welfare of each animal and its offspring their first priority. It is unfortunate that the negative publicity which unethical breeders engender, tarnishes the credibility of a legion of breeders who do a splendid job. A final word on ethics is perhaps that the "criminalisation of dog breeding is as wrong as indiscriminate dog breeding".

Chapter 2 Ethics of Dog Breeding

Chapter 3

Beginning and Evolving as a Breeder

3.1. Choosing a breed

In most cases the choice of breed is influenced by a prior association with a breed. However, if no such prior association exists; prospective breeders are encouraged to do research through digital media and books, before deciding on a specific breed. Once a shortlist of breeds has been established, breed-specific books should be consulted. Accurate descriptions of breed traits and breed requirements should be studied. The choice of breed will also depend on the life style of the prospective breeder and availability of space.

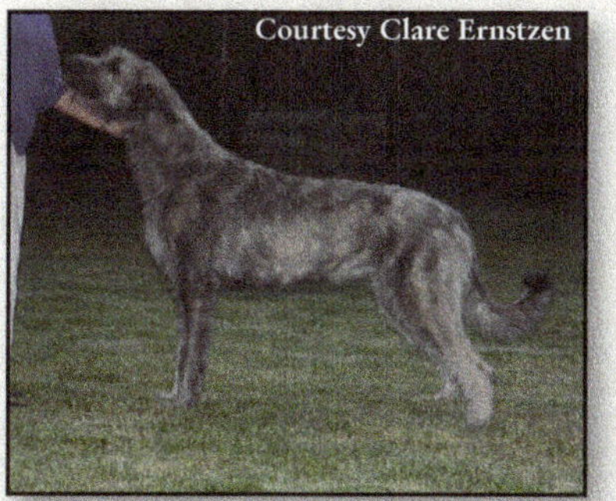

Irish Wolfhound 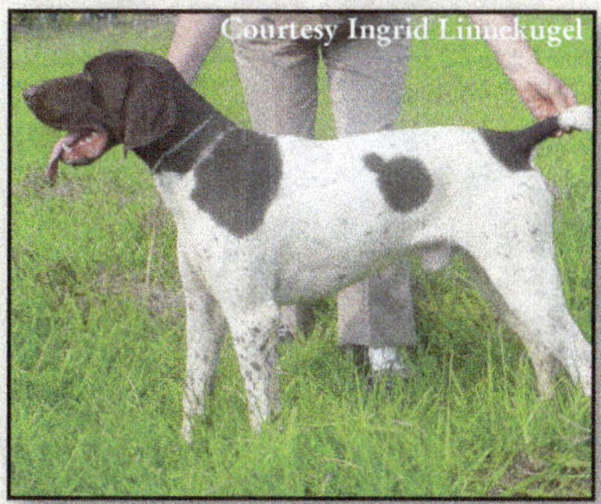   *German Shorthair Pointer* 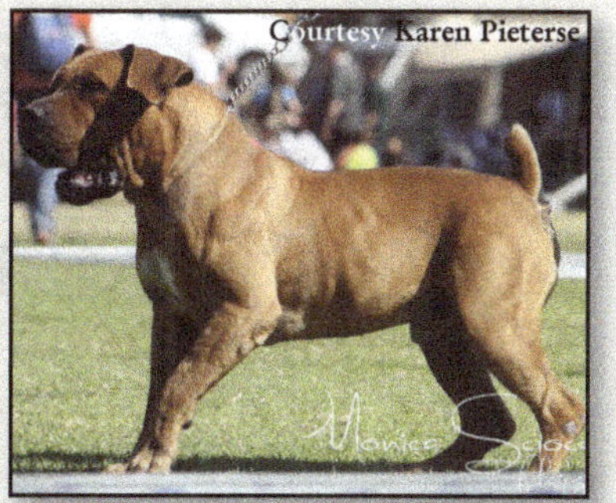   *Boerboel*

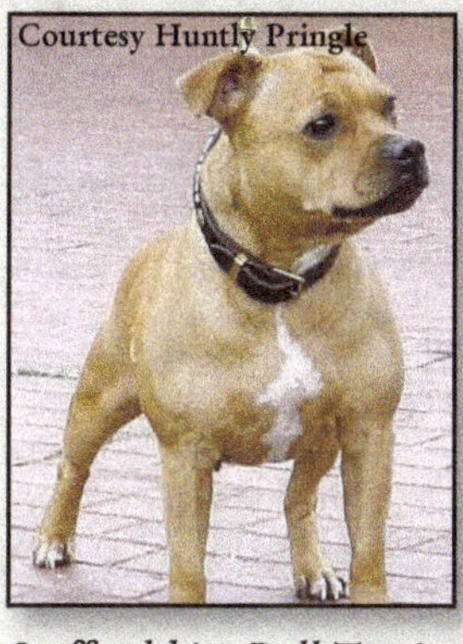

Staffordshire Bull Terrier 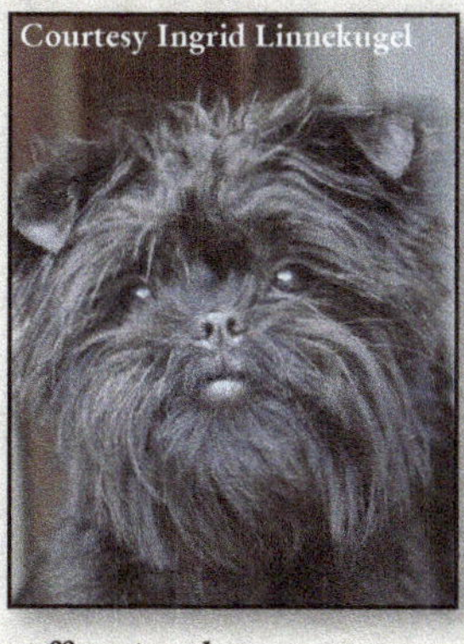   *Affenpinscher* 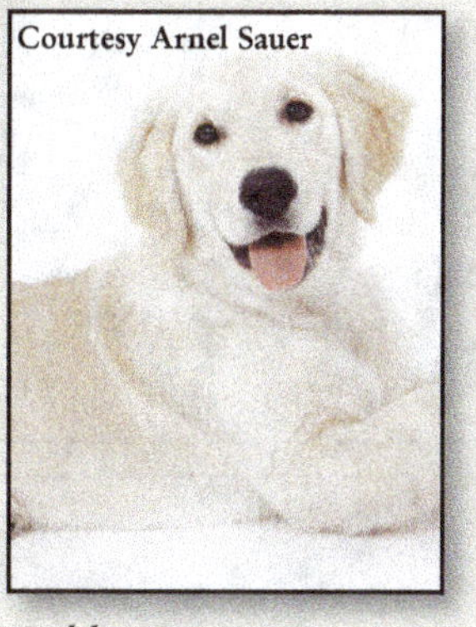   *Golden Retriever* 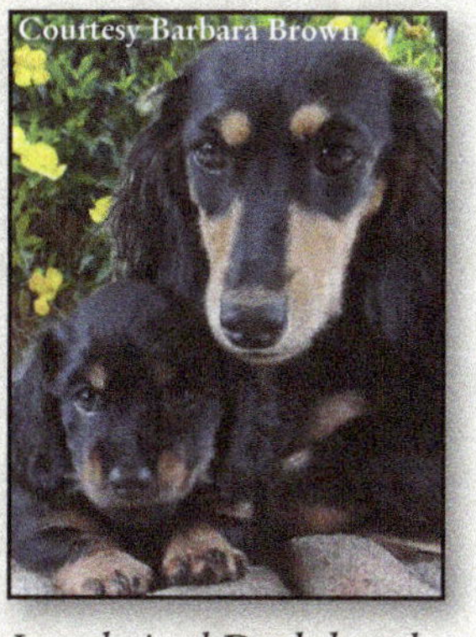   *Longhaired Dachshund*

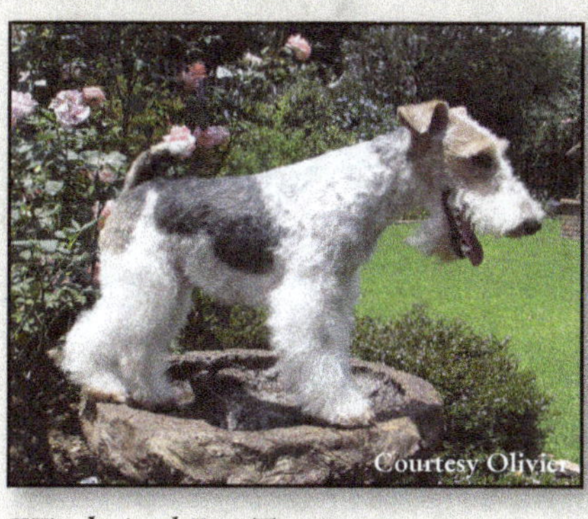

Wirehaired Fox Terrier 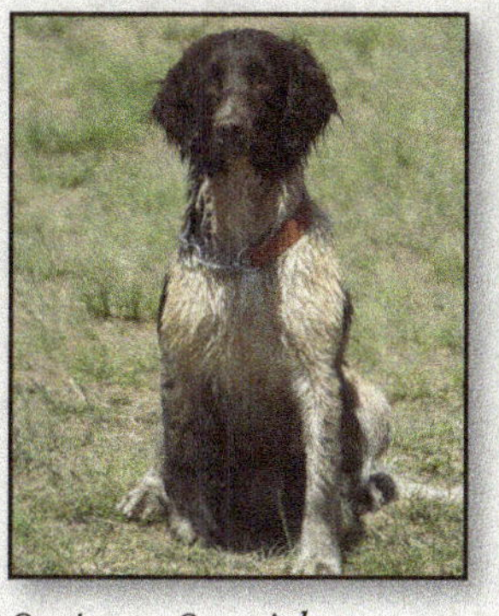   *Springer Spaniel* 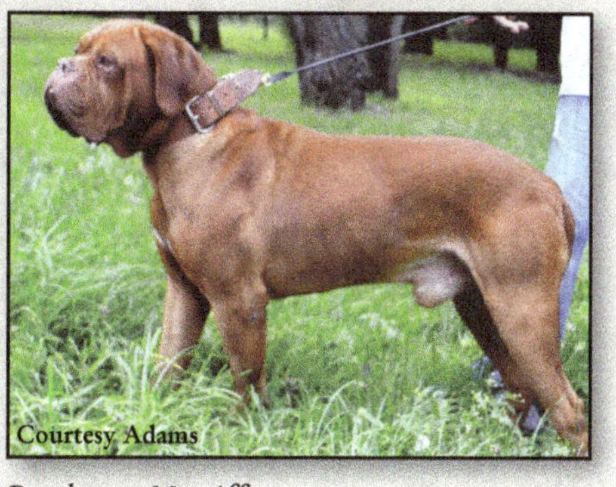   *Bordeaux Mastiff*

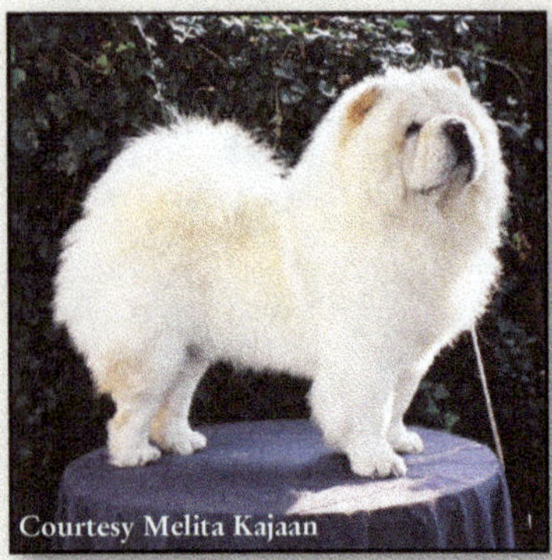

Courtesy Melita Kajaan	

Chow Chow — Courtesy Melita Kajaan

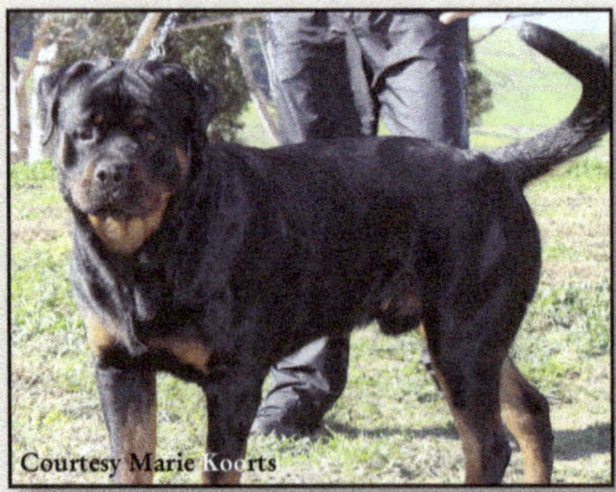

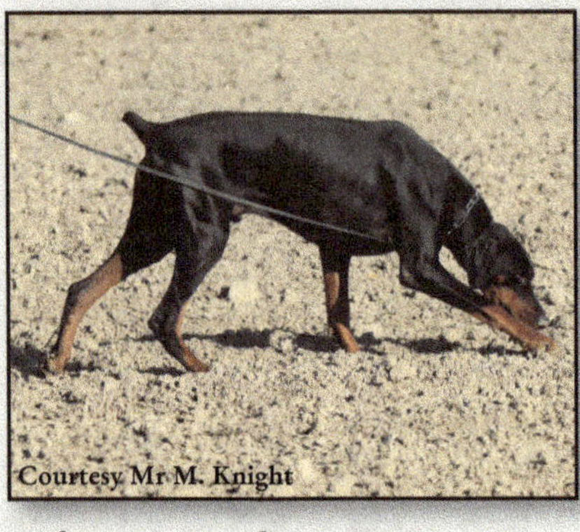

Rottweiler — Courtesy Marie Koorts

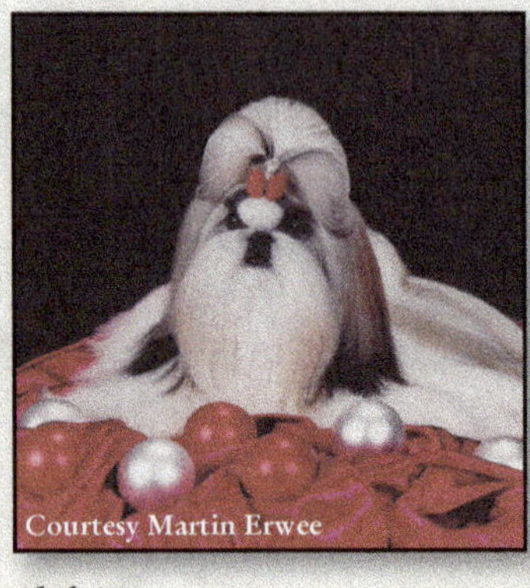

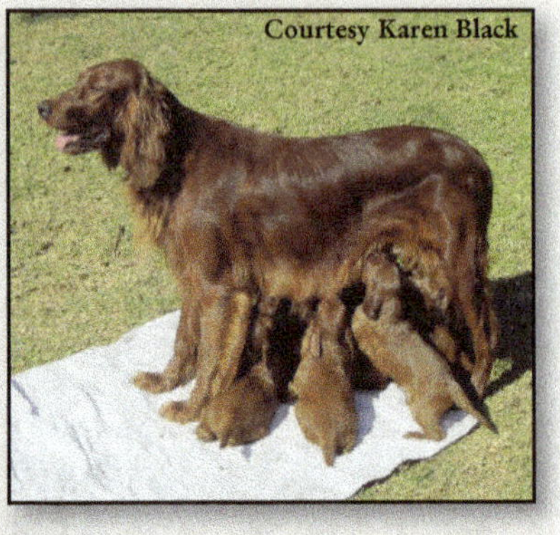

Vizla — Courtesy Ingrid Linnekugel

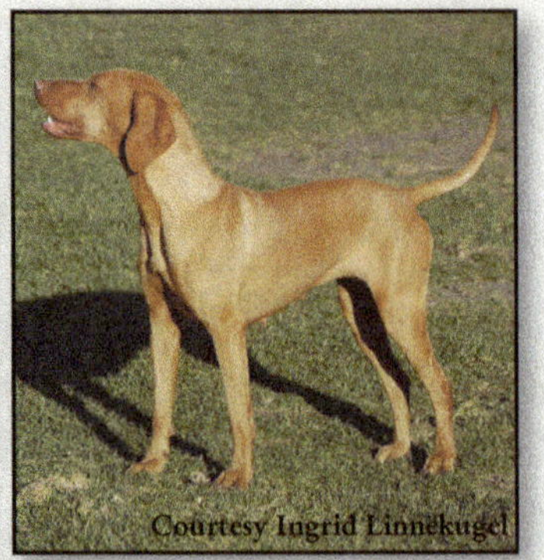

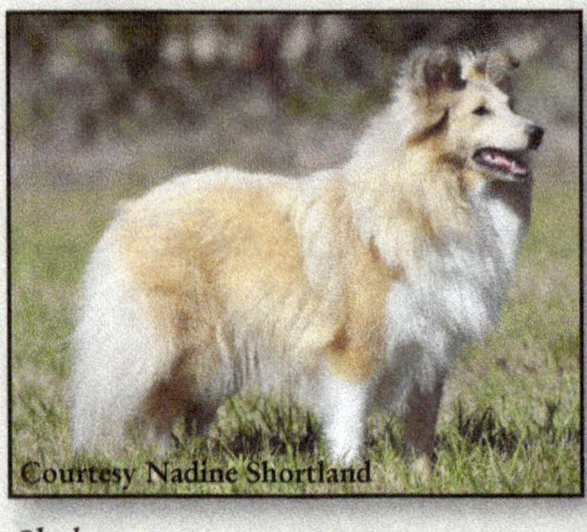

Doberman Pinscher — Courtesy Mr M. Knight

Shih Tzu — Courtesy Martin Erwee

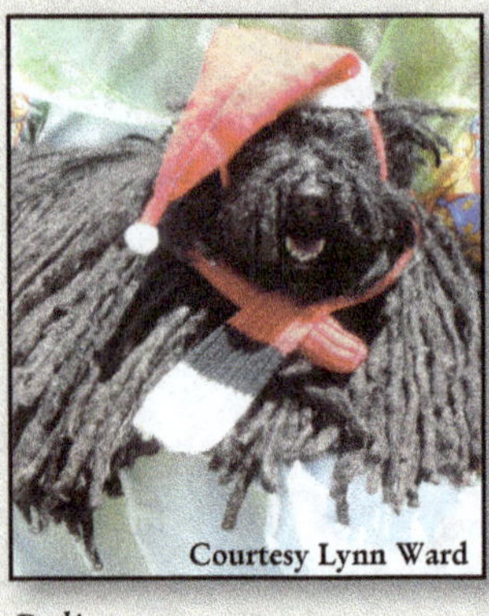

Irish Setter — Courtesy Karen Black

Shelty — Courtesy Nadine Shortland

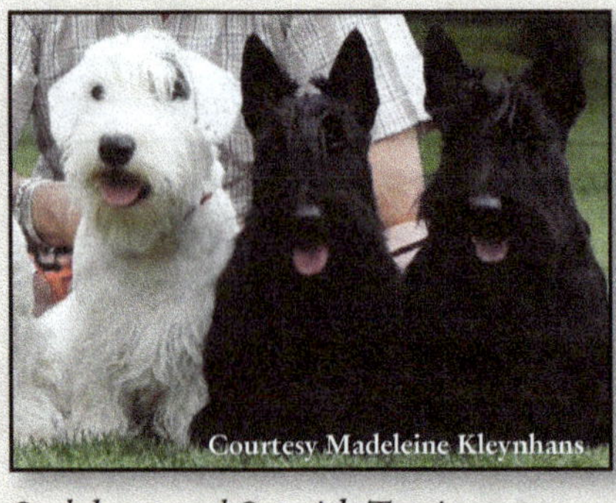

Sealyham and Scottish Terriers — Courtesy Madeleine Kleynhans

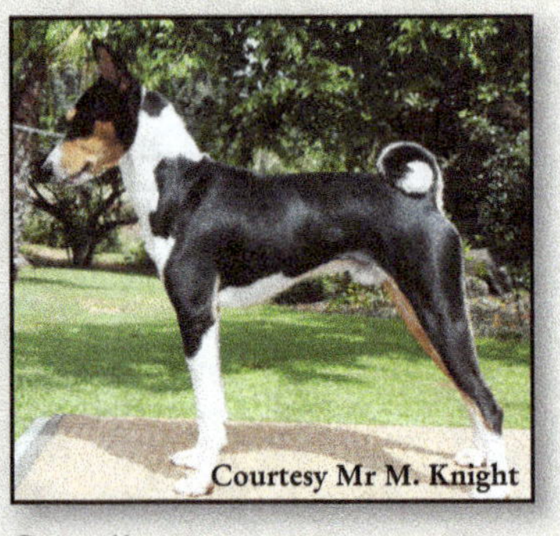

Basenji — Courtesy Mr M. Knight

Puli — Courtesy Lynn Ward

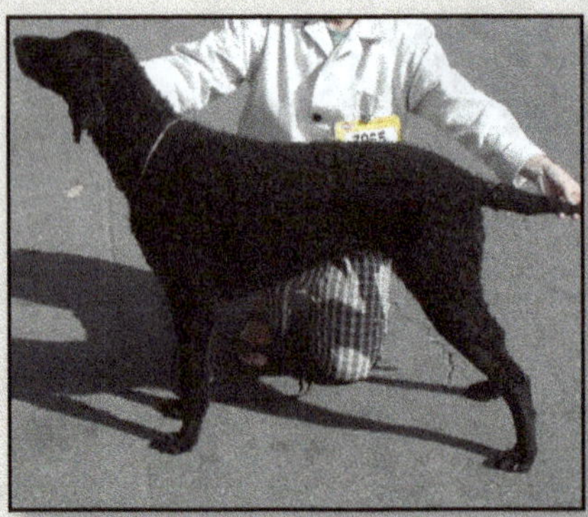

Portuguese waterdog at Birmingham show

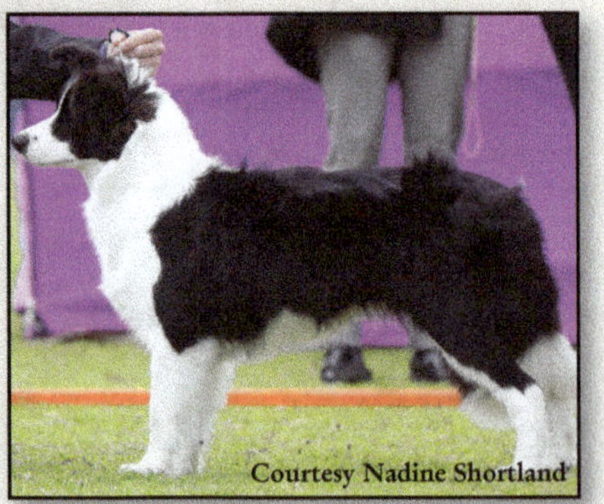

Border Collie — Courtesy Nadine Shortland

Active involvement with breed clubs and dog enthusiasts will help prospective breeders to make informed decisions. The popularity of a breed should also be taken into account. Popularity is driven by various factors such as: country of origin, patriotism, climatic conditions, security requirements and also through the popularisation of a specific breed by celebrities and the media. Some breeds might be popular in a certain part of the world but be relatively unknown elsewhere and vice versa. There are truly no rights or wrongs regarding the ultimate choice that the prospective breeder makes. However, the breeder should, at the very least, have an affinity for the breed. The choice should not be based on the possible financial gain which breeding might bring about for the breeder.

3.2. Purchasing stock

3.2.1. Purchasing foundation stock

Once the choice of breed has been made; the breeder must then decide where to buy foundation stock. It is wise to purchase dogs from a breeder who has already started the process of selection against undesirable traits as the prospective breeder then merely has to continue the good work of improving the breed. This does not imply that it is possible to acquire foundation stock which is genetically perfect. Neither perfect dogs or genetically pure dogs exist. It merely means that the reputable breeder will already have subjected his stock to stringent selection processes in an attempt to reduce the incidence of known faults and to increase the incidence of good heritable traits. It is also important to keep in mind that the quality of the progeny which a stud dog or a bitch produces is more important than the "looks" of the dog, i.e. whether it is a show champion or not. Local breed associations and veterinary surgeons should be able to help with referrals to reputable breeders.

3.2.2. Purchasing puppies

It is better for new breeders to purchase young puppies from established breeders, especially those who are involved in breed improvement schemes. Established breeders also need to augment their existing stock in order to improve it or to avoid excessive inbreeding. If the breeder already has a number of active brood bitches and wishes to acquire "new blood", the risk profile is different. The seasoned breeder, with existing breeding stock, is therefore advised to purchase older dogs.

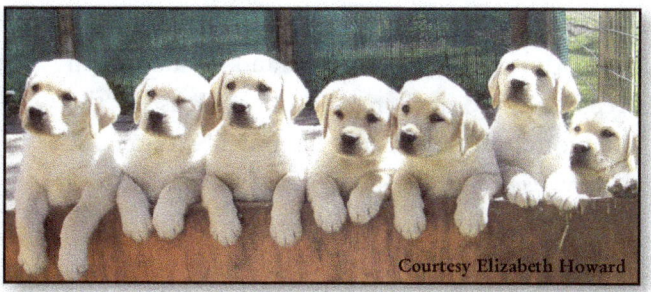

8 week old puppies all looking very much alike making selection at this age difficult at best

The main advantage of purchasing older puppies, young adults or even adult dogs is that they are less prone to disease. This is particularly important if the breeder already has a number of young puppies on the premises. Puppies under the age of 12 weeks generally have not yet been fully vaccinated and therefore the purchase of young dogs (over 16 weeks of age) is less likely to result in mortality or disease transmission to existing stock. Introducing newly weaned puppies to premises where there are new-born puppies or bitches which are about to give birth, presents a serious threat of disease introduction. Another advantage of acquiring a young adult dog is that the good and not so good characteristics of the dog are already observable unlike young puppies where choosing really is a shot in the dark.

3.2.3. Purchasing adult brood bitches

Purchasing adult dogs is normally more expensive and the price escalates if the dog comes with a list of achievements. It is advantageous to buy an adult bitch because they can be bred as soon as they come into season. Purchasing a pre-pubertal or pubertal bitch carries with it some risk. This is because a reproductive history has not yet been established and one cannot know whether the bitch will develop reproductive problems or not. If a bitch is post pubertal, the reproductive history should be investigated. From a reproductive point of view, the bitch which has had a number of cycles (2-3), was bred and has produced a litter of normal size, is the ideal bitch to buy. Bitches which have not been bred for 4-5 heat cycles are more likely to develop reproductive problems.

Purchasing a pregnant bitch is another option. This at least confirms that the bitch is fertile and it ensures an immediate return on your investment. Bitches, whose offspring have already been subjected to progeny evaluation, are the ideal. The buyer can see what the bitch looks like (phenotype) but also what the bitch is capable of producing (genotype). Of course it is important that a bitch should be phenotypically correct, however, genotypic soundness is even more important. The ideal of course would be to purchase a bitch which is phenotypically and genotypically sound. Unfortunately these bitches are not easy to come by and even if one is lucky enough to find one, it will most probably come at a premium price.

3.2.4. Purchasing an adult stud dog

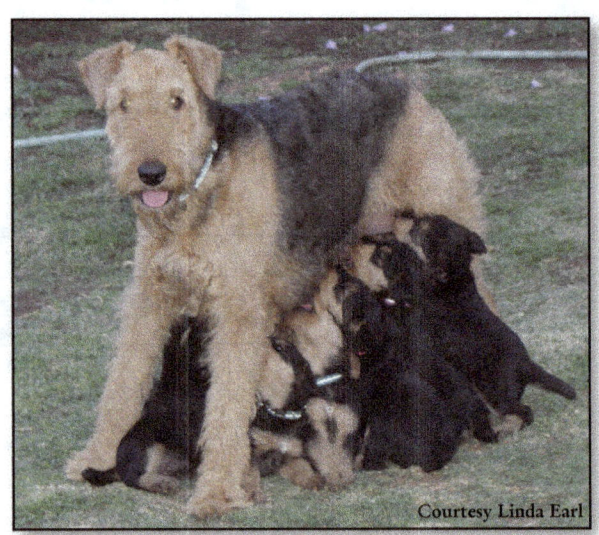

Purchasing adult brood bitch makes it easier to evaluate quality of the bitch as well as allows new owner to confirm fertility as in this case

A reproductively healthy bitch may produce up to half a dozen or so litters in her lifetime. In contrast, a stud dog will sire far more litters in its' reproductive career. A stud dog therefore makes a significantly larger contribution to the gene pool of a specific breed and to individual breeding colonies and for this reason the selection criteria should be much stricter. A widely used stud dog, carrying an undetected negative genetic trait, will pollute the genetic pool more intensely than would a bitch carrying the same trait. Likewise, the genetically sound stud dog has a much more profound effect on the genetic pool than the best bitch can ever have. What this all translates into is that more time, effort and money should be spent on acquiring the "right" stud dog. A cheaper alternative is to make use of outside owned studs dogs of proven superior quality.

It is advised that the following be investigated before a stud dog is purchased:
- Breeding soundness that includes semen evaluation
- Examination for venereal disease, depending on the country of origin
- Hip and elbow evaluation at the appropriate age by a specialist veterinary radiologist, if it is relevant to the breed.
- Eye tests by a veterinary ophthalmologist if relevant to the breed
- Relevant genetic tests for the breed
- Veterinary examination to eliminate obvious disease around the day of purchase

A breeder's ultimate goal should be to achieve genetic superiority in the dogs which are bred. Genetic superiority means that a dog possesses desired genetic traits and lacks genetic defects. Equally important is the dog's ability to consistently transfer the desired genetic traits to its offspring. This ability is often measured by performing progeny evaluation. Despite a breeder's best intentions, true genetic purity cannot be achieved. No one can guarantee genetic purity, in other words, no one can guarantee that a dog will not have genetic defects. Notwithstanding this limitation, a breeder should make every effort to breed with genetically superior dogs and only purchase stock from breeders whom do the same.

3.3. Pre-purchase veterinary examinations and certification

The pre-purchase veterinary examination requires more discussion. Experienced veterinary surgeons who examine a dog for purposes of issuing a health certificate will factually report their findings made on the day. The use of words such as "healthy and sound" should not be used in these certificates as there may be many "hidden" health problems present on the day of examination. A veterinary surgeon may for instance be requested to examine an apparently "healthy" dog. Upon examination the dog appeared lively, had a good appetite, was in a good condition, its coat appeared glossy and its rectal temperature, respiration rate and heart rate were within the normal range. Auscultation of heart and lung fields revealed no abnormalities. The veterinary surgeon would therefore have issued a report or certificate which reflected these exact findings. However, on closer examination, the following was noticed:

- Early signs of pannus (inflammatory condition of the cornea which affects vision)
- Early signs of perianal fistula
- Blood clotting defect
- Enlarged heart

For the purposes of this example, a German Shepherd Dog was selected randomly. The above dog was anything but healthy, yet a normal examination did not reveal this. The conditions mentioned above are rare, two of which can be detected with the naked eye, requiring very close examination and the others only with specialised tests and examinations. The problem is compounded by the fact that some conditions may be latent. This implies that they are indeed present on the day of examination but have not manifested themselves and may do so later. Some of these conditions can be detected following specialised examinations, others cannot.

Veterinary surgeons normally take care not to use inappropriate wording on these certificates as it may have legal implications. A factual report must be written and generalizations such as "fit for breeding", "healthy" and "sound" must be avoided. If veterinary surgeons are careful to protect their own interests, so should breeders. This can only be achieved by compiling a list of defects, conditions or diseases which the breeder wishes to have the prospective breeding animal specifically screened for. It is not possible, in this book, to compile a checklist for each breed. Such a checklist should be discussed with the breeder's veterinary surgeon as it will be different for each breed. It is also important to understand that all these efforts merely reduce the risk of buying a dog with a problem; it does not eliminate all the risks altogether. Breeders and veterinary surgeons should consult dog breeder associations which provide checklists for individual breeds as well as a checklist of genetic tests which are available in the respective breeds.

3.4. Number of dogs kept

As time goes by the number of animals kept on the premises may increase and become problematic. The first problem which can arise is the one of aggressive interaction or fighting. Depending on the breed, a breeder may be able to keep 2-3 bitches and a stud as a breeding "harem" and essentially keep these dogs, in harmony, as freely integrated pets sharing a single confinement. With small breeds a larger number of bitches and males are sometimes kept together without any real problems. For most breeds however, this is impossible.

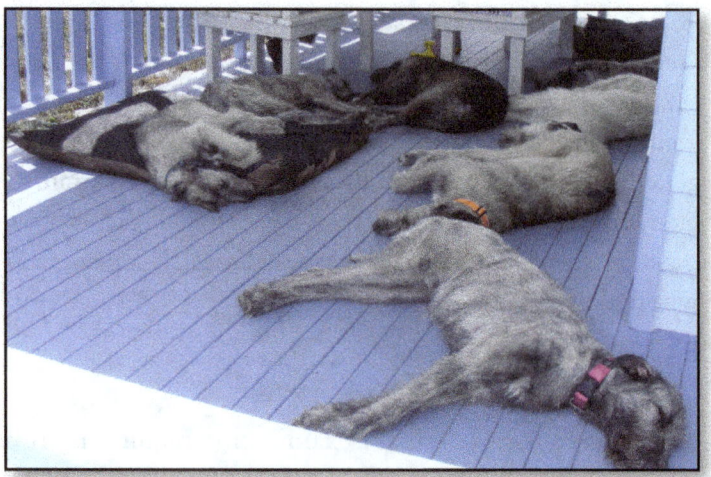

In an active dog breeding colony, fighting amongst males will necessitate their separation. In most breeds, this is also true of bitches. Bitches may be kept in small groups with a male but the temperament of each individual bitch will be the deciding factor. The tendency to fight usually increases when bitches come into season. With experience, the breeder will be able to establish the critical number of

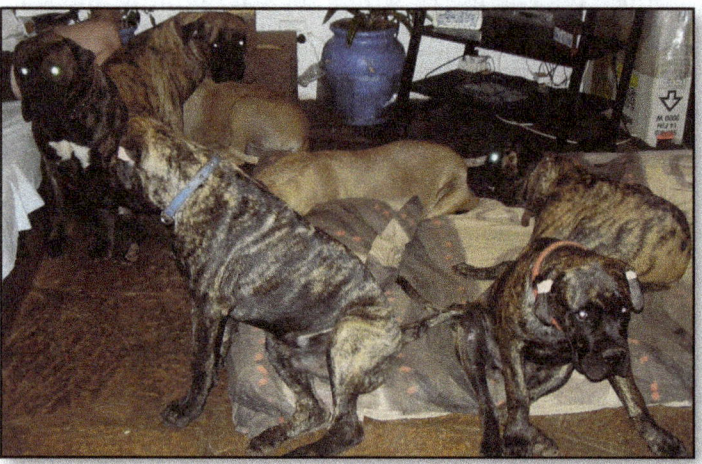

Several dogs of large breeds of both sexes living together, seemingly in harmony

individual dogs they can keep together. This critical number will vary depending on breed, individual temperament of dogs and the way in which these dogs were socialised and disciplined by the breeder.

It is important for breeders to acquaint themselves with the behavioural aspects and instincts of dogs before an attempt is made to put them together. Dogs in groups will form so called packs with each dog having a specific rank or hierarchal position within the pack (pack order). True and lasting stability in the pack does not exist but an uncomfortable truce may. This "pack order" is dynamic with individuals constantly challenging one another for a higher status. These battles may lead to serious injuries and even fatalities, not to mention injury to human beings during efforts to separate fighting dogs. It is also important to know that dogs may adopt a "mob mentality". This involves dogs ganging up against the apparent loser in a fight. This show of solidarity has manifested in packs of puppies as young as 4 months of age, with fatal outcome. Keeping dogs in kennels and rotating them in runs or camps is sometimes the only solution.

The ratio of males to bitches kept is also important. The ideal male to female ratio is about 1:4-6. Males can easily mate daily for a number of consecutive days without adversely affecting fertility provided the stud is sound (see section 10.10). It is important to understand that if brood bitches are kept together, the dormitory effect will in time synchronise their heat cycles. This means that they all come into season at the same time. This effect and the consequent synchronisation of the heat cycle complicate the management of the animals. It often forces breeders to seek outside studs as they may not have enough stud dogs to cover all their bitches. It also results in a large number of puppies, of similar age, present in the kennel, at the same time. This can create housing problems; it increases the risk of disease outbreak and brings about too many puppies to home and care for at the same time.

The number of dogs kept will influence the decision whether to make a transition from a hobbyist breeder to a larger scale breeder because more dogs will have a greater impact on the breeder's lifestyle. The number of dogs kept therefore requires careful consideration because time constraints, financial constraints and an inability to attend to the essential day-to-day care of breeding stock, will end up in poor results.

Breeders who keep large numbers of dogs are sometimes labelled as puppy farmers and or back-yard breeders. These labels are normally attached to a breeder who, in the opinion of other breeders or the public, is a breeder who:
- breeds inferior specimens
- breeds animals with temperament problems
- has "too many" different breeds on the premises
- has "too many" dogs on the premises
- does not actively show or work the dogs
- breeds for the money
- has been in the unfortunate position of having bred a dog with a problem
- has been visited by infectious disease
- has dogs on the premises that appear in poor condition

This text will refrain from such discourteous labels. Just the mere fact that a breeder has a large breeding population, per se, is no grounds for this label. However, the following is true! The larger your dog colony, the more likely it is that your problems will increase, not in a linear manner but exponentially.

Due to the increased expenses when a large dog colony is kept, breeders may be tempted to skimp on nutrition or implement disease control measures sparingly. The unmeritorious labelling of breeders based purely on dog numbers or the number of puppies they sell is not justified. True, some breeders may be deserving of such a dreadful label but in many cases, the same problems which led to one breeder being labelled might call on the next breeder irrespective of the size of their breeding enterprise. Dog breeding, by definition, equates to working within a biological system that is subject to numerous problems and variables which are often impossible to predict or prevent. Parasites and pathogens (infectious agents which may harm your animals) are successful organisms which have developed survival strategies which are especially successful in larger dog populations. These infectious agents have the potential to cause havoc within a kennel environment and it is for this reason that large-scale dog breeding is not recommended for everyone.

3.5. Animal hoarders

Most veterinary practices, at one time or another, have had to deal with an animal hoarder. These individuals are usually very passionate about their cause, which is to do the very best for the animals in their care. They feel the need to collect and keep any animal which is in need. Many animal hoarders attempt to re-home some of these animals. Animal hoarders, by nature, usually have a strong objection to euthanasia.

Re-homing adult dogs is not easy and therefore hoarders usually end up with a large numbers of dogs which they have to care for. They frequently do not have enough financial resources to feed, keep and provide veterinary care for these large dog colonies and as a result are subject to potential disasters. Although most fulfil an essential function in society, usually at animal welfare organisations and rescue clubs, it is important to note that some animal hoarders will pursue their animal hoarding at the cost and detriment of themselves, their families and others. Ultimately, the very animals they take in may suffer. As with breeders, these individuals are cautioned not to keep more animals than they can afford.

3.6. Breed rescue organizations

Breed rescue organizations are important role players in animal welfare. These organizations have an interest in the welfare of dogs of a specific breed. They are run by very passionate individuals with an exceptional love for the breed. Rescue organizations are instrumental in finding the owners of lost dogs and the re-homing of lost or abandoned dogs. Breed rescue organizations are frequently more successful in re-homing adult dogs than any other animal organization. This may be because people are more comfortable with adopting an adult dog of which the breed characteristics are known. Breed rescue organizations usually insist on the sterilization of any animal which they home. The identification of animals using transponders (microchips), greatly assist breed rescue organizations and animal pounds to reunite owners with their lost dogs.

3.7. Closed kennel concept

The concept of a closed kennel involves ensuring that there is no uncontrolled contact between the core breeding population and outside dogs and people. The idea is to keep the breeding population relatively stable. Normally dog breeding kennels have a stable population of adult breeding animals and a transient number of puppies. The only disturbance to the stability is visiting dogs for mating purposes or the occasional "new blood" purchased.

Dog breeders, who train outside dogs or perhaps board dogs on the same premises, will find it difficult to maintain a closed kennel. In these instances the population of dogs varies from day to day as trained dogs leave the premises and new ones arrive. The risk is aggravated if younger puppies which have not yet been fully vaccinated are allowed on the premises.

As already mentioned; it is good practice not to introduce puppies younger than 4 months of age to a stable breed population, as this can introduce disease. If a new puppy is introduced, it must be fully vaccinated (at least three vaccinations in most areas), dewormed and treated for external parasites. It is strongly recommended that new introductions be isolated in a quarantine area for a period of 3-4 weeks to prevent any illnesses, diseases or parasites from spreading to the breeders own stock. A small quarantine facility is ideal. The closed kennel concept also applies to people who can introduce pathogens which are carried on their hands or feet. A system of disinfecting hands and footwear will help to limit disease transmission in this way.

3.8. What to do with non-productive stock?

Over time, a dog breeder invariably accumulates dogs which are not suitable for breeding or those which are well beyond breeding age. These dogs may have become beloved pets in the breeders' home. Some dogs have sentimental value; to which much is owed because they have served the breeder well in the show ring or may have produced many champions. There may also be puppies or young dogs with minor defects or faults which render them unsuitable for breeding. The breeder might opt to attach a breeding restriction and sell these puppies to pet homes. Some defects may be of such a nature that they might cause future health problems, resulting in expenses for the puppy's new owner. A puppy may for instance present with a severe heart murmur at the time of its first vaccination. The breeder then has a dilemma in deciding what to do with such a puppy. Some breeders elect to euthanize the puppy immediately; others elect to donate the puppy to a loving home. If a puppy is donated the breeder has to inform the new owner of the problems which the dog has and what the implications are for its future health.

Euthanasia is an option but for most breeders it is the absolute last option. For others it is not an option at all. To aggravate matters, there are people who just cannot bear to part with their dogs. They have great difficulty in placing a dog in a new home no matter how good this home may be. Whatever the emotional nuance, if a breeder decides to keep "passengers and pensioners", they must be able to afford to do so. These dogs deserve the same attention as their active breeding dogs do. Far too often breeders find themselves forced to save costs on their productive stock in order to keep and maintain unproductive stock. Eventually the breeder does neither properly with potentially disastrous effect. Breeders should be honest and realistic regarding the keeping of unproductive stock. If limited resources are a factor, re-homing or euthanasia may be the logical decision otherwise the breeder will be forced to neglect the sum total. Breeders are advised to only keep as many animals as they can afford to keep.

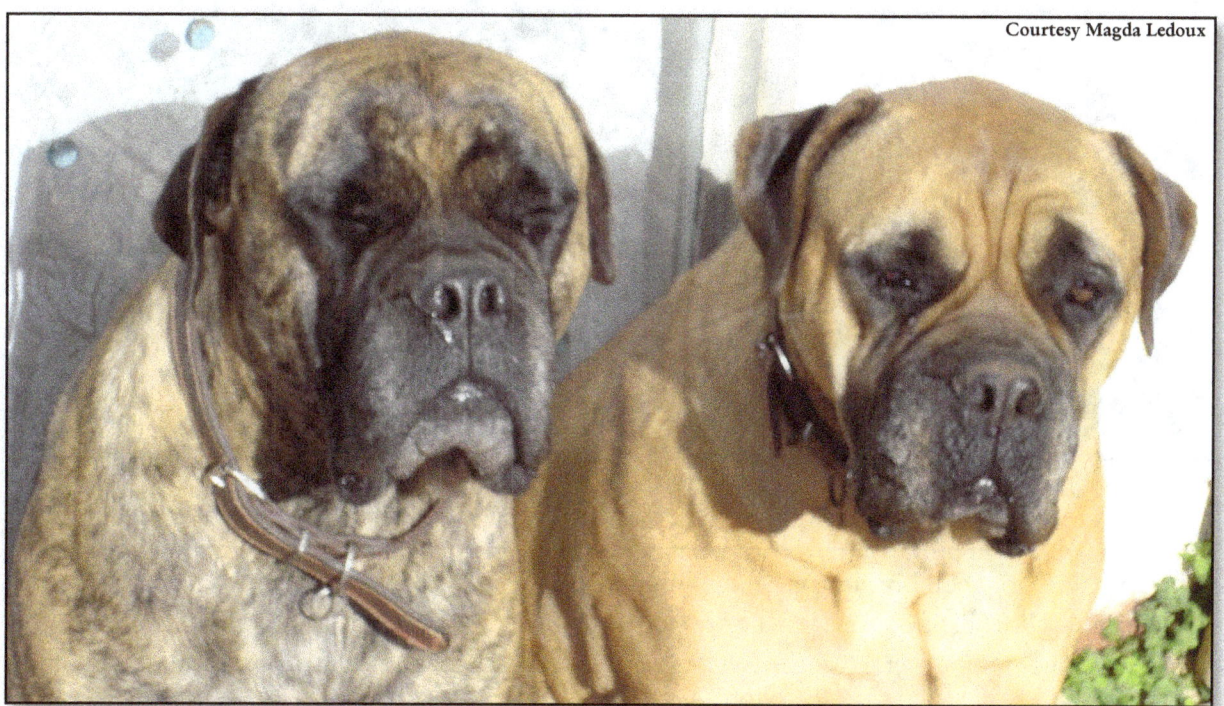

Dogs that have become "senior citizens"

Chapter 3 Beginning and Evolving as a Breeder

3.9. Showing dogs

The importance of showing dogs cannot be overemphasised. Breeders cannot breed in isolation without measuring breeding success against a breed standard and other breed specimens.

A breed standard describes observable qualities for each specific breed, i.e. conformation, movement and temperament. It is a detailed "word picture" of what the ideal dog of a specific breed should look like. Breed authorities also set additional requirements for health testing, genetic testing and work testing specific to the dog breed in question.

The goal of a conformation show is to identify breeding stock for the breed and the breed standard is the measure against which conformation judges evaluate each dog. The conformation judge evaluates the dogs to identify those that most resemble the ideal breed type and then places them in rank order. Those dogs that are frequently placed at the front of the class become the champions. These champions, by virtue of their excellent conformation, are highly recommended for breeding to improve the overall quality of a breed.

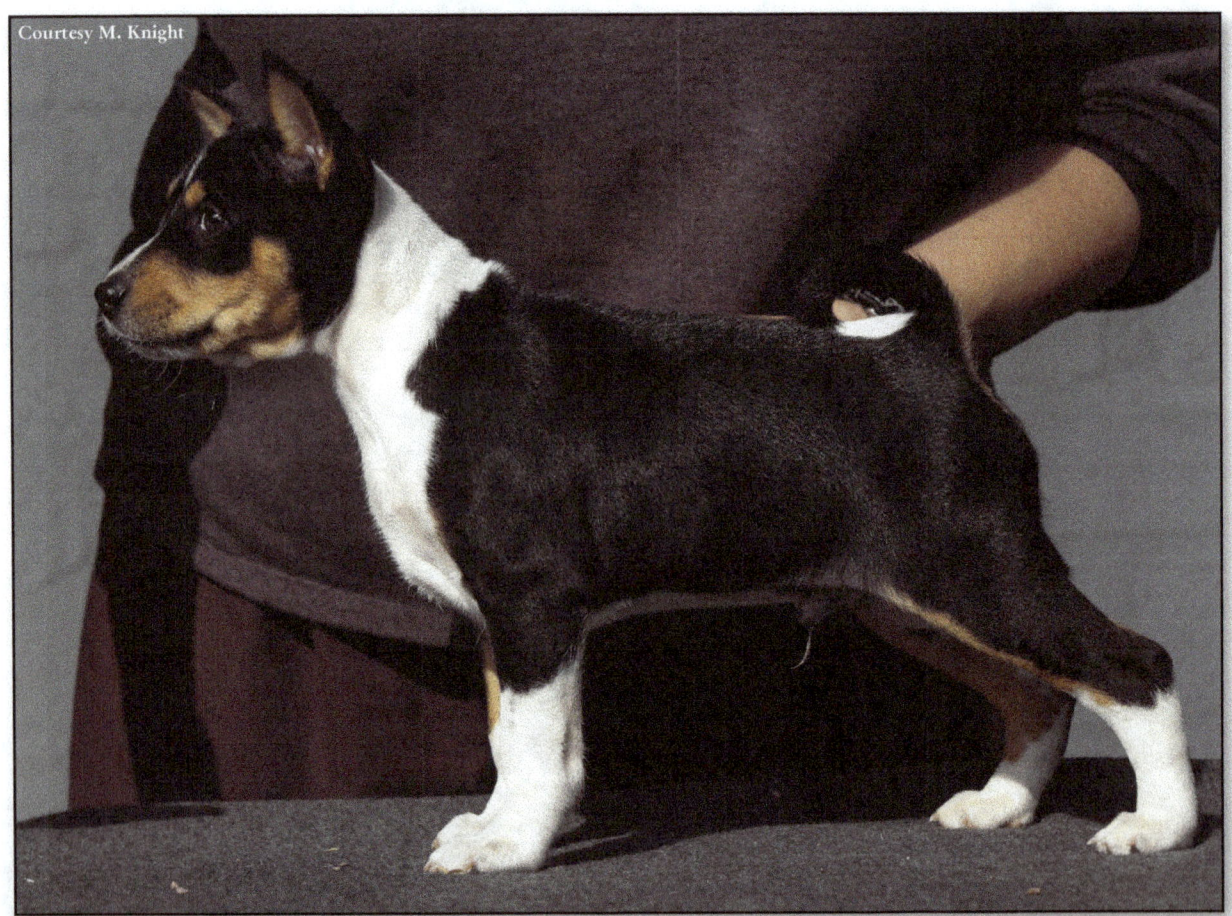

Basenji Puppy assuming a "Show stance". Many breeders claim they can already identify a champion at a very young age.

The death knell of good breeding is kennel blindness. This refers to the inability to identify faults in one's own stock whilst frequently being very critical of other's. Breeders who do not show are easily afflicted because they never expose their dogs to outside assessment and in so doing remain blind to the faults which might be evident in their dogs.

Chapter 3 Beginning and Evolving as a Breeder

The lure of breeding lies in the possibility of what might be. Most good breeders have one goal in mind; to breed a champion. In order to achieve this elusive goal a breeder has to breed with the best breeding stock available. Collectively, if many breeders do this, the overall quality of the breed is raised.

The sport of dog showing can become rather expensive. Breeders cannot spare expenses when it comes to nutrition because show dogs have to be in optimum condition and this is best achieved by feeding a premium diet. These diets, whether commercial or natural are expensive, especially if large breeds are involved. Over and above feeding costs, health costs and training expenses, there are a myriad of additional costs involved. These include travelling costs, accommodation, grooming equipment, entry fees, handling fees, food and beverages, to name but a few.

Nevertheless, dog showing can be a fulfilling hobby, especially for those breeders who go to great lengths to do justice to their breed through uncompromising observance of good breeding practices, hard work, and dedication. It brings about just rewards, either by way of accolade or personal satisfaction.

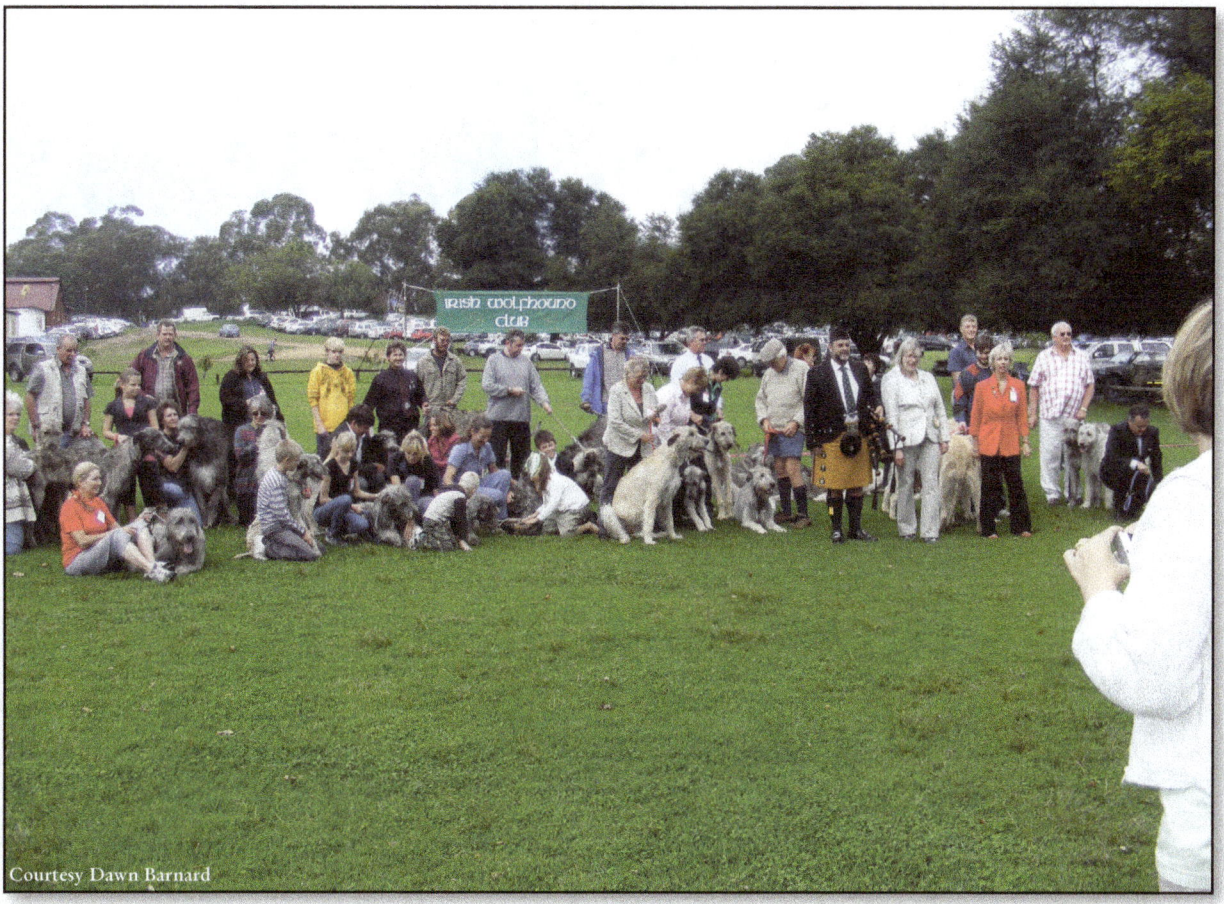

Irish Wolfhound Show

Chapter 3 Beginning and Evolving as a Breeder

Chapter 4

Nutrition

Considering that the single greatest expense in keeping and rearing live stock is nutrition, it is warranted that time and effort is expended on the subject.

4.1. History of commercial pet foods

The ancestors of the domesticated dog were most probably strictly carnivores and later developed into opportunistic omnivores by eating table scraps which were left behind by humans in and around their dwellings. In modern times, dedicated dog foods became available.

The first commercial dog food was made from vegetables and meat; either in cans or as dry meat based food. In all probability these early attempts were far from perfect and must have resulted in numerous health problems. Since those early days there has been significant progress in animal food science, which in turn, resulted in the development of the balanced diets which we have today. Over time, the market for animal food became very competitive and diverse, which led to the production of a wide, sometimes confusing array of foods, supplements and snacks.

Dog food products can be bought from a variety of outlets such as road side vendors, agricultural co-operations, grocery stores, pet shops and veterinary retail outlets. These products differ significantly regarding digestibility, palatability and nutrient quality; depending on the measure of quality control which is applied during the manufacturing process.

Foods which adequately meet the requirements of the different life stages, the breed differences and specific needs during acute or chronic illness have been developed. Research and development is on-going, notwithstanding severe price resistance by the consumer. The high-end dog foods are substantially more expensive than the lower-end foods and the average family, with a number of pets would have to spend a significant amount of their disposable income on pet food if they want to feed a better quality dog food. This leaves the pet food industry with the dilemma of maintaining the quality of the food at a price which is affordable.

Knowledge of a dog's nutritional requirements is necessary to formulate a balanced ration. These requirements may differ for the different life stages of a dog, the life style of a dog and to a lesser extent, for different breeds. The requirements and minimum standards have been extensively researched and on-going research ensures continuous improvement. Most developed countries have used these requirements to introduce minimum standards and quality control measures in their pet food manufacturing industry.

Commercial pet foods can be dry in the form of cubes, meal or pellets or wet as in canned foods. The advantages of commercial pet foods are clear. They are more convenient and likely to be cheaper than homemade food. This is especially true if the homemade food is manufactured to the same standard as commercial dog food, with an equivalent protein and mineral content and which is balanced and complete. A disadvantage of commercial pet foods may be that artificial additives have to be added to prevent contamination with mould and to prevent rancidity. There are many dog food products available which contain natural preservatives such as Rosemary extract, Vitamin E and others. Concerns are expressed about the use of the synthetic preservative ethoxyquin. No scientific evidence that indicate adverse effects has thus far seen the light regarding the use of ethoxyquin or any other synthetic preservative for that matter, if it is added at approved levels and in good quality food.

Canned dog food is a wet food which contains meat and vegetable products as the base with additives such as colour enhancers, carbohydrates and fillers as additional ingredients. Most breeders and dog owners will use canned food as a treat or to enhance palatability of dry food rations. If it is the only source of food, it can become quite expensive, and depending on the product, not fully meet the dog's nutritional requirements.

In some countries fresh commercially manufactured frozen dog food is available on the market. If fresh food is properly balanced, it is an alternative for those purists among us who insist on feeding natural and organic ingredients. With regards to manufacturing such a diet at home; even those who have a good scientific background, may find it difficult to prepare a fully balanced diet at home. It is also questionable whether it is economically viable. Some argue that homemade diets are more digestible than commercially manufactured dog food. This may only be true if the homemade diet is compared with cheaper commercial dog food brands. It is very difficult, if not impossible, for pet owners to prepare a balanced homemade dog ration. As a general rule, most breeders use commercial dry pelleted food or kibble for their dogs and therefore dry dog foods make up the bulk of pet food sales in most countries.

Dogs must like the food and therefore substantial research goes into the palatability of commercial pet food. Palatability and quality is sometimes erroneously equated. Pet owners mistakably rate a food to be of higher quality just because a dog prefers one food over the other. This leaves the food manufacturer with an additional challenge, to manufacture high quality dog food which dogs also enjoy.

Other factors besides protein and fat content which affect dog food are; raw material particle size, taste preferences of dogs and physical properties of the pellets including texture, density, size and shape. The method of processing and the equipment used in the manufacturing process, i.e. the extruder's capabilities, how the raw materials are processed and the cold chain process on raw meat ingredients also affect palatability. Enrobing is the last step in the dry food manufacturing process and entails the addition of fat and flavour enhancers to the outer surface of the kibble to improve taste and palatability.

In most countries, dog food packaging regulations require the inclusion of an expiry date on the packaging. Some companies also include the manufacturing date. As a rule, good quality dry food rations have a year shelf life and canned foods, two years. To maintain the palatability and nutritional value of dog food it should ideally be kept sealed and protected from sunlight; at room temperature in an area free from damp; in insect and rodent proof containers.

4.2. Homemade diets

Dog owners who cook for their dogs seldom succeed in providing a balanced and complete diet. Balance refers to the correct ratio of different nutrients in the food in relation to one another. Besides poor balance, the food might not be complete and require mineral and vitamin supplementation. "Complete" in the context of dog food means that it contains all the nutrients essential for good health and that it is not deficient in any of them. It is important to note that puppies are more likely to develop problems associated with poor nutritional balance than adult dogs. It is therefore even more difficult to achieve good results with a homemade puppy diet.

There are exceptions where it is justified to feed a homemade diet such as in allergy elimination trials. However, studies have shown that, in most cases of nutritional related allergies, commercially available protein diets render higher omega-3 fatty acids and are therefore better able to control an allergy. Some purists feed a homemade diet because they want food which is free from; anti-oxidants, chemical additives, colorants, fillers, flavour enhancers and preservatives. This is a goal which may not be realistically achievable in commercial diets because it reduces the shelf life. In extreme cases of purism, some even feed their dogs a vegetarian diet.

Despite overwhelming evidence to the contrary breeders of especially giant breeds still believe that top quality commercial dog food might not be appropriate for their dogs. They assert that commercial diets have too high protein content and that this excess can be rectified in a homemade diet. A homemade diet may be an appropriate option for sled dogs which work in extreme environmental conditions. These dogs have a very high caloric demand, which may not be available in all commercial diets. Specialised commercial options are however available which are appropriate for the energy requirements of canine athletes such as sled dogs.

A raw food diet is another option. It can be homemade or, in some instances, be bought at exclusive outlets. Raw food diets are often referred to as the BARF diet, which is an acronym for Bones and Raw Food Diet or Biologically Appropriate Raw Food. The appeal for raw dog food diets and its perceived benefits is mainly based on by "word of mouth" testimonials. No scientific studies have proven the benefits of feeding raw ingredients to pets. On the negative side, raw dog food can more easily become infected with bacteria such as *Clostridium*, *Salmonella* and *Campylobacter*, than dry dog food. Despite this negative, proponents of raw diets report good results.

It is not impossible to prepare a balanced homemade dog food and those wanting to do so must have sufficient scientific knowledge, access to laboratory assays but also the dedication and time to maintain a high standard of food production. Breeders should keep in mind that homemade food, if correctly balanced and complete, is likely to be more expensive than commercial dog food. Those who feed homemade diets should not advise their puppy buyers to do so, because they are unlikely to succeed at it.

Those who feed homemade diets should take care to provide chewable kibbles which promote dental health. This is important because homemade diets are often soft and do not require chewing. This contributes to tartar build up and ultimately periodontal disease and loss of teeth. Many commercial dog foods contain micro crystals in the kibble coating which reduces tartar build-up.

Most breeders and dog owners feed commercial diets because it is convenient and, in the opinion of the author, better. It is certainly also safer for both breeders and veterinary surgeons, to recommend to new owners of puppies, to feed commercial diets which are scientifically proven good diets.

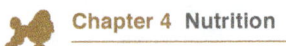 Chapter 4 Nutrition

4.3. The key nutrients in dog food

4.3.1. Fats

Fat is frequently perceived as an unhealthy source of energy in human nutrition. Therefore it is frequently erroneously regarded to be an unhealthy ingredient in dog food as well. It is however a very important nutrient in a dog's diet and healthy one too. The fat content of commercial kibbles varies between 9-22% on a dry matter base in puppy and adult dog foods, 20% in performance diets and up to 50% or more in sled dog diets. Dry matter base refers to a method of nutrient comparison and reflects the nutrient levels of the food after water has been removed. Fats provide energy and are more calorie dense than carbohydrates or proteins. It carries fat soluble vitamins and contains within it the essential fatty acids which are essential for hair and skin health.

The over-consumption of fat leads to obesity and may also cause pancreatitis or "garbage" disease in susceptible individual dogs. Over consumption of fat is frequently caused by excessive feeding of table scraps. Acute overdose usually occur when dogs gain access to garbage bins where fatty table scraps are discarded. Fats in dog food require preservatives and anti-oxidants to prevent rancidity. Rancid fats adversely affect palatability and causes gastritis (inflammation of stomach wall) and vomiting. Many people randomly add fat and oil to a diet, assuming that it will correct a dull and dry coat. However, only fats and oils containing the correct fatty acids in the correct ratio will have beneficial effects on skin and coat.

Some breeders add fat to commercial dry ration fed to individual dogs who fail to thrive. They add about 40-50 grams of fat for every 10 kg bodyweight on a daily basis. The fat fed is mostly beef fat (tallow). This practice appears to work well particularly in those dogs who fail to thrive on the normal commercial kibble and in dogs which are poor eaters. Dogs with nervous dispositions which are constantly in motion, and which burn up a lot of calories, fall into this category.

Fat supplementation is more likely to work well with dogs which are fed a marginal diet. Adding fat to a high quality dry food which already has a high fat content is less likely to have a dramatic effect. Despite this, there may still be dogs which do well on fat supplementation even if they are fed a premium diet. This is particularly true when dogs are subjected to prolonged exercise. Unlike humans, dogs derive most of the energy required for muscle contraction from fat metabolism and only a small amount from carbohydrate metabolism. Therefore, besides fitness, the fat content of food plays an important nutritional role to enhance stamina and performance.

It is suggested in some dog training circles that a high-fat diet predisposes a working dog to heat stress during work in high environmental temperatures. Studies have indicated that the opposite is true. Dogs metabolise carbohydrates and protein less efficiently than fat. More body heat is generated when carbohydrates or proteins are metabolised. Less body heat is generated when fat is metabolised and therefore less energy is expended in the process, which leaves the dog with more energy to perform its work and less heat stressed. High-fat diets are therefore more beneficial for hard working performance dogs which work in hot weather conditions.

4.3.2. Carbohydrates

Carbohydrates are present in all commercially manufactured pet foods. Most contain between 30% and 70% carbohydrates. It is acknowledged that wild canines do eat carbohydrates through

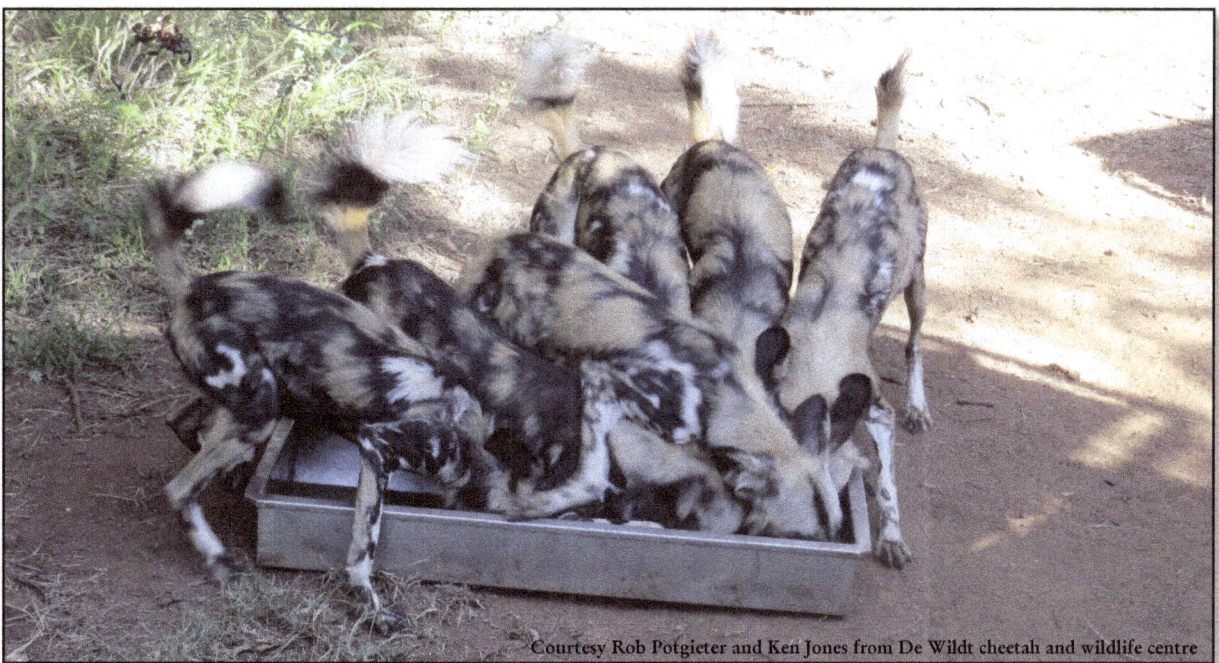
African Wild Dogs thriving on a premium commercial kibble

the consumption of fruit or the intestinal contents of their prey. The domestic dog has become an opportunistic omnivore or maybe it has always been partially omnivorous. Their wild cousin, the African Wild Dog, in captive breeding programs, does very well on high quality dry kibble that contains carbohydrates, without any adaptation.

The dog's energy and fibre requirements are met in part by the added carbohydrates. Carbohydrates are derived from plants and are therefore a cheaper source of energy than protein. Poor carbohydrate quality and composition may lead to flatulence, soft stools and even diarrhoea. Complex carbohydrates must be properly cooked before it is fed. Uncooked complex carbohydrates will often result in diarrhoea, flatulence and voluminous stools.

4.3.3. Proteins

Proteins are made up of amino acids. They are the building blocks in all animal tissues and are necessary for growth and structural development. Dogs can convert protein into stored fat in the absence of other energy sources. The stored fat is available as an energy source. Proteins are one of the most important nutrients in the diet and also the most expensive. Generally, animals require 22 amino acids. Animals can synthesize 12 amino acids themselves and these are called "non-essential" amino acids. There are however species differences. The amino acids that animals cannot produce by themselves are called essential amino acids and must be obtained from dietary sources. Taurine is an essential amino acid for cats but not for dogs. Dogs can synthesize taurine, and therefore, it need not be supplemented in their food. It is however an excellent antioxidant and supplementation may, for this reason, be beneficial in dog food as well. The saying, "dogs can eat cat food but cats cannot eat dog food" exists because dog food may not necessarily contain a source of protein which has taurine as a building block and thus lead to taurine deficiency in cats if they eat dog food.

Proteins with amino acid compositions which satisfy the animal's exact requirements are termed high quality proteins or proteins with a high biological value. Egg white has the highest biological value and for reason of comparison was given a biological value of 100 against which all other proteins are compared. Fish and whey protein have a biological value of around 90, chicken meat around 80 followed by red meat at around 75 and soy-protein at 65. Carcass meal and various plant proteins have a biological value between 40 and 50. The quality of the protein also depends on how digestible it is. For instance, hair, nail and hoof is high in the protein keratin but is virtually indigestible and therefore has very poor biological value (unless specially processed). Foods containing protein sources with poor digestibility and low biological value may indeed look good if the chemical composition indicated on the label is inspected whilst in fact they may be very poor diets. A food label may therefore not necessarily be a good indicator of quality. For instance, a dog food containing 14% protein of good quality may be vastly superior to one containing 20% poor quality protein.

Some breeders argue that certain dog foods simply have too much protein and contend that it is harmful. A harmful effect that is frequently cited as an example is kidney damage. Science has refuted these allegations. The kidneys have to rid the body of urea and other waste products following protein metabolism. Poorly functioning kidneys have a reduced ability to clear urea from the blood. High quality proteins generate less urea waste products which in turn reduces renal load. It is for this reason that dogs with reduced kidney function benefit from high quality proteins in the dog food. Restriction of protein in dogs with reduced kidney function is not the answer as it may further compromise the dog. Feeding moderate amounts of high quality protein renders the best results in these dogs.

The protein content (on dry matter base) in dog food generally varies between 17% and 30%. The minimum level according to a leading food regulatory body (FEDIAF) is 18% for adult dogs, 25% for dogs younger than 14 weeks and 20% for young dogs older than 14 weeks but not yet mature. The protein requirement varies depending on the growth stage, breed and life style of a dog. Puppy foods generally contain 25%-32% protein and adult dog foods between 19% and 30%. As previously mentioned, there are breeders of giant breeds who maintain that high end quality dog foods have too high a protein and fat content and that it leads to bone and joint problems including hip and elbow dysplasia. Research shows that the opposite is true. It is not the high protein levels in dog food but both too high energy and calcium intake which are the main culprits. The "too high energy" referred to in this context is essentially excess calorie intake achieved usually through overfeeding.

Food formulated for large breed puppies now has a lower fat and calcium content and unique calcium : phosphorous ratio. Although these changes may have reduced the incidence of skeletal problems it did not eliminate them altogether. The manifestation of these problems is not solely dependent on incorrect nutrition as genetic susceptibility also plays a role. Overfeeding is thought to be a major factor in the manifestation of skeletal problems in large and giant breeds. High end quality dog food brands are erroneously singled out as the main cause of skeletal problems in large breeds. Large and giant breeds have the genetic potential for massive growth and if these dogs are allowed to grow at the maximum rate, it can cause skeletal disorders such as osteochondritis dissicans, hypertrophic osteodystrophy and elbow and hip dysplasia, in genetically predisposed individuals.

When these breeds grow too fast, the bone supporting developing cartilage in the joints becomes weaker and less dense and therefore gives inadequate support to the overlying joint cartilage. To compensate for this weakening more bone is deposited in the socket making it more shallow and making the fit less snug and more unstable. Over-feeding these breeds during the critical growth stages (from weaning age until about 9 months of age in large breeds and weaning age until 12-15 months in giant breeds) can cause problems. The highest risk period is between 3-11 weeks of age, although clinical signs will only manifest later in life. The eventual size (height at wither) that a dog will reach is genetically predetermined and cannot be changed by how fast or how slowly the dog grows. Breeders need not be concerned that restricting food intake will affect the eventual size of a dog. It will just take longer to get to its genetically predetermined size. By virtue of the high digestibility and calorie dense nature of proteins it is much easier to over-feed with a high protein and energy dense dog food than with a poorer quality food. This may have led to the belief that high quality dog food brands are harmful, whereas the real culprit is actually overfeeding.

The incorrect calcium level in a diet is another important factor underlying skeletal abnormalities. Growing puppies absorb calcium from food through passive absorption until the age of 6 months. Adult dogs are able to regulate calcium absorption and stop absorbing if they have enough, but puppies are unable to do so. They keep on absorbing calcium and will in fact absorb almost all there is to absorb from the food. It is for this reason that the correct quantity must be added to puppy food; whereas if there was too much calcium in mature dog food for fully grown dogs, it would not matter. The quantity of calcium absorbed by a puppy is therefore directly proportional to the calcium concentration in the diet. As calcium affects skeletal growth, especially in giant breeds, the calcium level in puppy food is critical.

4.4. Choosing the right diet for your dogs

The phrase "one gets what one pays for" applies when buying dog food. The breeder should be able to recognise the difference between good quality dog food and dog food of lesser quality. Most breeders will recognize, early on, the value of good nutrition.

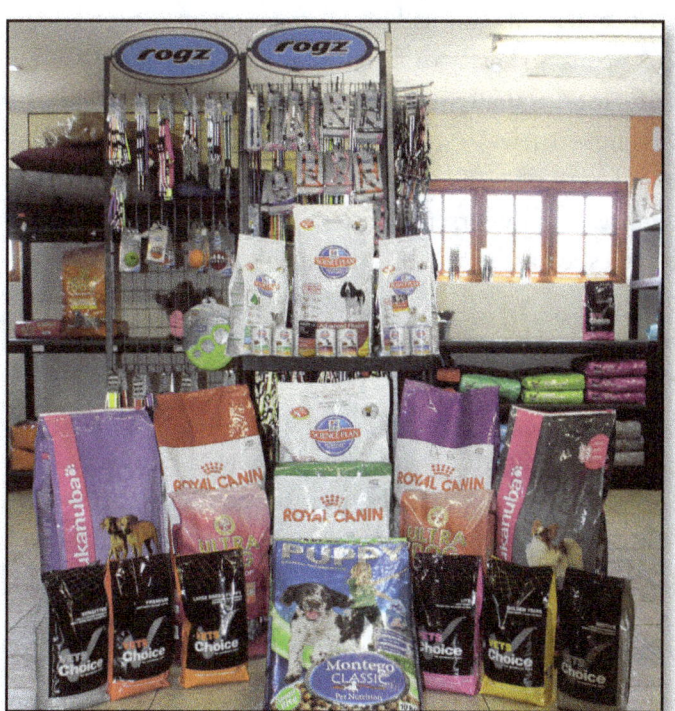

Breeders may get confused due to the very wide variety of dog food brands available

Generally, most breeders end up feeding their dogs a middle of the range dog food and will only consider high-priced foods for their active dogs, pregnant bitches, lactating bitches and their young puppies. In certain countries, the high end premium diets are only sold through veterinary outlets. This exclusivity has led many breeders to view the price with suspicion. The truth however is that these foods are usually priced the same in pet store outlets in countries where no exclusive retailing exists. The vast number of different dog foods on the market, the various brand names and convincing sales talk can leave dog owners very confused.

Chapter 4 Nutrition

The following factors must be considered when choosing dog food:
- Breed and size
- Life stages of dogs
- Quality of dog food
- Number of dogs to be fed
- Medical conditions which individual dogs may suffer from
- Money a breeder can afford to spend on dog food

It has already been established that dry food is the most popular choice for large-breed dogs. Breeders will justifiably be more conscious about dog food prices owing to and depending on the number of dogs they keep and therefore price per serving becomes an important factor in the breeder's budget. This is particularly true for breeders of large breed dogs.

Research has shown that various breeds have different nutritional needs. The smaller breeds tolerate caloric dense food (high in fat and protein) better than large and giant breeds. For instance, bone and joint problems occur if small breed dog food is fed to large breed dogs. Modern large and giant breed diets recognise these differences and therefore have a lower fat and protein content and an altered calcium and phosphorous ratio. It is important to look at the nutritional levels of certain nutrients in relation to the amount which is fed, especially to breeds which are prone to gastric dilatation and volvulus (GDV). Scientific studies have concluded that dogs that are fed larger volumes of food per meal have a significantly greater risk of developing GDV, regardless of the number of meals fed daily. For both large breed and giant breed dogs, the risk of GDV was highest if dogs were fed a large volume of food once daily as opposed to dividing the same volume of food into two meals.

Although vast differences exist between the nutritional needs of small breed dogs and large breed dogs, it is debateable whether the needs within each group are so vastly different that a breed specific food is justified. It is also debatable whether breed specific food actually does cater for the specific nutritional needs of the breed which it was designed for. It is nevertheless very popular with dog owners because it makes the choice of dog food easier for them and food manufacturers recognise this. However, dogs which have a nutritionally responsive disease, such as skin hypersensitivities, heart conditions, or renal disease, should be kept on a disease specific diet, irrespective of the breed concerned.

The quality of pet food is an important consideration. The concept of perceived quality versus true quality can be challenging for breeders, pet owners and even veterinary surgeons. High-quality ingredients are essential for a good quality diet. Dog food can be loosely classified in 3 categories; the economy brands, the semi-premium brands and the premium brands. The premium brands are the most expensive and are sold at exclusive outlets or veterinary practices, in most countries. As a rule, economy brands are made of less expensive ingredients. The problem here lies with digestibility and availability of nutrients to the dog. A practical measure to gauge the digestibility of dog food is the volume of stool which the dog passes in relation to the quantity of food which it has eaten. If the digestibility is poor, the stool will be more voluminous. The number of stools passed also has a direct correlation with the digestibility of the food; a greater number of stools will be passed if the food has poor digestibility.

Semi premium and premium diets are generally more expensive with better quality ingredients and greater digestibility. Breeders of small and medium breeds should calculate the cost difference between feeding a premium diet and a lesser quality alternative. The difference in cost might be negligible which may place a breeder in the position to feed a premium diet. The difference in cost between premium and economy diets is more apparent when feeding large and giant breeds.

An economy brand has lower digestibility, poorer bioavailability of protein and provides less energy, without it necessarily being evident on a food label. The bottom line is this; a dog has to eat much more of the economy brand food than the premium brand food in order to reach satiation and meet its requirements. Everything considered dog breeders are advised to feed the best dog food they can afford and should advise their puppy buyers to do the same.

4.5. Food for the different life stages and life styles

As dogs grow mature and age, their requirements also change and hence the development of dog food for the growing dog, adult dog and senior dog. The food which is fed should be appropriate for the life stage of the dog. Typically, puppy foods will contain proportionally more calories and proteins per unit of dog food in comparison to adult dog food. Likewise, specific diets are formulated to meet the requirements of older dogs, active dogs, lactating bitches and so forth. Not only are different foods manufactured according to specific life stage and life style requirements but also to satisfy the whims of dog owners.

The bulk of dog food consumed by breed dogs is commercial dry kibble as a maintenance diet. If the food is of acceptable quality, most dogs will thrive on it. In some multiple dog households the owners will communicate their unwillingness or inability to feed their dogs different diets as they are all fed together. These dog owners will therefore insist on feeding them one generic dog food. Breeders will usually not have this problem as many of their dogs are kennelled making individual feeding

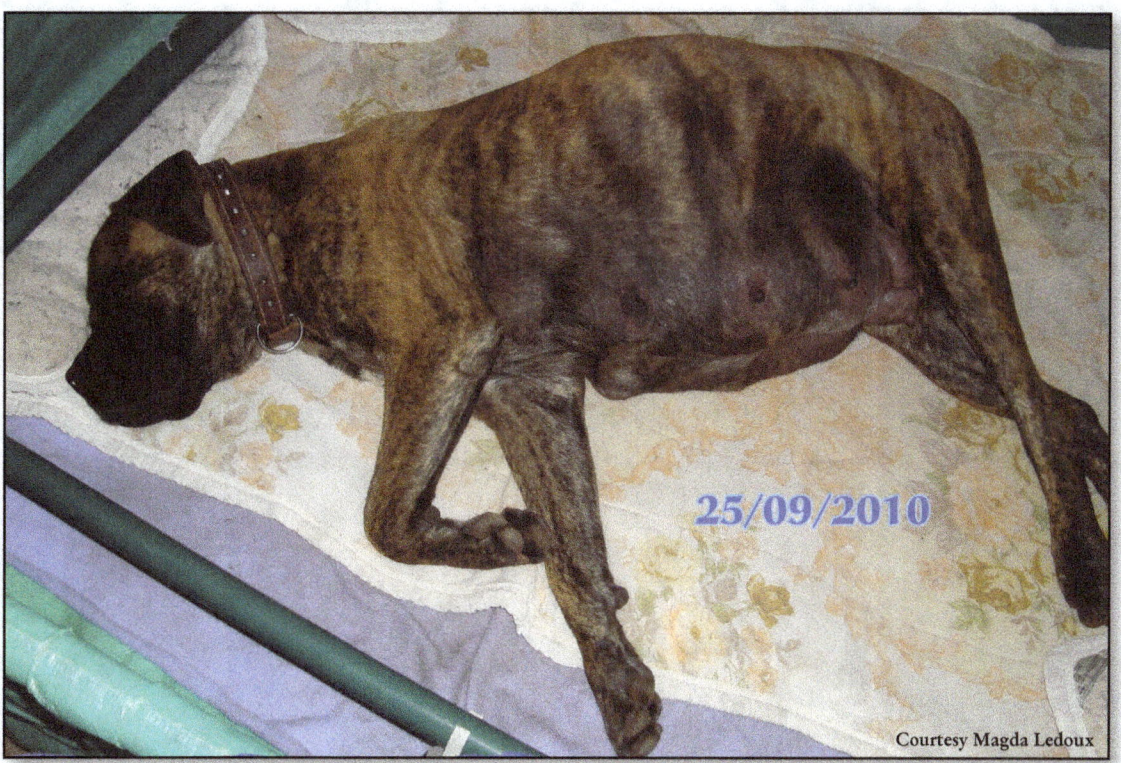

Courtesy Magda Ledoux

Obviously pregnant dam

practical. Although not advisable, dog owners and breeders who wish to feed one diet only, should consult their dog food retail specialists or veterinary surgeons to help choose the most appropriate dog food type that will best suit the majority of their dogs. The life stages of dogs are dependent on breed. Generally small breeds reach adulthood between 8-10 months; medium sized breeds at approximately 12 months, large breed dogs at approximately 15 months and Giant breeds between 18-24 months. The adult life stage spans from 12 months (24 months in large breeds) to 7 years of age, followed by the senior life stage from 7 years and older.

The lifestyle of a dog is determined by what the dog is used for. Breeds which are used as sport dogs, for instance, are selected for their high drive and willingness to work. Not unlike human athletes, these dogs benefit from special nutritional management. High performance foods cater for the special nutritional needs of these dogs and better results can be expected using these diets.

4.6. Feeding for pregnancy and lactation

Breeding bitches should be kept in optimal body condition. Bitches which are too fat may not conceive or develop birthing problems whereas underweight bitches may, in addition to poor fertility, have difficulty in providing enough milk to their offspring. During the early stages of pregnancy the bitch's nutritional requirements are no different to those which are not pregnant. There is however proof that most breeds benefit from folic acid and Beta-carotene supplementation, especially in the early stages of pregnancy. It is very important in the early stages of pregnancy, when implantation takes place (at around 11 days after ovulation) that there not be an event of starvation. At this stage even a short period of starvation (not feeding for a day or two) may cause failure to implant and thus failure to conceive. After implantation the risk of resorption is reduced but not excluded. Bitches that are starved will mobilize nutrients from fat stores and even muscle if her diet fails to meet her

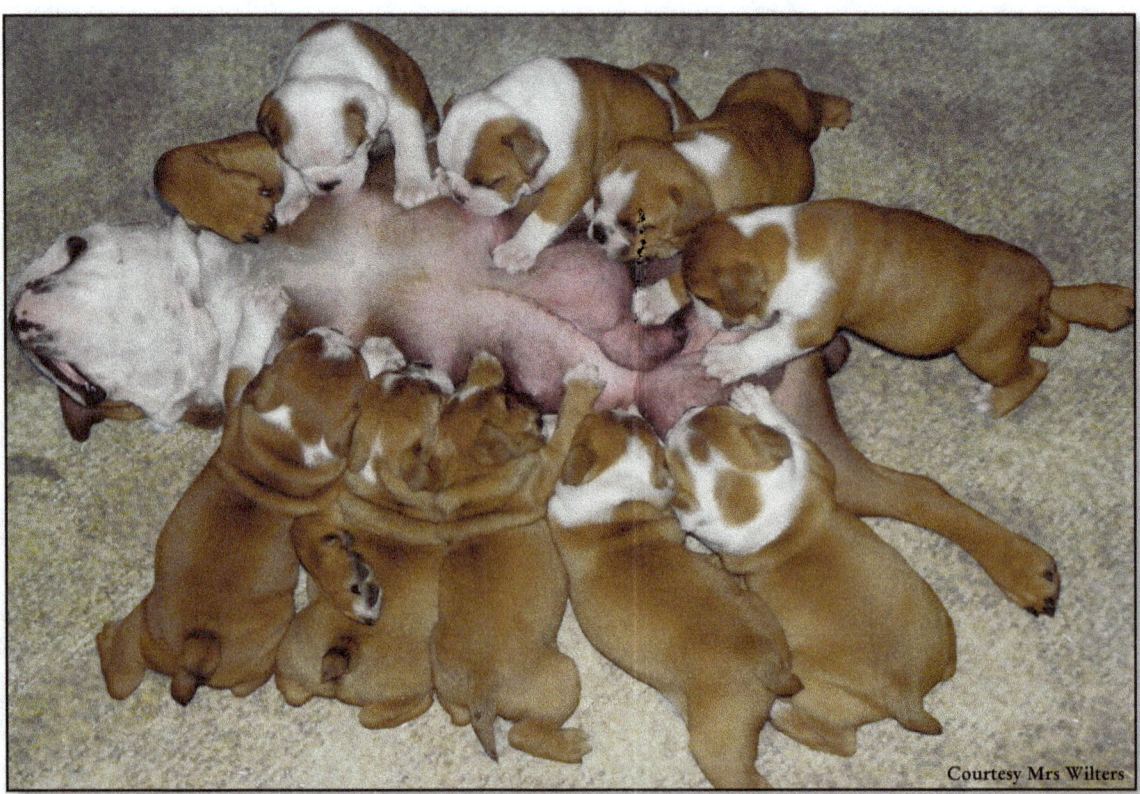

From the condition of the puppies it is clear that this bitch was well fed for lactation

nutritional requirements. If the nutritional shortfall is too great or lasts too long the bitch may resorb some or perhaps all the foetuses or abort them altogether. From about mid pregnancy, the nutritional demands placed on the bitch, start to increase and bitches require 20-40%(depending on litter size) more food towards the last trimester of pregnancy to accommodate the accelerated growth of the foetuses which takes place during this time. If the litter is large, the uterus and stomach compete for space in the abdominal cavity. Towards the end of pregnancy the stomach capacity decreases but the nutritional demands increase. More frequent feeding (2-3 meals per day) of a high quality energy dense diet makes sense during late pregnancy and low energy, bulky diets might be problematic.

It is common practice for breeders to feed puppy food to their bitches which are in late pregnancy or lactating. As a general rule this will do no harm and it is probably advantageous, if a marginal diet was fed up to that point. The ideal, during this critical period, is to feed the best possible diet that the breeder can afford.

Diets which meet the unique requirements of the bitch during pregnancy and lactation demonstrate distinct benefits and are manufactured by various leading companies. It is common for bitches to eat less during the last few days before whelping and some may even stop eating all together around 12 hours or so before whelping. It is also not uncommon for bitches to eat very poorly for two or more days following the birth of the litter. Breeders will often encourage their bitches to eat by adding meat and gravy to their diet. Healthy bitches will eventually resume eating once this post-natal anorexic phase has passed.

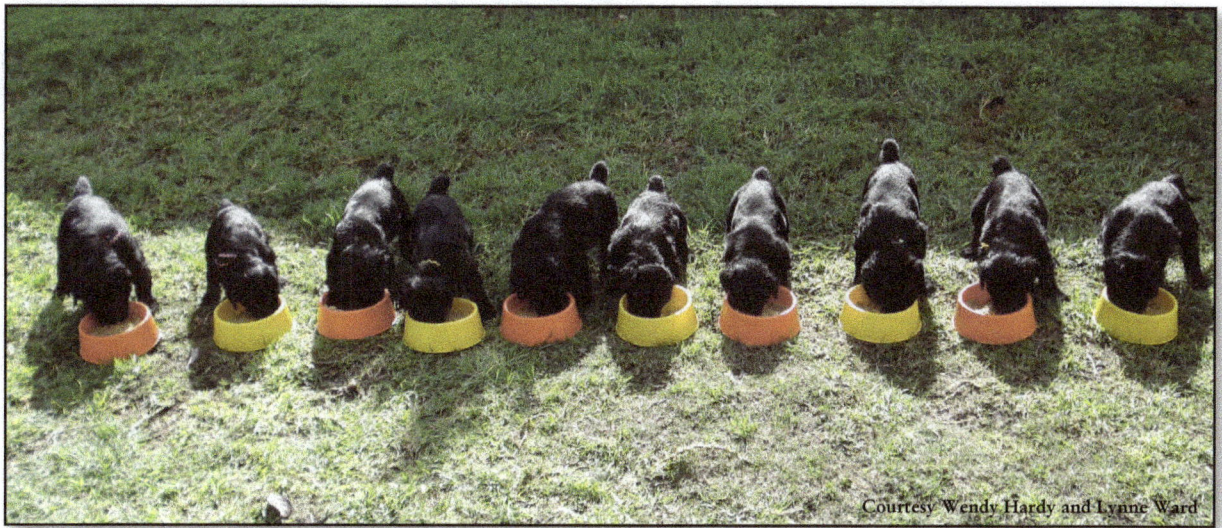

Individual feeding of puppies

In stark contrast to the slight increase in nutritional demands during pregnancy, the increase during lactation is phenomenal. An increase of 250-300% in food intake of bitches with normal sized litters is common and it is even greater in bitches nursing very large litters. The increase in nutritional requirements parallels the lactation curve which peaks at about 17-30 days post whelping. Breeders are encouraged to feed bitches to demand during this period and feed the best diet they can afford. Most breeders will soon realise that it is much cheaper to feed the bitch properly, enabling good milk production, than having to buy a milk replacer; not to mention the inconvenience associated with bottle feeding puppies.

4.7. How much and how often to feed my dog

4.7.1. Volume

Feeding ad libitum (ad lib feeding), is the practice of leaving out as much food as the dog wants, all the time. This is also known as free access feeding. An ad lib feeding regime, using self-feeders, is popular in some kennels. This is so because it is easier, results in less spillage and is less labour intensive. In these kennels, the dogs will control their intake relative to their nutritional requirements. Whether this self-control is dictated by breed is not known but it appears to work reasonably well in commercial kennels. In these kennels, very few dogs become obese. It must be pointed out that the vast majority of these kennels keep mostly dog breeds which are used as security dogs or service dogs and it is well known that these breeds are less prone to obesity. Also, in these kennels, the dogs are kennelled individually and the dogs are therefore not subject to dominance and food aggression. In pet households and breeding kennels ad lib feeding is generally not advised. There are many disadvantages to ad-lib feeding, whether from self-feeders or ordinary dog bowls, the greatest being the fact that dogs frequently become obese. If more than one dog feeds from the same bowl it becomes impossible to evaluate appetite or to establish what a dog's food intake is. The food in self-feeders can become contaminated with spray from hoses and faeces in back spray if pressurised water hoses are used to clean the kennels. Ad lib feeding of large breed puppies in particular, may lead to skeletal conditions as previously discussed.

Most dog owners and breeders try to feed the recommended allowance per day or per meal as accurately as possible. Some follow the feeding guidelines to the letter. Whilst this practice will work for most dogs, there are exceptions. Some individuals of any breed, may lose weight on such a program whereas others will become obese. The basal metabolic rates of dogs differ vastly and this accounts for the differences in maintenance requirements. The feeding instruction on the food bag gives the recommended amount to feed based on the growth stage and weight of the dog. In the end, the final ration which should be fed depends on the nutritional needs of each individual dog. The breeder or dog owner should therefore have an accurate record of how much the dog is fed so that they can adjust (tweak) the volume of food to suit the dog's individual needs. Feeding guidelines follow a normal distribution type curve and therefore the guidelines are for the average dog; there will be a small percentage of dogs which need either more or less food than what the guideline specifies.

Working dogs have increased energy needs. The maintenance requirement of normal adult dogs refers to the ration required to provide the dog with enough calories to maintain body weight and body condition. When weight loss occurs more should be fed. If dogs are worked they need to be fed more, to make up for energy expended during work. Dogs consume more food in winter to make up for energy consumption required to maintain body core temperature and to maintain body weight.

4.7.2. How often to feed

After weaning (at 6-8 weeks of age), puppies can be fed 3 times a day until about 5-6 months of age. Thereafter a dog can be fed twice a day if the breeder or dog owner elects to do so. Some breeders wish to feed once a day only. Pregnant and lactating bitches as well as active working dogs should however be fed at least twice a day. The question is often asked whether the single feed should be in the morning or in the afternoon. It really does not matter but many prefer to do so in the morning, as it gives early warning of a dog which is not eating. Owners of security dogs report that the dogs are more alert for their night time watch, if they are fed in the morning. Also, in large breeds where gastric dilatation and volvulus (GDV) (twisting of stomach) is common, early feeding is preferred as it allows the breeder to identify the early signs of GDV, at least during the day and not in the middle of the night when it can be missed, often with fatal outcome. Many breeders and dog owners elect to feed both young and adult dogs twice a day, which is the recommended frequency.

4.8. Obesity

Obesity occurs when a dog's food intake exceeds its energy expenditure. Excessive calorie intake due to overfeeding is the main cause of obesity and depends mainly on whether more food is made available to the dog than what it needs. It is easier to overfeed when the food is very calorie dense. Treats and table scraps fall into this category and is the leading cause of obesity in dogs. Lack of exercise is another contributing factor. Dogs who never exercise expend little energy; energy burns calories and so the lack of exercise reduces the dog's need to consume calories. Consequently, if the dog's diet is not adjusted to suit its energy expenditure level, weight gain problems will result.

Castration (neutering) and ovariohysterectomy (spaying) may lead to as much as a 30% reduction in metabolic rate and this should be taken into consideration when feeding sterilised dogs. Dog owners and breeders have the option, and are advised, to switch their dogs prophylactically (preventatively) to a diet appropriate for sterilised dogs. Such specialised diets are available in commerce and breeders and owners should consider using them as soon as they come off their puppy formula and are sterilised. The body condition score after castration and spaying must be closely monitored.

There appears to be an individual and/or breed related genetic predisposition towards obesity. Reduced activity levels associated with age may also play a role. Dogs in multi-dog households may be more susceptible to obesity because their "rival's" presence arouses the competitive spirit in them, which drives them to eat too much.

Breeders seldom have a problem with obesity because overfeeding is expensive. Obesity can also affect a dog's reproductive health which, from a breeder's point of view, is counterproductive. Obese bitches tend to have more problems giving birth than dogs which are at their optimum weight. Obesity can lead to a narrowing of the birth canal and fat infiltration of the uterine muscular (myometrium) wall which in turn impedes the ability of the uterus to contract. Obesity in stud dogs reduces their athletic ability to copulate and it adversely affects their libido (sex drive). Grossly obese bitches may also experience problems to conceive and have smaller litters. The exact mechanism by which this is mediated is unknown.

Obesity causes peripheral insulin resistance in dogs and dogs which are diagnosed with diabetes are usually obese. It is clear that obesity reduces the quality of life of a dog and negatively affects longevity. Breeders are also cautioned not to over-feed puppies. Some breeders and the public at large have the perception that a fat little puppy is a sign of good health. Dogs which are overweight at a young age are likely to become overweight as adults. Puppies which carry excessive weight are prone to skeletal problems and hip dysplasia as discussed before.

An obesity check can be performed by feeling over the rib area with the palm of your hand and to look from the top (dorsal view) to establish whether the dog pinches in behind the last rib. If the ribs are easily felt and the waist is clearly visible, the dog is of the correct weight; if not, the dog is obese. Dual-energy X-ray absorptiometry (DEXA) is a means of measuring bone mineral density but can also be used to measure total body composition and fat content with a high degree of accuracy. These methods are usually used for scientific studies where such accuracy is required.

Obese dogs should be on a calorie restriction program, regardless of the cause of obesity. Special diets are also available and may make the goal of weight loss easier to achieve because low-calorie dense food tends to produce satiety at a lower level of calorie intake. Simply feeding the dog less is perhaps the most practical solution for breeders.

4.9. Underweight dogs

If dogs are underweight the breeder should establish whether it is true of all the dogs in their kennel or limited to a few individuals. The breeder should also establish whether the underweight dog has a normal appetite (normal food intake) or a poor appetite. Some dogs are poor eaters and remain in a suboptimal condition for practically their whole life. Feeding meats and gravies in addition to their regular kibble may improve their food intake and therefore also their condition, but in some dogs, never to a level that can be considered normal.

Although the deep chested breeds are more prone to this, any dog of any breed can be affected. Affected dogs do not appear ill or listless and are sometimes even very energetic dogs. Extensive laboratory tests which include examinations for maldigestion, malabsorption, protein or glucose loss, endocrine disorders and so forth can prove inconclusive in certain individuals. Some of these dogs appear to be very nervous dogs and are usually low ranking and submissive. It may help to feed these individuals in a secluded spot, away from dominant pack members. Kennel confinement may be another option but many dogs resent it; in fact, any effort to improve their condition often fails. Breeders may consider retiring these dogs to a pet home where their condition often mysteriously improves.

Stud dogs may eat poorly or even starve themselves when a number of bitches come into season or if outside bitches in heat are introduced onto the premises. Although this is a temporary situation, it may affect their condition significantly, which may be more worrisome during the show season. Removing these bitches to another location will usually resolve the problem. Breeders should be mindful that dogs in poor condition draw unwanted attention to the breeder, leading the public to suspect there is something wrong with the breeder's stock or that there is neglect.

4.10. Feeding of bones

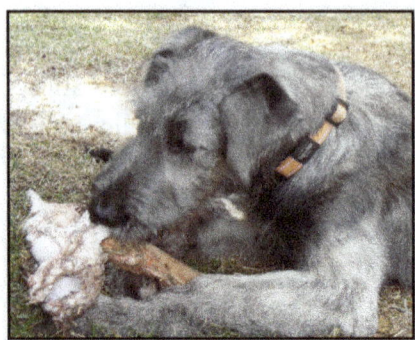

Despite controversy, many dog lovers feed their dogs bones and this dog is not complaining

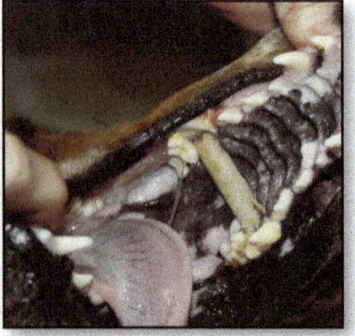

Piece of bone wedged in between the two rows of teeth on hard palate

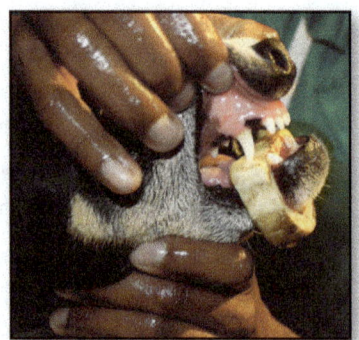

Bone caught in bottom jaw

It is true that bones make out a significant part of a wild dog's diet and for this reason, one might think that it is perfectly in-order to feed bones to domesticated dogs. Feeding bones is not recommended as it is not without risk. Bones may get stuck in the dog's palate between the two rows of teeth. If a dog attempts to swallow, a too big bone, it frequently gets stuck in the oesophagus, normally just before the heart or just before the diaphragm. This is a serious condition which may require surgical intervention. Once a single bone has entered the stomach, it is less likely to cause an obstruction lower down the intestinal tract. Dogs which are glutinous or ravenous feeders are more likely to develop an obstruction, either by swallowing a too big bone or for that matter, swallow any foreign object.

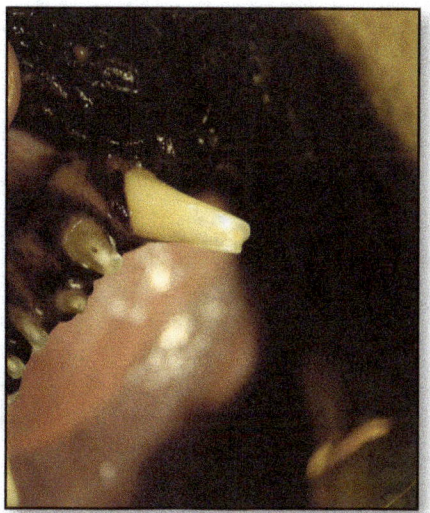
Tooth fracture

Another problem associated with eating bones is constipation. It is not the size of the bone which causes constipation but the number of bones consumed. Dogs which ingest too many bones of any size may get impacted with undigested hard bone delaying intestinal transit. The large intestine is the section of the digestive tract where the most significant part of water absorption takes place. When there is a delay in transit in this section, the stool gets increasingly harder and dryer resulting in constipation. The early onset of constipation can be corrected by performing an enema, advanced constipation is a different matter altogether. This is a serious condition which may require surgery to correct.

Bones can cause teeth fractures. Those who feed bones contend that given the options of an occasional tooth fracture and the discomfort of teeth loss associated with periodontal disease, they choose the lesser of the two evils, namely, the occasional tooth fracture. Scientists insist that there is sufficient evidence to prove that periodontal disease occurs in dogs independently of whether they eat bones or not. In conclusion, the safer option is most certainly not to feed bones of any description to dogs. Most will concur that the potential dangers far outweigh any faint claim of benefit. Lastly, bones have been the cause of fights amongst dogs that otherwise live together in harmony.

4.11. Dental care and diet

As a rule the accumulation of plaque and tartar is slower when dry, rather than wet food is consumed. Some manufacturers produce a kibble which does not disintegrate so rapidly, allowing it to cause enough lateral friction against the teeth crowns to mechanically help rid them of accumulated tartar and plaque. Some food manufacturers coat the food with polyphosphates in microcrystalline form. This helps to reduce tartar formation without the need for abrasive action on teeth crowns. Other than a genetic predisposition to periodontal disease, smaller breeds by virtue of their crowded mouth are more prone to plaque accumulation and subsequent periodontal disease. Home dental care is very helpful if dogs allow this intervention but unfortunately most dogs do not. Scaling and polishing teeth at a veterinary surgeon is sometimes the only option if the condition has deteriorated to a point where this is necessary. Dental chews may help but are not without risk. Cow hoofs have on occasion caused bowel obstructions whilst bones may cause obstructions, teeth fractures and constipation. Raw hide and gelatine based chews are generally safer but sometimes carry harmful bacteria. As a general rule, chews which are individually packed are less likely to be contaminated

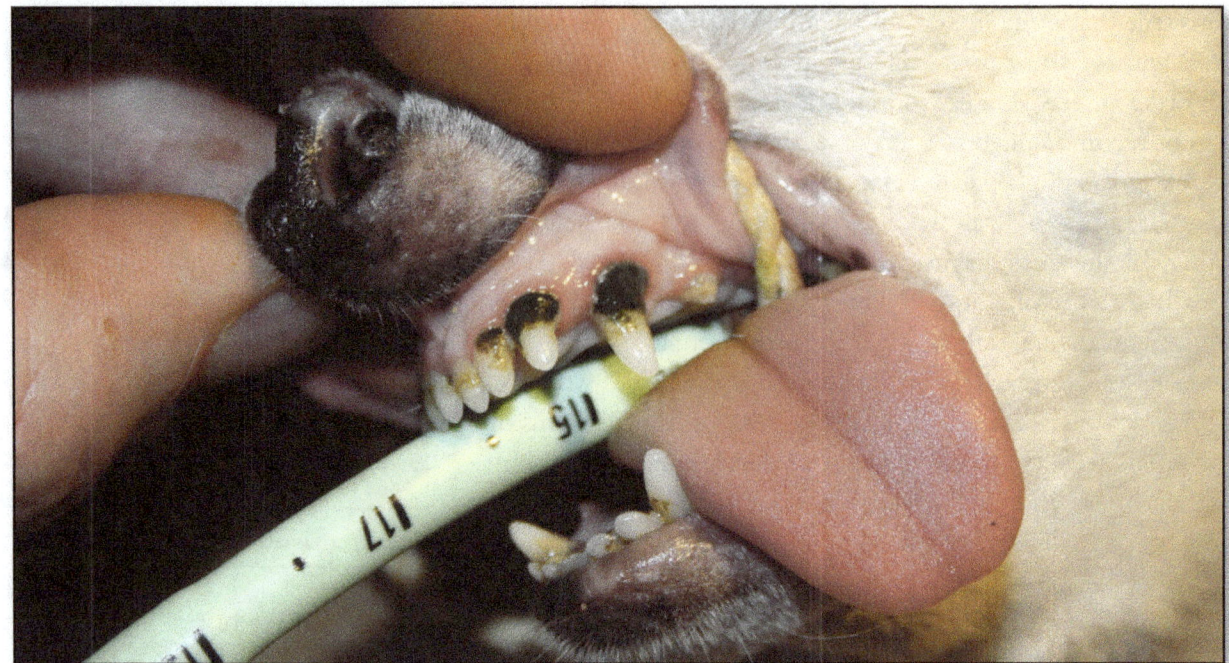

Tartar build up

and are considered to be safer. Chews satisfy the dog's need to chew and may even keep them from chewing valuables around the house, whilst at the same time, aid dental health.

4.12. Pica

Pica refers to the eating of foreign objects which do not have any nutritional value. These objects may be items such as stones, wood, clothing, cabling and so on. It can be harmful to a dog if the object is toxic or if it causes an obstruction, constipation or intestinal perforation.

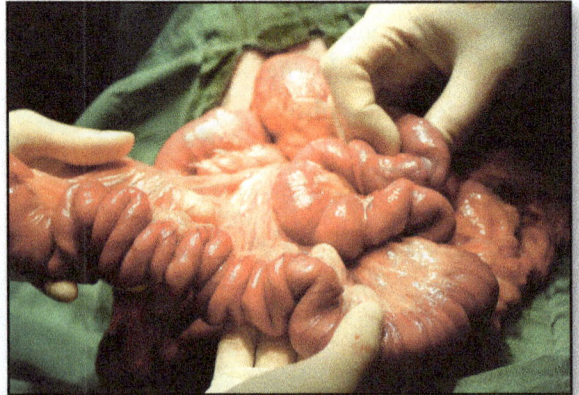

Linear foreign body in gastro intestinal tract

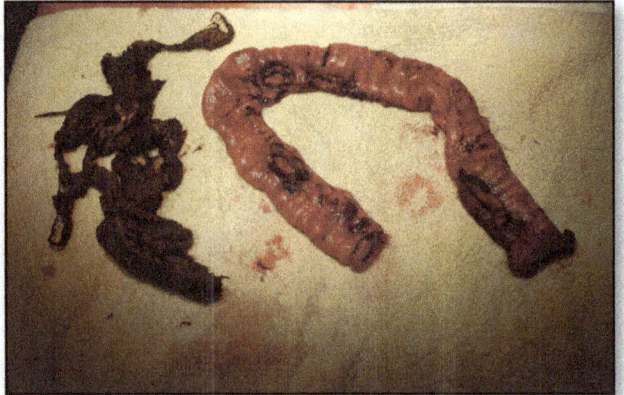

Resected piece of intestine as result of obstruction with cloth

Certain breeds are more prone to pica and especially puppies of all breeds are more likely to exhibit pica. Medical reasons for pica include dietary deficiencies, maldigestion, malabsorption and kidney disease. In most cases however, the cause is behavioural. Lack of exercise, boredom, stress, anxiety may all be contributing factors. In some dogs the cause of pica is considered to be an obsessive-compulsive disorder and anti-anxiety medication may be indicated. Pica should be investigated by a veterinary surgeon and the underlying causes must be addressed. If a medical cause cannot be found, behavioural modification should be attempted. Exercise will help rid the dog of excess energy and divert attention away from biting on objects. Providing acceptable chew items may also help. Spraying objects (which an individual dog favours to chew on) with taste deterrents may also help reduce interest in those objects.

Dogs frequently eat grass. Evidence suggests that the dogs are not necessarily unwell when they eat grass and unlike commonly believed, will not always vomit after the consumption of grass. Dogs cannot digest grass and therefore grass eating should, strictly speaking, be considered to be pica. Eating grass is however so common in dogs that some regard it as normal behaviour. We do not know the real reason why dogs eat grass. We know that wild carnivores eat grass on occasion and they do ingest grass when they consume the contents of their prey's ingesta. Opinions on this topic vary. Some experts report that wolves, predating on herbivores, will remove the rumen contents by shaking it. The intake of plant material from their prey's gut is therefore seen to be purely accidental and not intentional. African predators, on the contrary, are often observed ingesting the rumen contents of their prey, as do farm dogs when they eat the rumen content of freshly slaughtered sheep with the greatest relish. In arid regions, carnivores have been observed drinking the rumen fluid of their prey. It is interesting to note that all carnivores, domestic or wild, always chew fresh green grass shoots; never dry grass. The grass does eventually pass through the intestine (undigested) and can be clearly seen in the faeces.

4.13. Coprophagia

Coprophagia is the act of eating faeces. The dog may eat its own or another dog's stools or perhaps even other species' stool. As with pica; there may be a medical reason why a dog needs to "supplement" its diet, however, in most cases, the cause is seen to be behavioural rather than medical. The exact reason why some dogs simply enjoy eating faeces is not known. Regular removal of faeces, nutritional supplements which act as stool deterrents and aversion treatment should all be attempted to help control this behaviour. Verminosis (worm infestation) may result from this habit.

4.14. Appetite stimulants

A poor appetite may be a symptom of an underlying disease process and should be brought to the attention of the breeder's veterinary surgeon. A sure sign of illness would be if the poor appetite is sustained and the dog loses weight. During a recovery phase from disease, your veterinary surgeon might prescribe medication to stimulate the dog's appetite.

4.15. Supplementing commercial diets

Supplementing is the practice of adding something to the diet which may or may not have any nutritional value. Dietary supplements are not usually required to meet any quality standards as the industry is mostly unregulated. The concern is that consumers might not get what they are paying for. Manufacturers make unsubstantiated claims of benefits when using the supplement; the safety, purity, concentration, efficacy and potency can usually not be guaranteed. Adding supplements to balanced diets is a controversial subject. Some argue that considerable research has gone into the manufacture of high-end premium commercial dog food; that the food is balanced and complete and that it meets the dog's nutritional requirements adequately and therefore does not require supplementation. Others disagree and insist that supplementation can only benefit the dog. There are many breeders whom practice supplementation and they have many "well trusted recipes and secrets" which supposedly give them a "winning edge" in the show ring or working arena. Some swear by it whilst others think it is a waste of money.

Supplementation resonates with modern man because we frequently have an almost arrogant insistence on good health and youth and we want to believe in products and procedures that promise it. Some companies exploit this. It does not matter what evidence the scientific community may present to refute claims of benefits, people still believe in it and will continue to use supplements whether it is beneficial or not. This book will attempt to guide the breeders, who want to practice supplementation, to do so sensibly.

Because the practise of supplementing commercial diets is so common and widespread, considerable effort is spent on the subject in this text. It is probably true that the economy brands may benefit from supplementation, whilst with premium brands there is perhaps less benefit, if any benefit at all. Having said this; some breeders are very keen observers and will spot subtle differences in a dog's coat condition which others, including veterinary surgeons, may never notice. With regards to supplementation, it is important that our well-meant actions do not inadvertently harm our dogs. Breeders must realise that if they wish to supplement, they must do so judiciously. It is a fact that pet owners are more likely to supplement and give treats because their pet "likes" it so much and therefore it "must be" good for the dog. Breeders are instrumental in dictating opinions held by pet owners and should therefore act responsibly in advising their clients and future pet owners correctly.

Pet owners and or breeders may want to supplement commercial diets for the following reasons:
- They want to enhance the palatability of the food
- Their pet likes it
- They feel their pet's diet is monotonous
- They want to increase the calorie content by adding fat
- They want to increase protein content by adding meat or chicken
- They don't want to waste leftover food
- They want to improve the mineral balance and content of the food
- They want to treat a medical condition (therapeutic supplementation).
- They want to improve athletic ability
- They want to improve coat colour, thickness and lustre
- They themselves take supplements for their own health and deduce that it must be healthy for their pets as well

4.15.1. Calcium supplementation

Many years ago, when little attention was paid to the calcium : phosphorous balance in dog food (low calcium high phosphorous), dog owners supplemented calcium by adding either mineral sources of calcium or bone meal. At that time, this practice made sense. Dogs which were fed deficient diets often developed skeletal abnormalities (rickets), if their diet was not adequately supplemented with calcium. Today, calcium supplementation is no longer required and may actually be harmful. Unnecessary calcium supplementation together with overfeeding is linked to the development of skeletal abnormalities as previously discussed.

It is important for breeders to distinguish rickets from eclampsia (milk fever). The latter refers to low calcium levels in the blood during pregnancy and lactation. This condition will be discussed elsewhere (see 7.5).

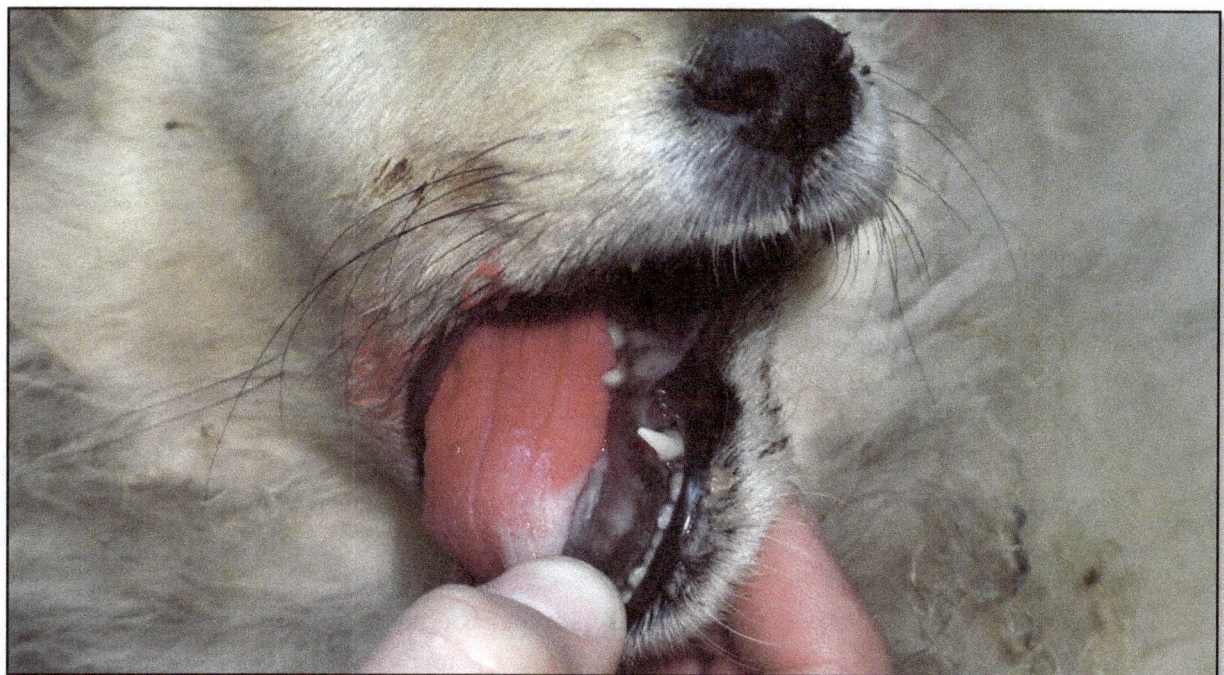
Puppy with rubber jaw as result of malnutrition but this may also be seen as result of renal disease

No supplement containing calcium should ever be given to puppies because they are unable to regulate calcium uptake and will passively absorb excessive calcium leading to the afflictions mentioned previously. Adult dogs are able to regulate the absorption of calcium, supplementation is therefore less likely to be harmful, but unnecessary.

The calcium balance and content of dog food can also be disturbed if excessive amounts of protein, carbohydrates or fats are added to the food. Although not recommended, giving a dog a meat only feeding, perhaps once a week, will do no harm, whilst doing so several times per week, could. Many dog owners add milk to their dog's diet because it is known to be rich in calcium. Although most dogs tolerate milk, many are lactose intolerant and develop diarrhoea if they consume milk. If a dog tolerates milk and if it is fed in moderation, it will do no harm.

4.15.2. Vitamin D
Vitamin D supplementation is dealt with in conjunction with calcium because they are intimately related. Vitamin D is referred to as "the sunshine vitamin" because the ultraviolet rays of the sun convert Vitamin D precursors into active Vitamin D, in the outer layers of the skin. Vitamin D plays a key role in regulating the calcium : phosphorous levels in the blood and also with calcium absorption. Deficiency of vitamin D therefore may resemble calcium deficiencies. Since the advent of modern diets, supplementation of Vitamin D is not required. Also, fat soluble vitamins like Vitamins A, D and E are stored in the liver and therefore have a much higher potential for toxicity than water soluble vitamins, if supplemented in excess.

4.15.3. Vitamin C
Humans supplement Vitamin C to recover from the common cold. It is however not clear whether it can actually prevent a cold. Evidence suggests that Vitamin C enhances the white blood cells' ability to fight pathogens, hence the benefit when used to treat respiratory infections. Vitamin C is often used as a urine acidifier and can be used to treat or prevent recurring bladder infections. Vitamin

C acidifies urine, making it hostile to bacteria, thus preventing their growth. With the exception of humans and certain rodents, most mammals do not require vitamin C supplementation as their bodies manufacture it themselves. Some argue that large and giant breed dogs grow so rapidly that their body's requirement for vitamin C surpasses its ability to manufacture it, and for this reason, it has to be supplemented.

Vitamin C plays an important role in bone formation, growth, mineralisation, formation of elastin and the formation of cartilage in mammalian tissue. For this reason, some deduced that vitamin C supplementation can help prevent hip dysplasia. Despite the fact that researchers have disproved this theory, vitamin C supplementation of puppies and young dogs, especially those breeds which are prone to hip dysplasia, is still common. Although its value has not been proven conclusively, it does not appear to do harm if supplemented in moderation. This is because Vitamin C does not accumulate in the body and excesses are excreted via urine.

Scurvy in humans is a well-known disease but is very uncommon nowadays. In large dogs, but especially giant breeds, a similar condition, known as hypertrophic osteodystrophy (HOD) occurs. Dogs with HOD exhibit swollen joints and may present with lameness. Some refer to this condition as canine scurvy. The cause is thought to be rapid growth and the inability of the bone to strengthen to keep up with rapid weight gain, leading to swelling and pain of long bones. Along with genetic factors, nutritional contributors are: high calorie food intake, overeating and too high Calcium intake. There are no controlled scientific studies which show that Vitamin C supplementation is indicated for the treatment of large breed skeletal diseases and therefore it cannot be recommended.

Rapid growth can also lead to inability of ligaments to lengthen in time leading to knuckling over.

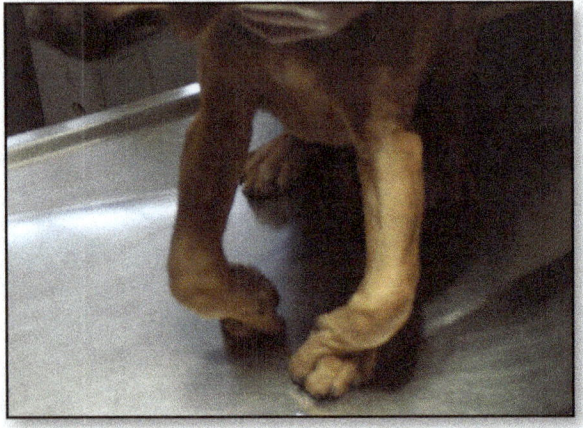
Bone growth surpassed ability of ligaments to keep up leading to knuckling over of carpal joints

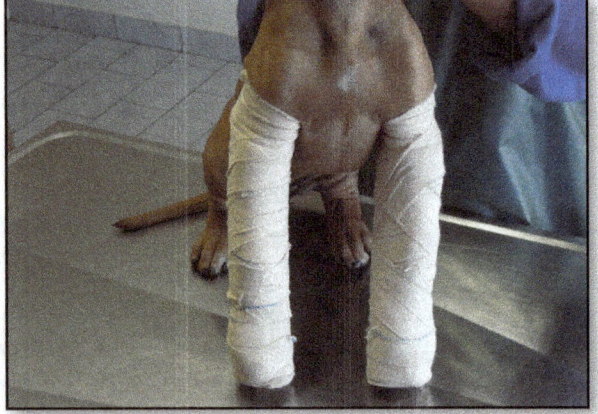
Corrective splinting for ligaments to lengthen

4.15.4. Vitamin B complex

It is common for people to take multivitamins and some insist that the occasional vitamin B-complex injection makes them more energetic, stimulates their appetite and really peps them up. In veterinary science, the therapeutic use of the B-complex vitamins are usually indicated during convalescence from disease especially when anaemia was present. Being water soluble, toxicities of these vitamins do not pose any concerns. The B-complex vitamins comprise of thiamine, niacin, riboflavin, pantothenic acid, pyridoxine, folic acid, cyanocobalamin, and biotin, commonly referred to as vitamin H. Brewer's yeast is a common source of B-complex vitamins. There are scientific papers which allude to the value of vitamin B-complex supplementation over and above what is available in the recommended daily requirements and that it can improve the dog's coat condition, its athletic ability and it also assists with muscle building and repair processes. To what extent these improvements are as a result of the supplementation of B group vitamins or as a result of good nutrition is not known.

4.15.5. Folic acid supplementation and pregnancy

Folic acid (folate) is a synthetic form of Vitamin B9 which, when combined with vitamin B12, helps to synthesise nucleic acids and neurotransmitters. Folic acid supplementation has been shown to reduce the incidence of harelip and split palate (cleft lips and/or palates) when administered to pregnant bitches.

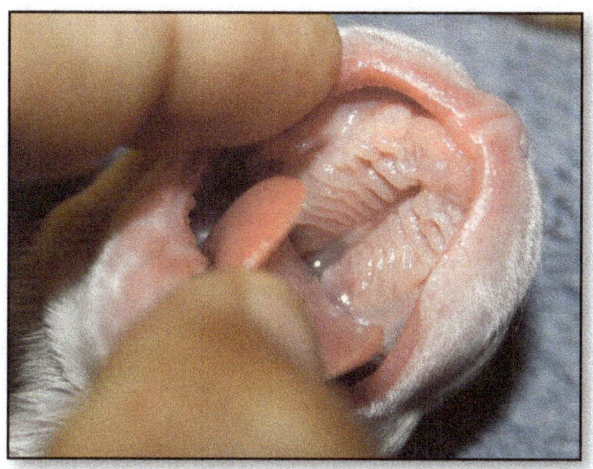
Split palate

These two conditions result when maxillary buds fail to fuse in the canine foetus, at around mid-pregnancy. Brachycephalic (short muzzled) breeds have up to a 30% chance of developing these conditions. A specific gene has been identified that controls this event and which plays a crucial role in the foliate cycle. Work is in progress to identify a specific marker so that carriers can be identified. Although the primary aetiology (cause) is thought to be hereditary, drug or chemical exposure, mechanical interferences with the foetus and some viral infections during pregnancy, have also been implicated. The supplementation of pregnant woman with folate, very specifically during the first month of pregnancy, reduces the risk of cleft palate by up to 50%. Studies in Boston Terriers and French Bulldogs have shown the same result. It is therefore justified to supplement folic acid, in at risk breeds, at doses of 5 mg, from time of mating until the last quarter of pregnancy. Some continue to supplement until time of weaning; the palates will have closed by then and additional folate is unlikely to make a difference.

Folic acid supplementation is also practised because it is thought to prevent cranial clefts (discussed elsewhere). There is no scientific evidence to support whether folic acid supplementation can indeed prevent cranial clefts in dogs or not. We do know however that moderate supplementation of folic acid cannot harm a pregnant bitch. More research is obviously required regarding this syndrome. Some breed specific diets contain additional folate to help prevent these birth defects.

4.15.6. Vitamin A

Vitamin A is seldom supplemented by itself; it is primarily included in a multi vitamin supplement. Vitamin A is a fat soluble vitamin and occurs in several forms, such as retinol, retinaldehyde, retinoic acid and retinyl palmitate. The main source of Vitamin A is the yellow pigment (carotene) found in plants; dogs can convert carotene to Vitamin A. Vitamin A is stored in fat cells mainly within the liver. Vitamin A is required for growth, reproduction and many other functions. Larger doses, above the normal recommended daily allowance, are indicated for artic breeds which suffer from Vitamin A responsive dermatosis. Either excess or deficiency is rare with the advent of brand name commercial pet foods. Because Vitamin A is stored in the body, toxicity resulting from over-supplementation is theoretically possible but only if very large doses are given for long periods of time.

4.15.7. Vitamin E

Normal reproduction requires a balanced diet which provides the breeding animal with enough calories. It is accepted that deficiencies in micro and macro nutrients can indeed adversely affect reproduction. There is a belief that Vitamin E supplementation above recommended daily allowance (RDA), improves fertility but evidence suggests that it does not. In contrast supplementing Vitamin E above RDA, to sled dogs, enhances endurance and reduces muscle damage. When supplemented, the vitamin E should be in the form of alpha-tocopherol and extreme doses should be avoided.

4.15.8. Glutamine

Glutamine (L-Glutamine) is classified as a nutritional supplement. It is a non-essential amino acid and can lead to decreased immune defence and endurance if deficient. Intense endurance exercise depletes glutamine stores and therefore many supplements include glutamine to enhance athletic performance.

4.15.9. Prebiotic and probiotics

A prebiotic is a non-digestible food ingredient. It is specific types of dietary fibre which selectively stimulates the growth and or activity of beneficial bacteria, especially in the large intestine. A probiotic actually contains live (viable) cultures of beneficial bacteria which present health benefits to the animal after ingestion. The promotion and addition of normal flora aids in the recovery from intestinal upsets. Some believe that it actually prevents intestinal upsets and therefore routinely give it as a supplement. Breeders usually limit supplementation with probiotics and or prebiotics to the recovery phase especially following antibiotic therapy or during stress associated events whilst others use it continuously, thinking to prevent intestinal upsets. It is debatable whether it can truly prevent intestinal upsets. Supplementation with prebiotics and probiotics is not harmful even when dogs do not need them.

4.15.10. Kelp and algae

Seaweed, algae and kelp are supplements which are rich in minerals such as iron, iodine, potassium, and various trace minerals. Polar bears consume sea vegetables probably for its mineral content and vegetable protein. Certain algae contain substances which adsorb toxins in the intestinal tract and also carcinogen (cancer causing) binding substances. Some breeders give chlorophyll containing supplements because they claim it improves the dog's pigmentation. Breeders will start supplementing months before a show even if the safety and efficacy of doing so, has not been established.

4.15.11. Table scraps

Table scraps are not really a supplement but dog owners often think it is a very healthy treat because it contains fats, oils and meat along with assorted carbohydrates. Feeding table scraps is not advisable but if a dog owner insists, they should make sure that it does not exceed more than 10-25% of the dog's total food ration. Exceeding this percentage may undo the balance of nutrients in the food. Negative aspects associated with feeding scraps are mainly digestive disorders, not to mention the irritating habit of begging at the table which most dogs develop. Obesity may also become a problem if the caloric requirement of the dog is constantly exceeded.

4.15.12. Treats

If pet owners insist on spoiling their dogs with treats they are encouraged to do so in a healthy way. Many of the leading dog food manufacturers recognise this "need" and have manufactured healthy treats accordingly. These treats should never account for more than 10% of the dog's caloric intake (which is not much in Toy breeds). Some treats may even keep dogs entertained and keep the teeth clean at the same time. There is a difference between treats and chews. Treats have nutritional value and chews normally do not. Lower calorie treats are also available for dogs which are on a diet. Treats are often used by dog trainers and animal behaviourists as a training aid (positive reinforcement).

4.16. Nutraceuticals

Nutraceuticals are synthetic or naturally occurring food supplements which have a beneficial effect on animal or human health. These products appeal to many health conscious people as they are natural products and have few or no side effects. Depending on the product their use promises anti-aging effects, longevity, vitality, disease resistance, arthritis and allergy control.

4.16.1. Glucosamine and chondroitin

Glucosamine and chondroitin are naturally occurring substances which are at their highest concentration in cartilage. The body synthesizes most of its own glucosamine from glucose. Normal healthy animals will not benefit from supplemental chondroitin and glucosamine but arthritic conditions may increase the need, and therefore make supplementation useful. Glucosamine and chondroitin provide the building blocks to synthesize glycosaminoglycans which, when combined with hyaluronic acid, make proteoglycans which together with collagen are the main structures of cartilage. Chondroitin and glucosamine are usually combined with Vitamin C, cobalt and manganese. There is benefit and merit in using these products but their cost is prohibitive. There is no indication that these products slow the progression of hip dysplasia or prevent it, but they do have therapeutic value. They are often given in combination with non-steroidal anti-inflammatory agents to dogs suffering from arthritis, with good results. For this reason, chondroitin and glucosamine are included in some joint support and geriatric diets.

4.16.2. Antioxidants

Antioxidants are beneficial because they combat free radicals in the body. Free radicals are chemically reactive compounds which result from normal metabolism and cause membrane damage to cells in our bodies. There are naturally occurring combatants (enzyme systems) of free radicals in our bodies and diet derived free radical scavengers which aid in the elimination of free radicals and prevent their build up. These include Vitamin E, and the carotenoids; beta-carotene and lutein. They have a positive effect on the immune system.

4.16.3. Omega-3 and-6 fatty acids

Omega-3 fatty acids include Alpha-linoleic acid, eicosapentoic acid and docohexaenoic acid (DHA), whereas Omega-6 fatty acids include linoleic acid, gamma linoleic acid and arachidonic acid. Most pet foods contain both but usually more of the omega-6 fatty acids than omega-3. The ratio, levels and types of Omega-3 are all important. DHA is needed during gestation and during puppyhood for optimal neurological development. Optimal neurological development can have a definite impact on the future trainability of the dog. Fish oils and some grains are rich in fatty acids. Omega-3 fatty acids can be incorporated in the cell membrane. When there is membrane damage the breakdown of the omega-3 containing cell wall results in less inflammatory metabolites. The benefits of omega-3 and 6 fatty acid supplementation include: the control of allergies, auto immune conditions and arthritis as well as yeast infections of the skin. It also prevents allergies in offspring, thromboembolic disease and hyperlipidaemia in some liver conditions. Fatty acids therefore form part of the treatment plan in mentioned conditions. It is particularly valuable in skin allergies because it often helps reduce the amount of cortisone required to ameliorate the condition.

4.17. Ergogenic aids (performance enhancing substances)

Ergogenic aids may be any substance, drug or procedure which improves athletic performance. In this section, only the supplements will be discussed. Performance enhancing drugs will be discussed elsewhere. When the ergogenic aid is a substance it is called a performance enhancing substance. These substances can be natural nutrients or synthetic drugs. A lot more is known about ergogenic aids in humans than in dogs. Illegal substance use, as an aid to enhance performance, is well known in the horse racing industry, where it is referred to as doping. Greyhound racing has also been implicated from time to time. It is the breeder's responsibility to familiarise themselves with the rules and regulations of the respective associations and dog clubs regarding the use of these products. It is however important to realise that the possession of scheduled drugs, without prescription by a registered physician or veterinary surgeon, is a criminal offence in many countries. How widespread the use of performance enhancing substances are in the show and dog sport arena is unknown, as little testing has been performed, if at all. Some over the counter substances can also be an ergogenic aid. Caffeine keeps us alert and it is used by athletes to improve endurance. Creatine is a popular nutritional supplement in humans and is a compound synthesized to fuel short bouts of energy production. Creatine increases muscle performance, size and strength and it improves the ability to recover from exertion. Ribose increases energy levels. Vitamin B complex and glutamine are sometimes considered ergogenic aids. There are many more but clear evidence of their efficacy is not always available.

4.18. Substances which are potentially toxic to dogs

Because a substance is safe for humans or other animals, it should not be assumed to be safe for dogs. Food which is edible for humans, and even other species of animals, can be hazardous to dogs because they metabolize food differently. Some substances may only cause mild digestive upsets, whereas others can cause severe illness and even death. General signs of a possible poisoning include: excessive salivation, vomiting, diarrhoea, abdominal pain, twitching, nervousness, weakness, poor balance, convulsions and finally coma. If pet owners suspect their dog might be poisoned they should immediately transport the dog to their veterinary surgeon. It is helpful to take the suspect container and its manufacture's insert with list of components or the suspected plant as it may help the veterinary surgeon identify the toxic component.

The following items should not be fed (intentionally or unintentionally) to a dog. This list is incomplete because one cannot possibly list everything which a dog should not eat. There are vast differences in the various potential intoxications in companion animals based on geographic locations and the plants which grow there or products and drugs they use. This list is compiled merely to alert the breeder against more common potential intoxications. Puppies are more likely to be poisoned due to their curious nature and tendency to swallow objects they chew.

4.18.1. Poisonous flora (plants, mushrooms and algae)

Common toxic plants are: berries of the Persian lilac or china berry tree *(Melia azedarach)*, Marijuana *(Cannabis sativa)*, Macadamia nuts, castor oil seeds *(Ricinus communis)*, Elephants ear (Alocasia *and Colcasia spp)*, Dumb cane *(Dieffenbachia)*, Delicious monster *(Philodendron spp)*, Arum lilies *(Zanthedeschia aethiopica)*, Oleander spp *(Nerium and Thevetia)*, Foxgloves *(Digitalis spp)*, Clivia spp, Cycads, Cycas, *(Encephalartos spp and Cycas spp)*, amaryllis, cyclamen, daffodil, day lily, Easter lily, English ivy, gladiolus, holly, hyacinth, hydrangea, iris, mistletoe, narcissus, poinsettia, rhododendron, tulip, yew, and yucca.

Food which humans consume on a daily basis may not be safe for dogs. Excessive intake of onion and garlic *(Allium spp)*, either raw, cooked, or in a powder form; all contain sulphoxides and disulphides, which can damage red blood cells and cause anaemia and jaundice. Although cats are more sensitive to its toxins, dogs can be affected if the intake is excessive. Some owners intentionally feed it because they erroneously believe that it will repel insects and prevent flea and tick infestations. Avocado can be toxic to dogs if consumed in large quantities. All the factors which lead to avocado toxicity are not understood but it is best avoided. Birds are a lot more susceptible to the toxin persin in the avocado than are dogs. Caffeine containing foodstuffs (chocolate, coffee, tea) and also caffeine containing supplements contain theobromine or theophylline, which can be toxic and if so, affect the heart and nervous system. Grapes and raisins are perfectly safe for humans; irrespective of the quantity consumed. Grapes contain an unknown toxin which can damage a dog's kidneys; even as little as a handful can be fatal. Grape seed extract, on the other hand, is perfectly safe. Fruits which have relatively larger pits (peaches, plums) can cause an obstruction in the digestive tract. Maize on the cob is eagerly consumed by dogs; the cob, on the other hand, is indigestible and can cause an obstruction. Potato, rhubarb, tomato leaves and stems contain oxalates, which if mouthed causes a localised irritation. Consumption, however, can affect the digestive, nervous, and urinary systems, but this is rare. Raw eggs contain an enzyme called avidin which decreases the absorption of biotin in the body and can cause skin and coat problems. Dogs would have to consume a very large quantity of raw eggs in order for this to pose a problem. Raw eggs may also contain Salmonella bacteria which causes high fever, vomiting and diarrhoea. If raw fish containing the enzyme thiaminase is consumed, a thiamine deficiency may develop that leads to a loss of appetite, seizures, and in severe cases, death. Large amounts of raw fish would have to be fed over a long period of time to cause a problem.

Dog owners should be aware that algae growing in ponds and lakes in some parts of the world may be very toxic and their dogs should not drink or even swim in water from these sources. The most common algae are the blue-green algae (Cyanobacteria) of which *Microcystis aeruginosa, Nodularia spumigena, Oscillatoria spp, Anabaena spp* are the most common. The toxicity of certain mushroom species should not be underestimated. The consumption of only one of the extreme toxic varieties *(Amanita spp)* may be fatal. Mushrooms which grow underneath trees are more likely to be of a toxic variety than those growing in open grass, but there are exceptions, and only experts should be trusted to identify edible mushrooms.

4.18.2. Pesticides

Accidental ingestion of pesticides is common in dogs. Pesticides should always be kept out of range of animals and children and kept in closed containers. Containers holding pesticides are frequently stored on shelves in pantries, store rooms, garages and sheds. Rodents might knock them over and when they fall to the floor, dogs gain access to them. Dogs sometimes eat rodents poisoned by rodenticides; fortunately secondary poisoning does not occur and dogs will not come to harm.

Chapter 4 Nutrition

A dog would have to consume a substantial number of rodents in order to consume sufficient poison to have an adverse effect. Dogs may be poisoned accidently by ingesting pesticides which are left around the house. Dogs should be kept away from an area where insecticides are used. Instructions and preventative measures, as indicated by the manufacturer's insert, should strictly be adhered to. Malicious poisoning is very common in parts of the world, where the keeping of guard dogs is necessitated by crime. Aldicarb is frequently the poison of choice in many of these countries because it is readily available, it is tasteless and odourless and requires miniscule amounts to have an effect. It kills or incapacitates a dog in less than half an hour. Many dogs are poisoned unintentionally by their owners following the incorrect application of tick, flea, louse, mite or fly control measures. In cases where an external toxin is suspected; washing the product off with copious amounts of water and soap is indicated before taking the dog to a veterinary surgeon.

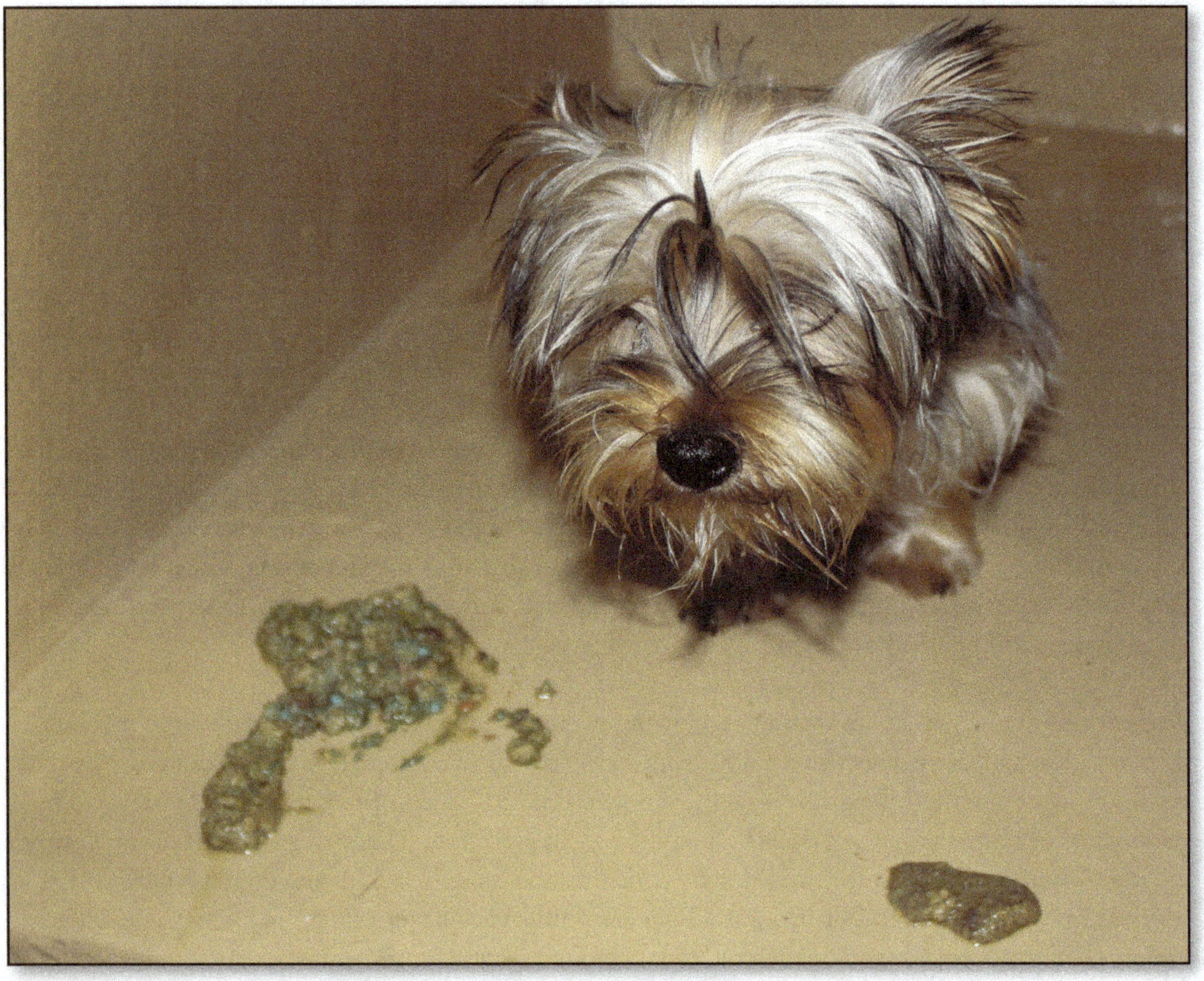

Dog was treated with an emetic (agent to induce vomiting), because of ingestion of rat poison

4.18.3. Prescription and over-the-counter drugs

Self-treatment by dog owners is a frequent cause of poisoning. Some pet owners assume that household remedies which are perfectly safe for their children, are also safe for their pets. Sometimes these products are indeed safe for dogs but are administered as a massive overdose because the pet owner neglects to adjust the dosage. An average lapdog is likely to weigh 14 times less than an average person, and for this reason the dosage must be adapted accordingly. Anti-inflammatory agents are frequently involved. Acute poisoning occurs when a dog gets hold of a packet of anti-inflammatory tablets such as paracetamol, aspirin, phenylbutazone or others. Dogs are very sensitive to anti-inflammatory agents and may suffer from gastric ulcers, renal or hepatic impairment following extended use. There are anti-inflammatory agents registered for chronic use in dogs suffering from arthritic conditions. Because they are quite expensive, dog owners change the prescribed anti-inflammatory agent to a common household one, with serious health consequences for their dog. Accidental overdose of other commonly used drugs such as anti-depressants, anti-hypertensive drugs, contraceptives, sedatives and sleeping pills frequently occur.

4.18.4. Commercial dog foods

Albeit rare, intoxications have been reported in commercially available dog foods. Aflatoxins are toxins produced by fungae *(Aspergillus spp)*. It is a mould which is ubiquitous and often grows on seeds, nuts and grains when it is stored. Aflatoxin is produced by mould on the seed which is later used in the manufacturing process. Routine testing for the toxin will usually reveal its presence and prevent the toxin from entering the dog food. Ionophore antibiotics are commonly used in the manufacture of feeds for poultry, cattle, pig and sheep. Accidental contamination of dog food, also made in these factories, can occur. Melamine poisoning of dog food has also been reported. Rancidity of fats in dog food occurs when the food does not contain appropriate anti-oxidants. Although not fatal it may lead to severe gastritis, vomiting and diarrhoea.

4.18.5. Common house-hold hazards

Disinfectants, detergents, cleaning agents, acids and soaps can accidently be consumed by dogs. Ethylene glycol (Antifreeze) is a frequent culprit because it is so often used in some parts of the world and dogs consume it readily. A dog might accidentally consume alcohol or it is deliberately fed by irresponsible owners. Lead and other heavy metals found in lead toys, paints, fishing sinkers and batteries are often ingested.

4.19. Water

Although not a true nutrient, water is fundamental to life. Round the clock access to good quality water is therefore essential. In most countries there are strict rules in place which govern water quality for human consumption; this water is also safe for your dog. Water can however be contaminated by bacteria, viruses, protozoa and parasites or have excesses of nitrates, irons, phosphates, sodium, fluorides, magnesium and other minerals. Borehole water (pumped water from underground natural reservoirs) is likely to contain such excesses and should therefore be tested annually if it is used as drinking water for animals and humans. Water bowls should be kept clean.

Dogs will roughly consume between 60-100 ml of water per Kg bodyweight per day, depending on the climatic conditions, the type of food which is fed and the activity level of the dog. If a dog consumes excessive amounts of water, it should be brought to the attention of your veterinary surgeon. It is helpful if one knows how much water your dog drinks over a 24 hour period. It can be established by leaving out a large bowl of water with a known volume of water in it; after 24 hours the difference in volume is determined.

Some diseases like kidney failure or diabetes can cause dogs to drink more water and to urinate more frequently. It has been established that healthy working dogs which are well hydrated, perform better and are more energetic. Keeping a dog well hydrated can therefore act as an ergogenic aid. This is important for dogs which compete in shows and or working trials. Because hydration is so important, competitors encourage water intake by flavouring the water and warming it a bit. Unlike food, water intake should never be restricted.

Chapter 5

Reproduction in the Bitch

To keep this text simple, scientific nomenclature and reference to complex endocrine events (hormonal fluctuations) has been avoided where possible. This section on reproduction is, however, central to the book. A thorough understanding of unique features of the canine reproductive cycle is needed in order to discuss many important concepts and topics. Veterinary surgeons and reproductive specialists reading this book will have to forgive the deliberate use of layman terms as if synonymous with scientific terms, which strictly they are not. This sacrifice in accuracy is made in order to simplify otherwise complex explanations. Those who have read extensively on reproduction in the bitch may be left somewhat confused after encountering different terminology which seems to refer to the same events, in different books. The following paragraph should clarify this confusion.

Generally, the word 'cycle' refers to events which follow cyclical patterns and thus repeat themselves. The words "reproductive cycle", therefore, may be misunderstood. In strict terms, the bitch only has one reproductive cycle which starts at puberty with the first heat followed by continued heat cycles until the end of the reproductive cycle when they exhibit no more heat cycles. The length of this reproductive cycle of the bitch, therefore, refers to her reproductive life span which starts at and encompasses puberty followed by repetitive heat cycles and ending in a reduced frequency of heat or total absence thereof, signalling the end of both her reproductive cycle and her reproductive life span. However, many breeders use the words reproductive cycle as synonymous to the terms, oestrous cycle, sexual cycle and heat cycle, because it makes sense to them. This should be respected by scientists. The words, "in heat" and "in season", refer to the bitch exhibiting typical external visible signs of heat. What the breeder thus commonly refers to as "in heat" or "in season", should be construed by scientists as a combination of two phases of oestrous known as pro-oestrus and oestrus combined. This will be discussed in more detail later.

The period between heats is referred to as the interoestrus interval. The average duration of the interoestrus interval is 6-8 months but may vary widely (6-12 months). Small breeds may have a shorter interoestrus interval (6 months) compared to large breeds (8 months). Breeders may notice that some individual bitches tend to have successive heat cycles of similar lengths and intervals. There are however some distinct breed differences which are perfectly normal for the breed. Basenjis, Wolves, some wolf hybrids, Tibetan Mastiffs and some lines of Greyhounds are amongst those which cycle once a year. In contrast, certain lines of German shepherds often have interoestrus intervals of 4.5-6 months. Interoestrus intervals shorter than 4 months or longer than 11 months (18 months in breeds where 12 months is normal), may be associated with infertility. Dogs may cycle throughout the year but very subtle peaks in numbers of bitches cycling may occur during spring and autumn. These peaks may be influenced by circadian rhythms dictated by daylight length. Bitches transported from one hemisphere to another may have disturbed circadian rhythms and need some time (2 months or so) to adjust before cyclic activity is resumed.

5.1. Puberty in bitches and age of first breeding

On average, bitches reach puberty at the age of 7-12 months (extremes are 6-24 months). Small breeds tend to reach puberty sooner (6-10 months) than larger breeds and bitches of the same breed slightly

Chapter 5 Reproduction in the Bitch

earlier than males. Breeders are cautioned not to keep "puppies" together at ages approaching puberty to prevent unwanted pregnancies. Dogs usually reach puberty shortly after they have attained 90% of their adult shoulder height. The question is at what age should the breeder start breeding? Many breeding authorities have very clear guidelines on this. The minimum age at which a bitch is allowed to be bred varies from 12-24 months. Some breeding authorities prohibit registration of puppies whose dams have not yet reached the required minimum age. Bitches should not be bred at their first heat, but rather, it is suggested to breed for the first time at 12-18 months old, which usually coincides with their second or third heat cycle. Recommendations by breeding authorities may clash with those from reproductive specialists who advise not to start breeding too late. Similar to humans, dogs should not produce offspring too old as the likelihood of reproductive problems are increased.

Some breeders particularly of working and show dogs often want to complete the bitch's show or working career before breeding, by which time she is 4 years or older. These bitches will by then have had 6-8 oestrous cycles and may already have a compromised uterus which is unfavourable to embryo implantation and is more susceptible to uterine infections. Considering the age at which a bitch's fertility may start to wane, it is unwise to start breeding for the first time so late. Large and giant breed bitches are more commonly affected by these limitations. Their breed authorities will only allow breeding after 2 years or even later. They also age quicker and have shorter life and reproductive life spans. These factors should be taken into account when determining restrictions on minimum age of first mating in the respective breeds by breeding authorities. These recommendations should be evidence-based and scientifically sound.

5.2. Delayed puberty

When a bitch is older than 15 months (small breed) and 24 months (larger breeds) and has never been in heat, then the bitch may suffer from delayed puberty. Aberrant cycles, which will be discussed later, must first be excluded, as must the use of heat suppressing drugs. After thorough investigation, induction of heat can be considered by the breeder's veterinary surgeon.

5.3. The oestrous cycle (reproductive cycle or heat cycle) of the bitch

A bitch is referred to as being polytocous, a spontaneous ovulator and non-seasonally monoestrous. Polytocous refers to this species as having multiple offspring in a single pregnancy. Spontaneous ovulator means that this species does not require coital stimulation to ovulate (release egg from ovary). The monoestrous (mono = one and oestrous = "in heat") means that she shows one or two oestrous (heat) cycles per year irrespective of whether she conceives or not. In contrast, animals which are polyoestrous (poly = many) will show many oestrous cycles during the same season. Therefore, animals which are polyoestrous (e.g. ewe), will keep on cycling until they conceive or until the season is over for them (if seasonally polyoestrous). Seasonal or non-seasonal respectively refer to a heat (oestrus) which is exhibited during a specific season only or a heat which is not bound to season at all. An animal with a non-seasonal heat thus exhibits oestrus cycles throughout the year and only stops cycling while she is pregnant and lactating, or once she reaches the end of her reproductive age and stops cycling due to senility or ovarian quiescence. For example, a cow cycles every 3 weeks and thus a farmer has many opportunities to ensure that his cows conceive. If insemination or mating to a bull fails on one cycle, he can try again 3 weeks later. In contrast, the dog breeder only has one or two opportunities a year to achieve the same goal in his bitches.

Chapter 5 Reproduction in the Bitch

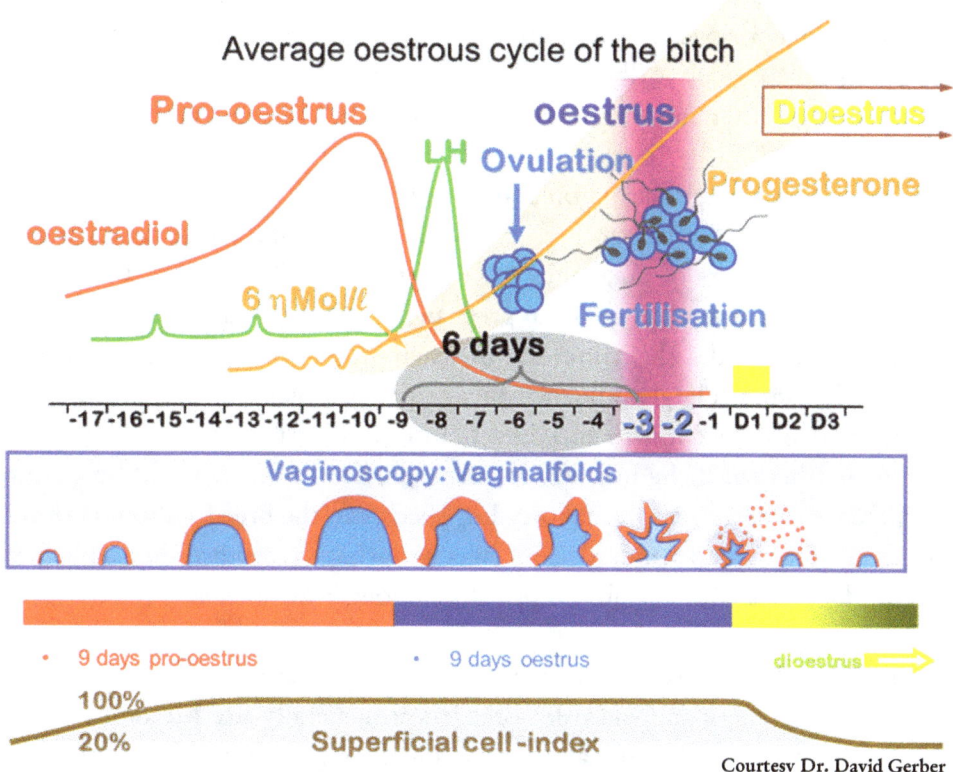

Courtesy Dr. David Gerber

Reproductive events in many species are in perfect synchrony with nature. This is to ensure that offspring are born at a time that the environmental temperatures are not too harsh and that food is available. The mother needs access to enough energy, enabling adequate milk production for her offspring. Also, in many animals, the timing of the birth season for that species is synchronized with conditions most favourable to their offspring's survival. Environmental influence of the reproductive cycle in many animals is intriguing. Some species stop cycling during unfavourable conditions, for example, drought. This prevents pregnancy and lactation during times when the mother would be unlikely to successfully support and raise her offspring. Another interesting adaptation in some herbivores is the ability to vary the length of pregnancy (gestation length) and synchronise it with weather conditions favourable to their offspring, availability of food at time of birth and the birth of other group members. Pregnancy is a lot less demanding on the body than lactation (milk production) and the synchronization of births minimises loss of vulnerable offspring to predation. Because canids in nature have evolved as cunning and resourceful hunters and scavengers, they were able to access food throughout all seasons. This probably led to season having minimal effect on their cyclicity.

As mentioned, the reproductive life span of the bitch starts at puberty and ends when she no longer is able to reproduce. A bitch's fertility peaks at about 3-4 years of age and may begin to wane from 4-8 years onwards. Peak fertility is characterised by a high pregnancy rate (in excess of 85% of bitches mated conceive) as well as litter sizes fitting the breed average. The first sign of declining fertility is usually noticed from 5-6 years of age characterised by decreases in litter size. In addition to litter size, bitches (6-8 years) and older, may show seriously lowered fertility, characterised by increased interoestrus intervals, increased incidence of suboestrus (silent heat), increased incidence of anovulatory follicles and low pregnancy rates, increased incidence of difficult births (dystocia), increased number of stillbirths and increase in neonatal (soon after birth) deaths. Some old bitches may stop cycling altogether. Bitches that show lowered fertility other than smaller litter sizes, at an early age around 4-5

Chapter 5 Reproduction in the Bitch

years, are said to suffer from premature ovarian failure. It is very important for the breeder to realise that there are many other reasons for small litter sizes other than waning fertility. The exact age at which fertility wanes varies widely. Albeit rare, it is not impossible for an 11 year old bitch of a large breed to still whelp a large litter and raise them successfully.

Many breeders ask until what age they should and may breed an aging bitch. This may become an ethical question. The general objection to breeding older dogs is the notion that older bitches should not be subjected to the stressors of pregnancy for the breeder's selfish gains. It remains speculative whether older animals have more discomfort in pregnancy than do younger individuals. It is however true that declining fertility and a slight increase in whelping problems in older bitches is a reality. Breed and condition has a much larger influence on whelping problems than age. From a reproductive point of view, there is no objection to breeding the old bitch irrespective of age, provided she is in good condition and health. If the breeder, for instance, has a nine year old brood bitch in good condition that happens to be an exceptional breeding specimen, the breeder should not feel guilty for wanting to breed her. There is no standard age at which one has to stop breeding a bitch. The old dog naturally starts producing less if she is physiologically no longer capable.

Another question is how frequently a breeder should breed the bitch? The ethical considerations are a frequent topic of debate amongst animal lovers. Breeders are generally advised to mate a bitch on every alternate cycle. Indeed many breed associations prohibit the registration of more than one litter per year. It is the author's opinion; however, that there is no harm in mating a bitch on two consecutive cycles and then skip her once. This frequent breeding or "back to back breeding" is sometimes frowned upon. It also raises ethical concerns and accusations of overbreeding and exploitation of dogs. Again, biologically, there is no definitive number of litters after which a bitch should not be allowed to breed again, provided she is in good condition and health. Reproductive health in the bitch is to some extent correlated with her parity (number of times she has produced offspring). There is a positive correlation between the number of consecutive non-pregnant cycles and the occurrence of uterine disease, which may end the bitch's reproductive career. Infrequent breeding may also increase incidence of pseudopregnancy which is, in turn, correlated to increased risk of mammary tumours. It seems that bitches which do not contribute to the genetic pool are naturally eliminated from reproducing through the non-pregnant bitch's uterus being more prone to infection after a heat cycle. This infection is also called pyometra. Bitches with untreated pyometra would eventually die.

There are countries where dog breeding ages and number of litters are regulated and breeders must acquaint themselves and comply with such regulations.

5.3.1. The stages of the oestrous cycle of the bitch

The breeder understands the heat cycle (oestrous cycle) to be the time that the bitch is ready to mate or in-preparation for mating. Scientists have however divided the oestrous cycle of the bitch into 4 stages namely; pro-oestrus, oestrus, dioestrus and anoestrus. The word oestrus (estrus in US), should not be confused with the word oestrous as in oestrous cycle. Oestrus is merely a phase in the oestrous cycle. The exact transition from one stage to another differs depending on what criteria are used to differentiate the stages. It makes sense for most breeders to use a method which is visible to them. The word 'heat' is often used by breeders and refers to the period during which the bitch's vagina is swollen, has a vaginal discharge of varying colours, attracts males and later accepts mating. The layman term "heat" therefore refers collectively to pro-oestrus and oestrus combined. Not unlike the breeder,

Chapter 5 Reproduction in the Bitch

the veterinary surgeon may use the outwards signs of heat as clues but will use other methods to differentiate the stages more accurately from each other for reasons which will become evident later.

Schematic illustration of stages of the heat cycle of the bitch

| **Proestrus** May vary from 2-24 days but averages 7-9 days | **Oestrus** May vary from 3-21 days but averages 9 days | **Dioestrus** Lasts 65 days in the pregnant bitch and a week longer in non-pregnant bitches | **Anoestrus** This phase may last 4 - 10 months depending on breed and is the phase that dictates the interoestrus interval (period between heat cycles) |

a) Pro-oestrus

Pro-oestrus starts with the first outward signs of activity of the reproductive system, namely, widespread oedema (swelling) of the vulva (vaginal lips), a bloody vaginal discharge and attractiveness to males, usually without allowing coitus (mating).

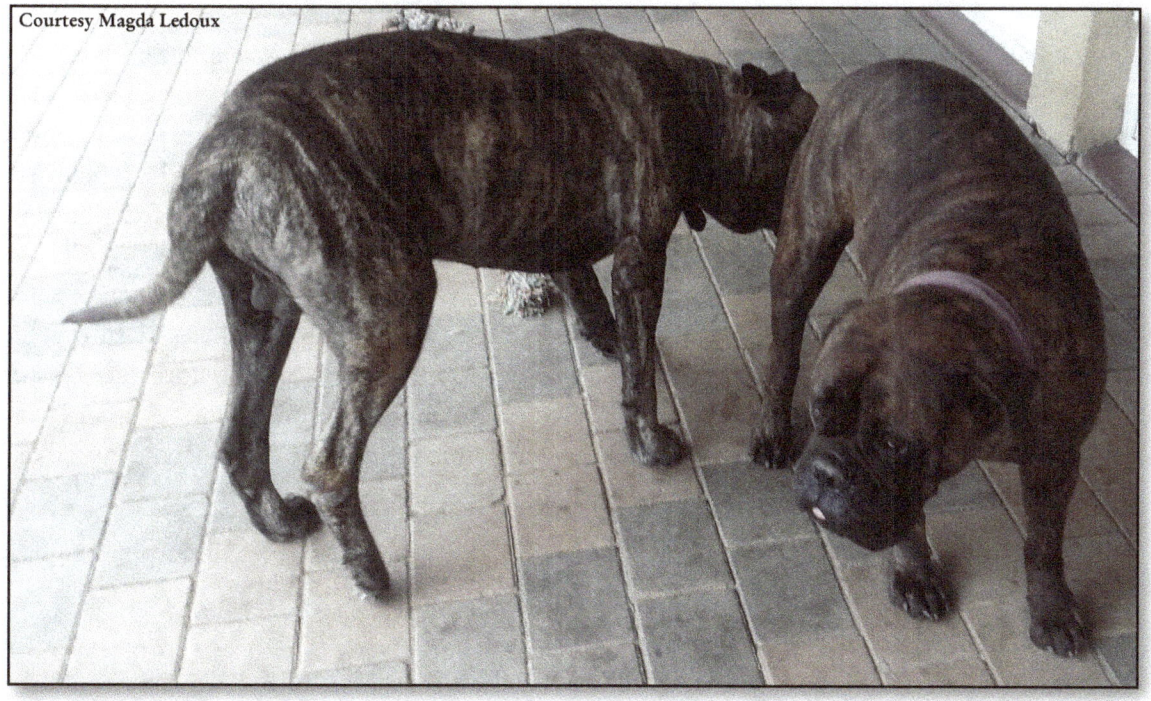

Stud sniffing bitch

Any of these three signs signal the onset of pro-oestrus or heat. Pro-oestrus, on average, lasts about 7-9 days, but may vary from 2-24 days. Breeders should take note of this very wide variation as it has important implications in planning and success of matings.

During pro-oestrus, follicles start developing on the ovaries and the cervix opens slightly to allow semen in and uterine discharges "bleeding" out. Oestrogen is the dominating hormone during pro-oestrus and peaks at the end of this phase.

b) Oestrus

The term oestrus refers to the outward signs of receptivity which leads to attraction and subsequent acceptance of a male. The first sign of the bitch's willingness to mate indicates the onset of oestrus.

Chapter 5 Reproduction in the Bitch

Oestrus ends when the bitch does no longer accept the male. Oestrus usually lasts 6-12 days, averages 9 days, but may be as short as 3 days or as long as 21 days. Again, breeders should take note of this very wide variation as it has important implications in later discussions.

During oestrus, the discharge from the vulva usually decreases and may change from a bloody discharge to a straw coloured discharge. There are, however, bitches that may have a bloody discharge until end of oestrus. The volume of the bloody vaginal discharge may also vary significantly during both pro-oestrus and oestrus. Some bitches have only scant discharge which is barely visible as slight "spotting" of the floors in the bitch's living quarters. Some breeders will take some adsorbent paper, wipe it against the external genitalia of the bitch and inspect it to identify the earliest signs. In contrast, other bitches may "bleed" heavily. In exceptional cases, the bloody discharge may accumulate in the vagina and discharge when the bitch squats, measuring volumes of up to 30 ml or more at a time. If there is a resident male on the premises, he is sure to point out the bitch by excessive sniffing and licking of her vagina and attempts to mount her. Some kennels with large number of bitches may employ the services of a vasectomised male to help detect "in heat" bitches.

During oestrus, the bitch will respond to the male by playing, presenting her hind quarters to him. They will typically stand for the male and allow him to lick her vagina, flagging the tail towards one side (tail reflex) and lifting her vagina (vaginal or vulva reflex) also referred to by breeders as pouting. Some bitches may mount other bitches or allow other bitches to mount her. The lordosis reflex refers to the contraction of the cutaneous muscles over the bitch's croup and lower back area. This reflex may be absent in many bitches and therefore not well known amongst breeders.

Oestrus is the phase during which, the follicles complete their development, follicles mature, follicles ovulate, the ovulated eggs (ova) mature and finally fertilization takes place. The hormone oestrogen declines and progesterone increases as oestrus progresses. As the oestrus phase can be rather long the time of real importance to the breeder is that time during which the fertile eggs become available and ready for fertilization. This is the fertilization period.

The fertilization period

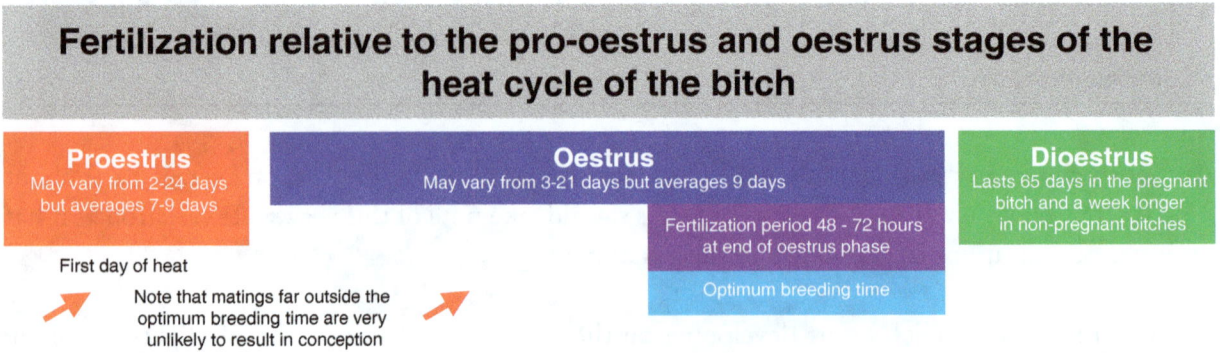

The breeder needs to understand that the time span during which the bitch is in heat and the period during which fertilization is possible (fertilization period), overlap but are not equal in length. The fertilization period is normally considerably shorter than the heat period and occurs in the last couple of days of standing heat (the oestrus stage) but not right at the end. The fertilization period starts at about 48 hours after ovulation when the eggs have fully matured and are ready for fertilization. It lasts for about 48-72 hours after which the eggs age and the cervix closes, making fertilization impossible. Clearly it should therefore be the breeders aim to breed the bitch from just before (12-24 hours) the fertilization period until the end of it. This period is also termed the optimum breeding time. The fertilization period thus occurs in late oestrus, lasts for 2-3 days and ends 1-2 days before the end of oestrus and beginning of dioestrus. The fertilization period is therefore that limited 2-3 days of the heat period during which there are eggs available for fertilization. Monitoring the oestrous cycle by various means can give the veterinary surgeon accurate clues as to the beginning and end of this period.

c) Dioestrus

In some texts, the stage described as dioestrus is referred to as metoestrus. This text only uses the word dioestrus and for our purposes, the two terms should be considered synonymous. In simple terms, dioestrus starts when the bitch no longer allows mating until the pregnancy hormone (progesterone) returns to its normal (basal) levels. In all dogs, irrespective of breed, the length of dioestrus is the same. In the pregnant bitch this is approximately 65 days and in the non-pregnant bitch approximately a week or so longer. By making a vaginal smear of the vaginal cell wall using an ear bud, the veterinary surgeon can use vaginal cytology to establish the first day of cytological dioestrus also known to veterinary surgeons as D1. The exact day that dioestrus starts is important to any veterinary surgeon with a keen interest in canine reproduction. Knowledge of this day retrospectively reveals whether matings or artificial inseminations were done at the correct time and it will give them a good indication of whelping date. The whelping date is usually 57 ± 1 days after D1. During dioestrus, the uterus responds to the pregnancy hormone by hyperplasia of uterine glands and the mammary glands enlarge and milk production may start.

It is important to note that the breeder will not be able to distinguish dioestrus from anoestrus in the non-pregnant bitch nor will the veterinary surgeon unless they perform a progesterone assay. This is because during this phase there are no outward signs of sexual activity.

d) Anoestrus

Anoestrus starts at the end of dioestrus and ends at the start of the next heat cycle or next pro-oestrus. During this phase, there are also no outward signs and no sexual interest is evident. This period may last from 4-10 months. The length of anoestrus determines the length of the interoestrus interval. During this phase, the progesterone levels are baseline and there are low concentrations of sex hormones.

To the breeder, separating the time occupied by the dioestrus and anoestrus phases is not of any practical importance. To breeders, these phases are collectively the "off heat" period or "interval to next heat" period. They may become concerned when this interval becomes longer than expected for their breed.

5.4. Aberrant heat cycles in the bitch

5.4.1. Split heat

A bitch exhibits split heat (also known as split oestrus) when she appears to come into heat (enters pro-oestrus) and her heat cycle appears to progress normally. She may or may not allow mating. The bitch then goes out of heat abruptly. At that stage, the breeder has every reason to believe that all is well and normal. However, following a period of 3-12 weeks later, the bitch comes into heat again. The first of these two heat cycles in these bitches is not fertile and bitches will not conceive on this heat even if mated with a fertile male. The second heat in this split heat cycle may be fertile but not in all cases. Lower fertility is thus usually associated with these cycles. Split heat is most common in pubertal bitches but may also occur in older bitches. In these it may reoccur on subsequent heat cycles. The exact cause of split heat is not known but it is suspected that it happens because of incomplete follicular development and failure to ovulate. As the condition resolves spontaneously, we do not treat it and breeding is advised during second "true heat".

5.4.2. Silent heat

Silent heat refers to a cycle where the bitch exhibits very little to none of the external signs of swelling or bleeding normally associated with heat. The breeder may often miss this cycle and erroneously assume that the bitch has very much extended intervals between heats. These cycles are also sometimes called suboestrus or even "shy" heat. If the breeder has a stud on the premises, this dog is likely to notice this bitch. Examination by a veterinary surgeon may confirm that the bitch is indeed on heat, based on vaginoscopy, vaginal smear or even blood results. These bitches are not abnormal but usually require monitoring by a veterinary surgeon to determine the optimum time of breeding.

5.4.3. Persistent heat

Persistent heat is characterised by a bitch that is either showing signs of heat continuously for longer than 4 weeks or intermittently for approximately a week with intervals varying from 3-6 weeks between. The cause may be ovulation failure, cystic ovarian disease or tumours. Few of these bitches will respond to treatment, many develop pyometra and require ovariohysterectomy.

5.5. Bitches which do not cycle at all (anoestrus)

Anoestrus is the term scientists use to describe a condition in the bitch which does not cycle after she had previously shown apparent normal heat cycles. There are numerous causes including endocrine disorders and cystic ovarian disease. It is important that the breeders opting to breed from such bitches realise that extensive examinations are required to establish the cause and that fertility will not be restored in all of these bitches. Sterilization should be seriously considered unless the bitch is of exceptional value to the breeder.

5.6. Short intervals between heat cycles (short interoestrus intervals)

Intervals between heat cycles shorter than 4 months are considered aberrant and are usually associated with infertility. This is because the uterine wall needs to prepare itself for pregnancy following a cycle and if insufficient time is allowed to complete this process, the uterus cannot maintain pregnancy. The exact cause of shortened cycle intervals is not known. It is important to note that some bitches of the German Shepherd dog breed have inter heat intervals as short as 4.5 months and this should be considered normal for that breed.

5.7. Dormitory effect

The effect that one oestrous bitch has on other bitches in synchronizing their cycles, is termed the dormitory effect. This effect leads to synchronization when bitches are co-housed. It is assumed that this phenomenon is mediated by pheromones. Some believe that the presence of a vigorous male with bitches will have a similar effect. It is important to realise that this phenomenon is likely to impact on the management of the breeding kennel.

5.8. Excessive vaginal haemorrhage during heat

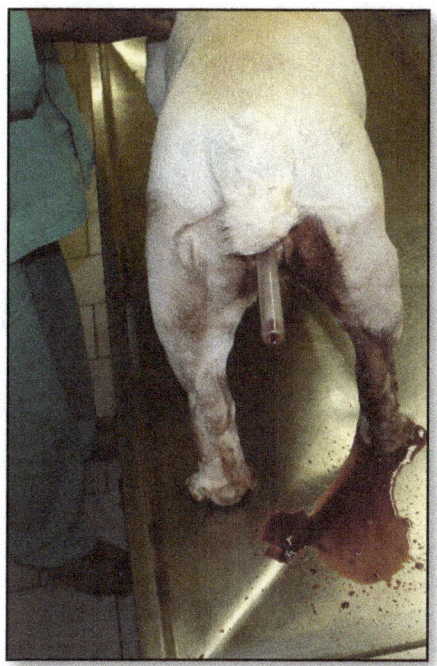
Excessive vaginal haemorrhage during heat

The extent and duration of the bloody vaginal discharge during heat can vary considerably between bitches and heat cycles. Some bitches may have almost no discharge whereas others may have a lot of spotting and dripping of blood. There are, however, bitches which bleed excessively leaving puddles of varying size on the kennel floor. When a speculum is passed in these bitches up to 100 ml of bloody vaginal discharge can flow from the speculum. This extent of vaginal haemorrhage should be regarded pathological. The exact cause of this phenomenon is not known but is suspected to be due to high oestrogen levels (hyperoestrogenism) or increased sensitivity to oestrogen during heat. Heat cycles characterised by this excessive discharging are frequently infertile and bitches are prone to vaginitis during such cycles. Bitches which exhibit excessive vaginal haemorrhage during heat are likely to repeat it at the next cycle. Management of these cycles involves frequent vaginal drainage and flushing followed by artificial insemination and antibiotic treatment.

5.9. Vaginal fold prolapse (vaginal hyperplasia)

This condition is also known as vaginal fold oedema or vaginal hyperplasia. It may be seen in any breed, but is especially common in brachycephalic breeds as Boxers, Bulldogs and many Mastiff-like breeds. It is unknown whether the condition is hereditary or not, although a strong breed predisposition suggests a hereditary nature. The condition occurs because of excessive swelling of the vaginal wall under the influence of oestrogen during early stages of heat. The condition is characterised by a pink, fleshy mass bulging from the floor or, less commonly, from the whole circumference of the vagina whilst in heat. Rarely, it may also occur during late pregnancy. Usually the condition recurs during subsequent heat cycles. The bitch does not necessarily have to show vaginal hyperplasia at her first heat. In most cases it will manifest before her third heat cycle. The mass may interfere with natural mating and artificial insemination is advised in these bitches. Different grades of the condition exist depending on how much of the vaginal wall actually protrudes from the vagina.

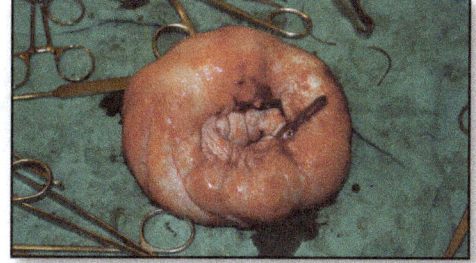
Vaginal fold that has been surgically resected

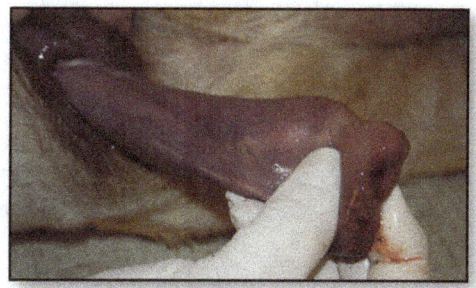
Prolapse of vagina in a pregnant bitch

Grade I vaginal hyperplasia consists of an enlargement of the floor of the caudal vagina which protrudes into the vestibulum and, from the outside, appears as a swollen vestibulum. Inside the vagina, a round bulge can be seen. Grade II hyperplasia is similar to Grade I but protrudes through the vulva. Grade III involves prolapse of the whole circumference of the caudal vaginal wall through the vulvar opening and appears outside the vulva as a pink, doughnut-shaped mass. As a bitch will not necessarily show vaginal hyperplasia at her first heat or every heat for that matter, it is difficult to certify any bitch free from the condition. Also a bitch cannot be presented for examination of vaginal hyperplasia unless she has been in heat for at least a couple of days. A veterinary surgeon may only certify that on the day of examination the bitch was free from any signs of vaginal hyperplasia and certify that she was indeed in heat at that time. Whilst the debate about heritability is ongoing, some breeders elect to sterilize affected bitches whilst others wish to breed. It is the opinion of some breeders and veterinary specialists that even if conclusive evidence of heritability emerges, the benign nature of this condition does not warrant selection against it until more serious conditions have been addressed. For those wishing to breed the bitch naturally, surgical correction is possible. Once the wounds have healed, it may be very difficult if not impossible to check whether a bitch has undergone an operation for vaginal fold prolapse. Although very unlikely, a bitch which has been operated may still get vaginal fold prolapse at a next cycle (and then, usually in a much reduced form).

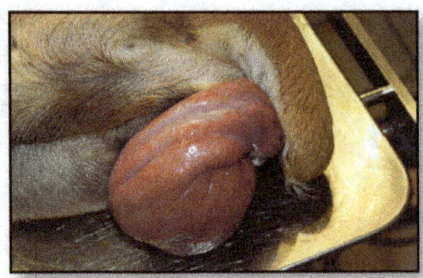
Vaginal Hyperplasia

5.10. Vestibulo-vaginal strictures

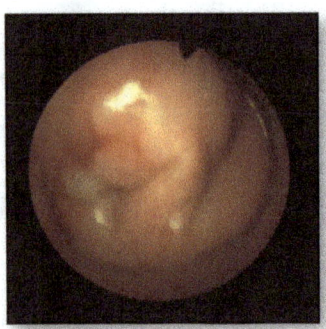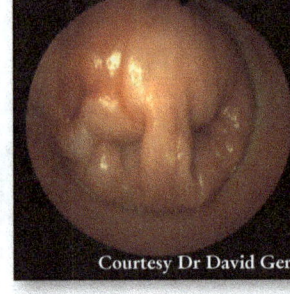

Vestibulo-vaginal band

Vestibulo-vaginal stricture is a collective term used in this text for any defect which leads to a narrowing or any form of obstruction of the vagina. The vestibule is the first part of the canal that leads into the vaginal canal. Vestibular stricture or stenosis is a narrowing in the first few centimetres of the vagina which restricts the introduction of the penis. These strictures can easily be palpated with the index finger although strictures deeper in the vagina can only be diagnosed using endoscopy. Other forms of obstructions include dorsoventral bands (band stretching from top to bottom in vagina), vaginal septae (bands of tissue dividing the vagina into two parts) and segmental aplasia (a missing portion of the vagina). Considering that some of these abnormalities appear more in certain breeds than in others, heritability cannot be excluded. Irrespective of the cause of narrowing, the bitch will object to penetration by the male due to pain or space constraints. Even if the problem is surgically corrected, the bitch may still refuse the male due to previous association of mating attempts with pain. Artificial insemination is the method of choice to ensure that these bitches conceive. Paradoxically, many bitches with vaginal strictures will whelp normally, probably due to the influence of the hormone relaxin at the time of labour. The stricture then returns preventing coitus during her next season. It is thought that these bitches have a lower pregnancy rate than normal bitches. This is believed to be due to improper drainage of the vagina with fluid retention in the anterior vagina and a low-grade vaginitis. Draining of the fluid using a speculum and antibiotic therapy appears to improve results.

The hymen is discussed separately as it is a normal feature in some dogs. Some dogs have a hymen which may still be intact at the time of her first mating and it is then referred to as a persistent hymen. The hymen can be distinguished from dorsoventral bands in that the former is a very thin and flimsy vertical web of tissue across the opening which breaks easily with a speculum. In contrast, dorsoventral bands are thicker strong bands of tissue requiring surgical removal. The hymen can easily be felt with a gloved index finger in medium to large breeds but in smaller breeds a speculum examination is required.

5.11. The genital lock

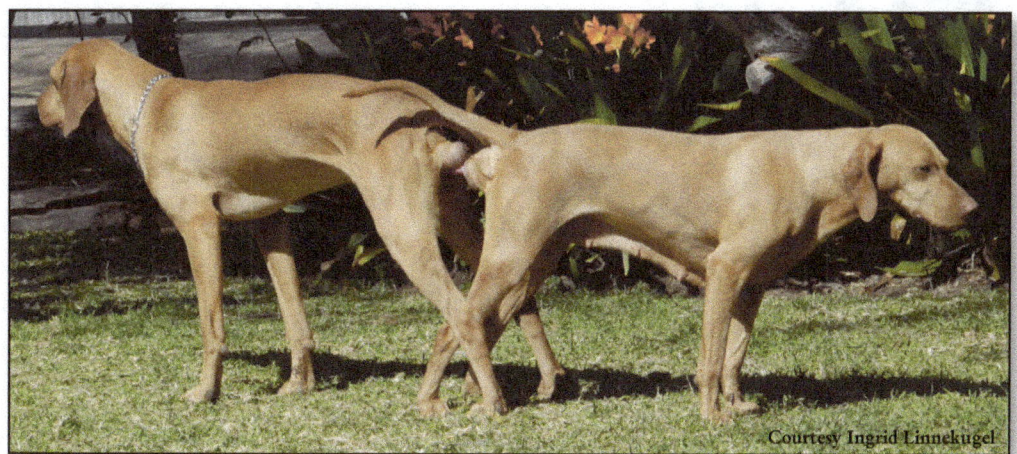
Genital lock

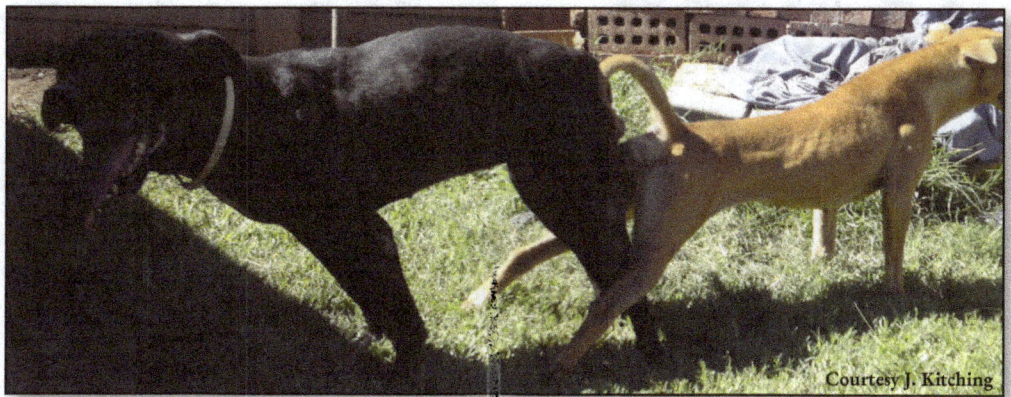
Some dogs are very dextrous and may mate with partners of extreme size differences

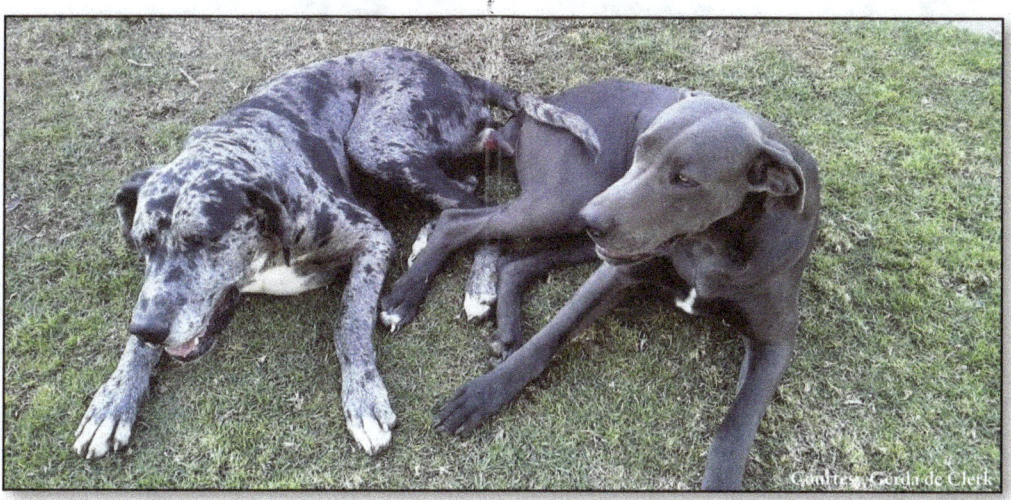
Copulatory tie lying down

Chapter 5 Reproduction in the Bitch

The genital lock is also known as copulatory lock or tie (genital tie) in the domestic dog and basically entails the stud and the bitch getting stuck at mating. This tie is possible because a part of the dog's penis situated at the base of the penis named the bulbus glandis engorges to several times its normal size in a ball shape and gets stuck in the vagina soon after full erection is attained following penetration.

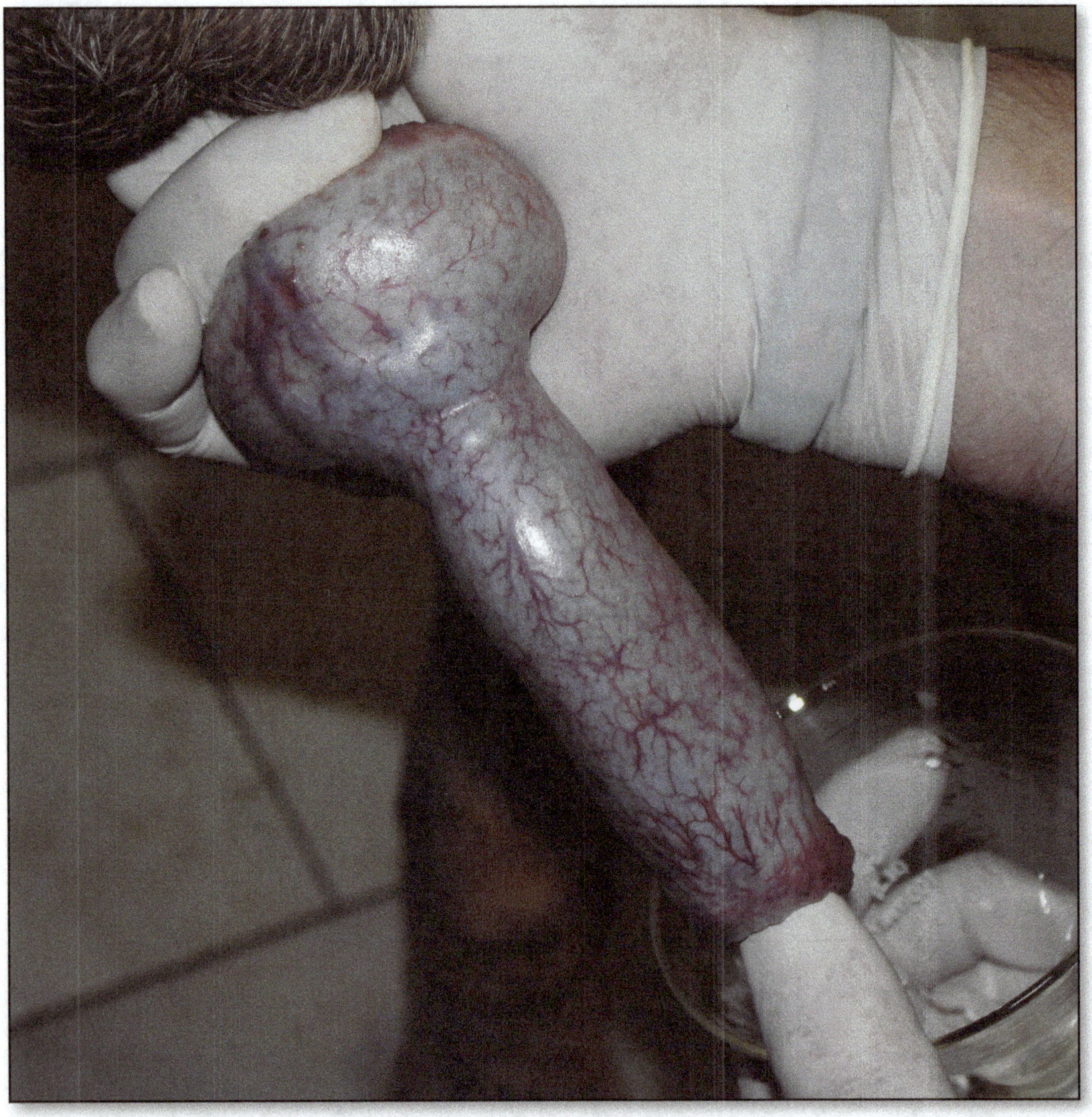

Engorged penis clearly showing the bulbis glandis enabling the dog to tie

The normal process is as follows: The male mounts the bitch and thrusts whilst attempting to penetrate the vagina. As soon as the male has entered the vagina he normally thrusts harder and it is at this point that the penis enlarges and gets stuck. As soon as the copulatory lock is achieved the male will dismount the bitch and lifts one of his hind legs over the bitch. They may stand side-by-side or more frequently back-to-back. In some cases they may even lie down facing away from each other. During the copulatory lock, the penis tip and cervical opening to the uterus are aligned in close proximity thus increasing the chances that a larger number of sperm will traverse the cervix to reach the eggs and prevent leakage of the ejaculate. It is the stud that determines the duration of the genital lock. The tie may last a couple of minutes to 45 minutes or even longer. The duration of the tie in most studs remains fairly constant. There is no correlation between duration of the tie and fertility outcome. It is important that a tie actually took place, as this is a strong indication that ejaculation occurred. The bulbus glandis may engorge prematurely before entering the vagina, thus preventing intromission. There are factors relating to bitch and stud which may lead to failure to lock properly. In the bitch, anatomical abnormalities and acceptance of stud can play a role. A bitch which does not stand willingly and continues to squat during mounting attempts will prevent intromission. Some studs may be inexperienced, overeager, suffer from erectile dysfunction or lack mating dexterity and athletic ability. In these cases, the stud may get excited and develop a full erection thus preventing penile intromission. The stud may then ejaculate outside the bitch. In these cases, breeders sometimes assist the stud and manually guide the tip of the penis in the bitch's vagina. The stud will then usually thrust and ejaculate. Matings achieved in this fashion are referred to in breeder slang as a "slip mating" or an "outside tie". Slip matings are not ideal and a bitch may or may not conceive following this type of mating. Therefore, accomplishment of the genital lock is not a prerequisite for achieving pregnancy in the bitch but certainly is considered to increase the chances of conception. Slip matings are generally unreliable because it remains uncertain whether the stud, ejaculated, ejaculated completely, ejaculate actually entered the vagina or whether enough prostatic fluid aiding as transport medium for the sperm was deposited.

Because mating in many mammalian species is a very brief affair, ejaculation in these species occurs soon after penile intromission. Also, the ejaculate in these species will be emitted in one fraction. This means the prostatic fluid and sperm rich fraction and if applicable (depending on species) other accessory gland excretions, all are emitted almost simultaneously during ejaculation lasting in the order of seconds. The dog, however, has a prolonged coital process. The dog's semen consists of three separate fractions which are ejaculated one immediately after the other. The first fraction is the pre-sperm fraction and is usually emitted before and at the time of intromission. The second fraction is the sperm rich fraction and this is emitted soon after thrusting and achieving the genital lock. The

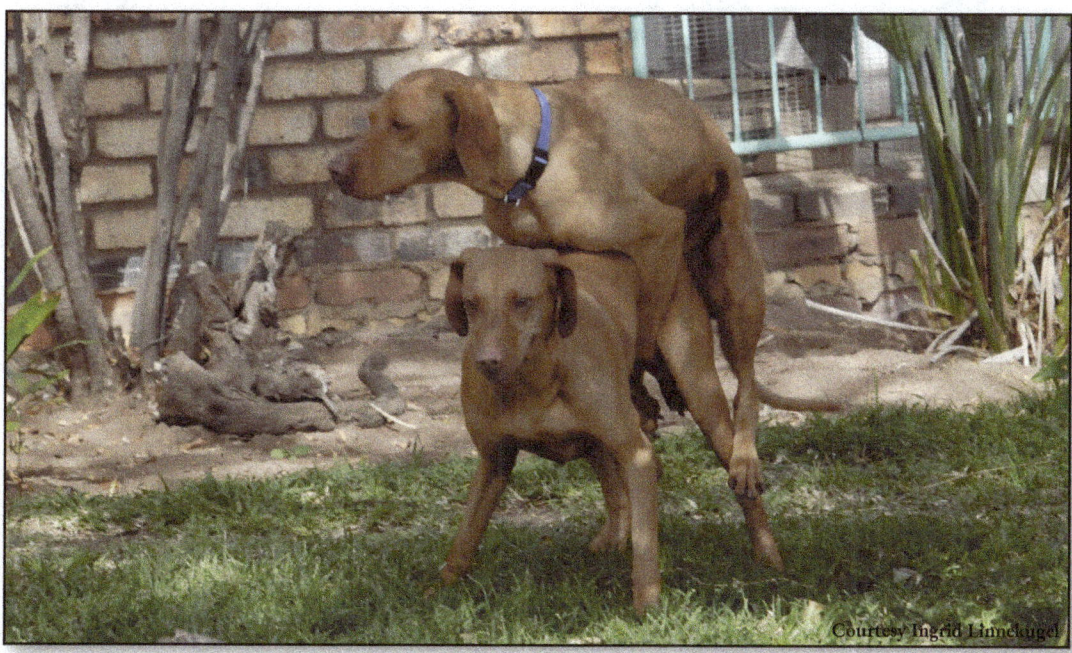

Stud thrusting to achieve intromission and genital lock

Chapter 5 Reproduction in the Bitch

third fraction is the prostatic fraction and may be emitted for the entire duration of the tie. Some dogs may however have an ejaculation pattern that is not as well fractioned as described above.

Interestingly, the genital lock occurs in most wild canids as it does in domestic dogs but in areas where there are many larger stronger carnivores threatening these canids, the copulatory tie is short and where the threat is less, the duration of the copulatory tie is much longer. For instance the Golden jackal in Eurasia may have a copulatory tie which lasts 15 - 20 minutes whereas in the African Golden jackal it may last only 4 minutes average. Likewise, the copulatory tie in the African wild dog *(Lycaon pictus)* seldom lasts longer than a minute. The copulatory tie clearly makes the mating couple engaged in lengthy ties more vulnerable to predation. Wolves have no real threats in their native habitat and have copulatory ties with durations similar to those of dogs.

5.12. Vaginitis

Vaginitis refers to inflammation of the vagina usually caused by bacterial infections. Trauma, vaginal anatomical defects, polyps, tumours, herpesvirus, urinary infections and uterine infections can all lead to a vaginitis. Vaginitis should be suspected if the bitch has a vaginal discharge and licks the vulva continuously. Vaginitis in bitches not in heat may also attract males.

5.12.1. Vaginitis during oestrus

It might be difficult for the breeder to identify signs of vaginitis in bitches which are in heat. This is because during heat there will be a vaginal discharge varying from a watery discharge to a straw coloured discharge towards the end of oestrus. Excessive discharges and thick purulent discharges should alert the breeder and be examined for the presence of vaginitis. Bitches suffering from vestibulo-vaginal strictures are frequent sufferers of vaginitis due to improper drainage (See 5.10). In exceptional cases, Herpesvirus may cause vaginitis during heat. Yeast infections of the vagina are rare but may occur following frequent antibiotic use.

If vaginitis is diagnosed, the underlying cause should be addressed and the vaginitis should be treated using antibiotics. The routine use of antibiotics during heat in attempts to "prevent" vaginitis requires discussion because it is a common practice by breeders and is frequently recommended by veterinary surgeons as well as some reproductive specialists. Prolonged antibiotic courses are often administered to bitches in heat because of a history of conception failure, uterine infection or following results from a bacterial swab and culture. The latter is comprehensively discussed in 5.17.1. Urogenital infections may indeed lead to conception or pregnancy failure. The uterus is usually a closed and sterile environment and is only subject to invasion by ascending bacteria when the cervix is open. The cervix only opens during heat and during whelping. During heat, the cervix is expected to be open from the first signs of vaginal haemorrhaging until the bitch is no longer receptive. Therefore, if preventative antibiotic therapy is indicated, it makes sense to administer antibiotics during the entire stage that the cervix is expected to be open. Cases in which the use of preventative antibiotic courses is justified include bitches with a history of endometritis, history of treatment for pyometra, vestibulo-vaginal strictures, vaginitis and bitches which are confirmed to suffer from cystic endometrial hyperplasia (See 5.13).

5.12.2. Dioestrus vaginitis

A bitch may suffer from a mild vaginitis characterised by a scant slightly yellow discharge in the period soon after she is no longer receptive to the male and may occur in bitches whether they were bred or not. If it is a mild infection with little discharge (a couple of drops), it may be perfectly normal. If the discharge appears excessive, it is best to have this examined. Bitches with a very pendulous vagina (Brachiocephalic breeds) frequently show excessive signs of dioestrus vaginitis. This normally does not require treatment.

5.12.3. Skin fold vaginitis

Some dogs may acquire a skin fold above the dorsal commissure (vaginal slit opening) which results in a huge fold covering all or most of the opening of the vagina. In these bitches the lower part of the vagina is frequently also tucked in and hidden under skin. This often results in a chronic vaginitis and urine scalding (burn). Even though local treatment may temporarily alleviate the signs, long term resolution often requires surgical resection of the fold.

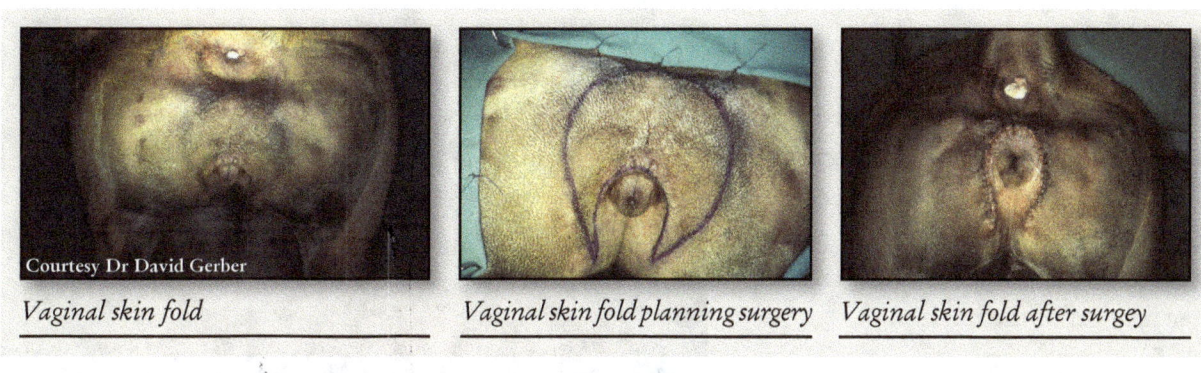

| Vaginal skin fold | Vaginal skin fold planning surgery | Vaginal skin fold after surgey |

This may be very difficult or even impossible if the bitch is obese and she may need to lose a substantial amount of weight prior to surgery. In some cases, obesity is the primary cause of the problem and weight loss may resolve the problem altogether.

5.12.4. Puppy vaginitis

This is an uncommon but very frustrating condition. It manifests as a chronic yellow purulent discharge which is usually poorly responsive to antibiotics. By definition it occurs in puppies from as early as 8 weeks onwards till puberty. The exact cause of the condition is not known. The disease is usually self-limiting and may only disappear as mysteriously as it came after her first heat cycle. Early spaying of these puppies is not advised as it will not resolve the problem.

5.13. Cystic endometrial hyperplasia

Cystic endometrial hyperplasia (CEH) is a term which is used to describe a condition of the uterus. The uterine wall is known as the endometrium. In CEH, the uterine wall becomes thickened due to both the abnormal increase in number (hyperplasia) and increase in size (hypertrophy) of the uterine glands within the wall of the uterus (endometrium). In summary, CEH is the development of cysts in the uterine wall and thickening thereof. Cystic endometrial hyperplasia may be cumulative and get worse following each cycle that a bitch does not conceive. In the normal uterus, during oestrus, the uterine glands have the function of secreting a fluid (known as uterine milk) in small quantities with the main function of feeding the embryos prior to implantation. It appears that pregnancy has a rejuvenating action on the uterine wall because bitches that have regular litters are far less frequently diagnosed with CEH than are those which are bred infrequently or never. It is speculated that pregnancy, the sloughing of the endometrial lining following birth and the involution process (recovery of uterine wall following pregnancy) all aid in preventing CEH. It is for this reason that the number of cycles prior to first breeding should not be excessive as discussed in 5.1. CEH can be diagnosed by high resolution ultrasonography of the uterus, hysteroscopy, uterine biopsy or uterine inspection via laparotomy (abdominal exploration).

Under normal circumstances, the healthy uterine wall is resistant to bacteria which enter the uterus during heat. The bitch that suffers from CEH will appear perfectly normal and have normal cycles. CEH is significant because it predisposes the bitch to low grade uterine infections, pyometra and indirectly to infertility. The combination of the low grade infections and a uterine wall unfavourable to implantation leads to poor conception in affected bitches. For this reason, preventative antibiotic therapy may be indicated in these bitches as discussed in 5.12.1. These bitches are also more likely to develop pyometra - 5.15.

5.14. Ovarian cysts

Numerous types of ovarian cysts exist and may cause infertility, predisposition to uterine infection, persistent heat or failure to come into season. Ovarian disease requires specialist attention and may result in sterilization of the bitch.

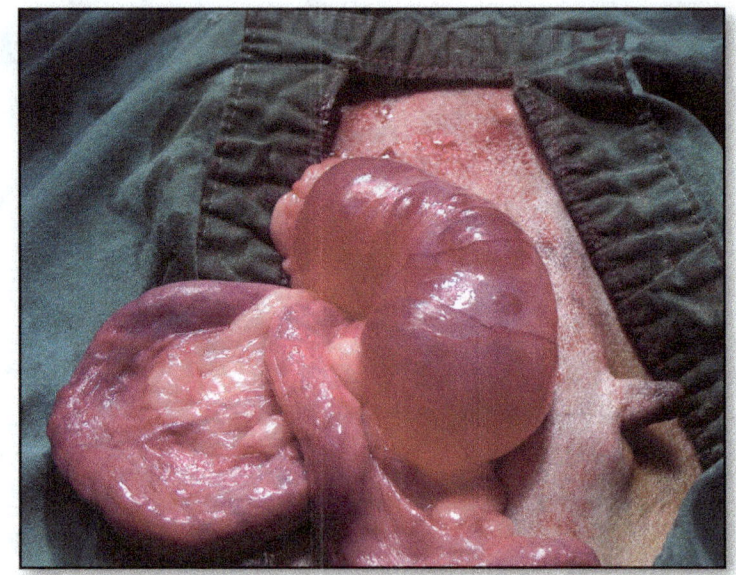
Ovarian cyst

5.15. Para-uterine cysts

Para-uterine cysts are frequently encountered in older bitches and although they appear rather dramatic, they have little influence on fertility and this condition does not require sterilisation. These cysts may be detected during surgery for caesarean section or on ultrasound as incidental findings.

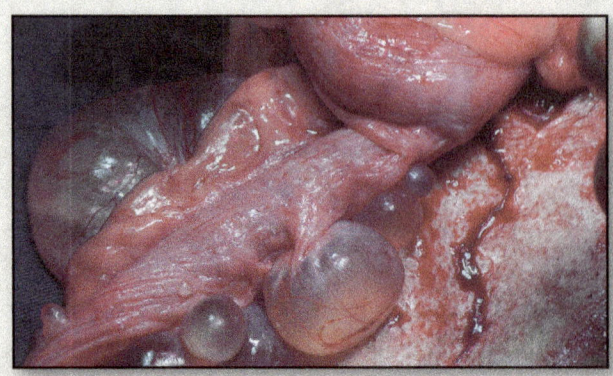
Para-uterine cysts

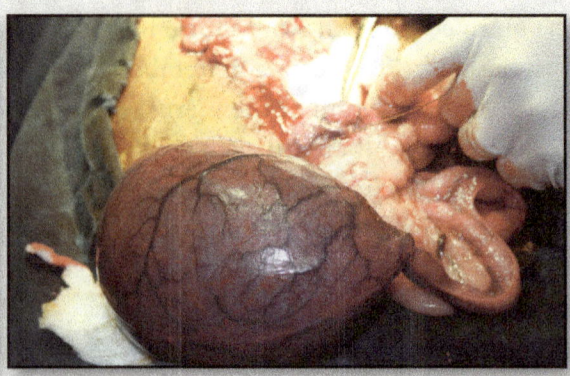
Uterine cyst

5.16. Pyometra

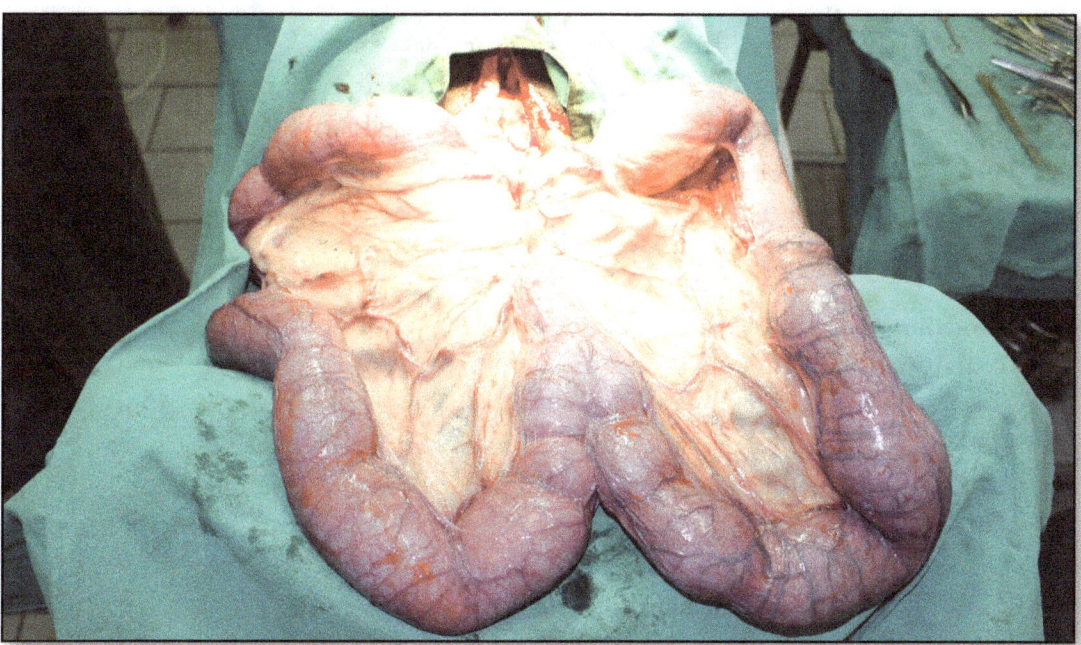

Massively engorged uterus filled with puss (pyometra)

The cervix only opens twice during the oestrus cycle. Once during heat to permit fluids escaping the uterus and semen into the uterus and the other is following pregnancy to allow for birth. During all other times, the cervix remains closed. Pyometra refers to an infection of the uterus with pus accumulation in the uterus which typically occurs in adult bitches several weeks following a heat cycle. The clinical manifestations may include excessive water intake, poor appetite, abdominal distension, vomition, weight loss, fever and anaemia. A purulent vaginal discharge may however be the only symptom in some cases of pyometra where the cervix is open. When the cervix is closed, no vaginal discharge is seen. Pyometra may be a life-threatening disease. Parity and age are significant risk factors in the development of pyometra. Bitches which continuously cycle without being bred, for example, show dogs and working dogs and which are only bred at 4 years or later, are at increased risk. In exceptional cases, younger bitches or even post pubertal bitches may be affected. The use of progestogens, oestrogens and other hormonal compounds to manipulate the heat cycle, may contribute to its occurrence. The treatment of choice by most veterinary surgeons is sterilisation. Although not entirely risk free, the condition can be treated successfully in cases where to owner wishes to regain reproductive capacity. Medical treatment involves drugs which promote emptying of the uterus combined with antibiotic treatment. Surgical flushing of the uterus may also be considered as it results in shorter recovery times and may prove successful in cases where medical therapy failed. It is of vital importance that the breeder has every intention to breed the bitch on her very next heat cycle following treatment for pyometra. Following successful treatment for pyometra, preventative antibiotic therapy is advised during the next heat periods.

Breeders sometimes assume that the bitch may have contracted an infection from the male. In the case of pyometra, this is highly unlikely as the development of pyometra is dependent on the presence of a compromised uterus. Also, bitches may develop a uterine infection irrespective whether they were mated on that cycle or not. Similarly, the bitch is unlikely to transmit a urogenital bacterial infection to the male.

5.17. Monitoring of the oestrous cycle and determining optimal breeding time

There are many reasons for breeders to want to monitor a bitch's oestrous cycles or ask their veterinary surgeon to do it. Clearly, breeders want to breed their bitches at a time when they are at their most fertile in order to maximise their chances of pregnancy and attain normal litter sizes. It is also important for breeders to determine when the bitch is off heat so that she may be reintroduced to her "social group" without her inducing the havoc of an "in season" bitch and to make sure that an accidental mating to another undesired male is no longer possible.

Veterinary surgeons, on the other hand, may be required to monitor the cycle if more accuracy is required. Accurate determination of optimal breeding time may be required if there is limited access to the stud or the intended stud is of reduced fertility. The breeder may also want to use frozen, chilled or poor quality fresh semen, which has a much shorter lifespan once inseminated in the bitch's genital tract, necessitating very accurate timing of events. Oestrus monitoring will also enable the veterinary surgeon to determine whether the cycle is normal and give an indication of when the bitch is expected to whelp. It is of vital importance that breeders requesting their veterinary surgeon to assist them with oestrous monitoring give them their full co-operation. Accurate timing of events during oestrous is only possible when the veterinary surgeon has regular access to the bitch being monitored. Before the breeder makes the decision to go ahead with this lengthy process, they must have completed the logistic planning. The options are that the bitch remains in the care of the veterinary surgeon in their hospital or the bitch is transported to the veterinary surgeon's premises for examination when required. Not unlike veterinary surgeons, breeders may have very busy lifestyles with many commitments. Therefore, even with the best intentions, breeders often find themselves in the position where they were unable to present a bitch on a given day/s for examination. This may jeopardise the veterinary surgeon's ability to render a professional service. The frequency of access to the bitch that the veterinary surgeon requires depends on the accuracy required. In cases where compromised semen (semen of poor quality, frozen or chilled semen) is expected to be used, daily access is required. In cases where natural mating using a known fertile stud, or fresh semen insemination using good quality semen are the intended method of breeding, every alternate day access to the bitch may be sufficient. Because the veterinary surgeon may want to determine the first day of dioestrus, they may require having access to the bitch for a couple of days after the last breeding. This is important because this date helps with predicting the whelping date and it also confirms that the bitch is no longer in heat and in danger of mismating.

The vast majority of pregnancies in breeding bitches all over the world are achieved by breeders themselves determining the optimal time of breeding without help from their veterinary surgeons. The reason that their methods appear to work so well in many cases is not because it is accurate, but rather because fresh sperm of excellent quality may remain viable in the female reproductive tract for as long as 6 days (2-3 days is the safe accepted norm) after a single copulation. Also, when there is unrestricted access to the stud, the accuracy of their timing method becomes less important because the breeder can compensate for this by increasing the number of matings. Breeders therefore, usually only seek veterinary assistance for bitches where they do not achieve good results or in those where assisted reproductive techniques are planned.

5.17.1. Methods used by breeders to determine optimal breeding time

a) Counting method

The most basic form of determining "optimal breeding time" practised by breeders is the counting method. This involves monitoring the bitch daily for the first signs of heat. The first signs most commonly noted are swelling of the vagina and a bloody vaginal discharge. The first day that bleeding and or swelling was noticed is then known as the first day of heat and used as chronological landmark in timing events by breeders. The breeder starts counting from that day and allows mating on days 9, 11 and 13. Most breeders will report good results with this regimen provided the bitch exhibits a heat period of average length. There are many variations of this counting method with the exact day of mating after first signs of heat or number of matings allowed varying somewhat, e.g. matings on day 10 and 12. This method will fail in those bitches which have long or short cycles. The breeders' ability to accurately determine the first day of heat may also be questioned. This is because some bitches are very fastidious and may keep licking themselves clean whereas others may have little noticeable bleeding. This method is better than no method and may work for the breeder who either has easy unrestricted access to a stud or have their own stud. Breeders may use this method in most bitches and present other bitches which fail to conceive this way for more accurate monitoring of the heat cycle. The main reason for failure using this timing method is the considerable variation in the beginning of the fertile period in relation to the onset first signs of heat. This method is not suitable for assisted reproductive techniques.

b) Mating on alternate days during standing heat

This method involves timing of mating based on behavioural signs of the "in season" bitch and the stud's response to her. This method makes perfect sense to most breeders because it resembles what they expect would happen in a pack of dogs in nature. In this method, the breeder presents the bitch to the stud and observes her behaviour. On the first day that the bitch shows acceptance by a male, the breeder allows mating with the intended stud. The breeder will then normally mate the bitch every alternate day until she no longer allows mating. In the absence of alternatives and when access to the stud is not limited, this is an acceptable mating protocol. Although this method may be successful in an acceptable number of bitches, it has many drawbacks and limitations.

This method cannot work in cases where there is restricted access to the stud. Many normal bitches may remain in standing heat for 12 days and even longer. In these cases, 6 or more matings would then be required. This is a very wasteful use of the stud. Some studs will lose interest in a bitch which remains standing for this long, leading the breeder to believe that it is "all over". When not using their own stud, breeders are reliant on another breeder as stud owner. As a norm, stud owners will generally only allow 2 matings. In exceptional cases they will allow more matings depending on the stud's mating schedule. Stud owners of very "in demand" studs, may even restrict the number of matings to two or even a single mating. In the latter cases, it is advised that the breeder seek the assistance of their veterinary surgeon to monitor events in order to achieve good results.

This method does not work well for a bitch which displays an individual dislike for a particular male. In these cases, the bitch displays typical signs of heat but continues to refuse to allow that stud to mount and copulate whilst allowing another. It is important for breeders using this method to exclude idiosyncratic dislikes displayed by bitches. Failure to recognise this oddity will erroneously lead the breeder to assume that the bitch is "not ready" and the bitch's refusal will continue until the bitch is no longer in heat. Breeders whom are aware of this will often evaluate the response of a bitch to another stud before assuming

Chapter 5 Reproduction in the Bitch

she is not "ready". The exact reason for some bitches displaying this individual dislike is not known. Fear, dominance, inexperience and aggressive behaviour on behalf of both parties are believed to play a role.

Some bitches which are confirmed in peak season may attract the males but not allow them to mate. In contrast to the bitches described above they will not allow another stud or any other stud to copulate. In many cases the reasons for this behaviour are not known. Some breeders have observed that young maiden bitches which had experienced pain and fear during their first sexual encounter were more likely to develop an aversion to copulating attempts by a stud. This accentuates the importance of a serene mating quarters (honeymoon quarters) and a gentle and calm approach of a virgin bitch to her first sexual experience.

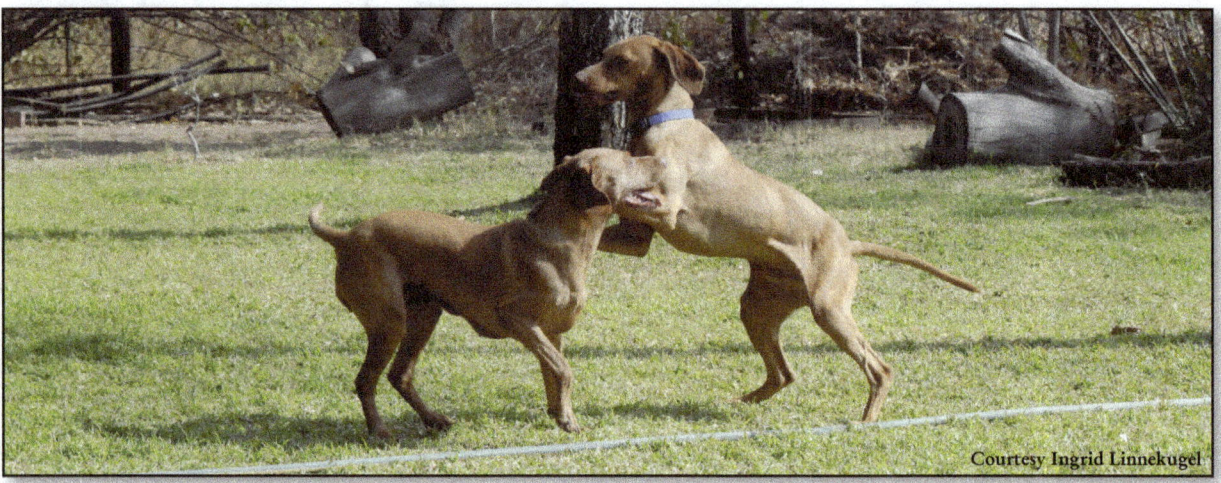

Dogs engrossed in foreplay

Rough handling of the bitch, busy surroundings and presence of other exited dogs may all contribute to negative connotations. Some studs are aggressive, dominant and rough in their approach to mating bitches and breeders should avoid these studs with young inexperienced bitches and rather select a gentler stud. Some bitches with vaginal pathology (vaginal stenosis, stricture, bands or other pathology) may experience pain during penile intromission and show sexual unwillingness despite being in peak oestrus. These bitches should be examined by a veterinary surgeon for correction of the problem, where possible. As bitches are likely to repeat this behaviour at the next heat, it is best that her cycle be monitored by more accurate means and artificial insemination be considered.

The stud may also have an idiosyncratic dislike for certain bitches. The stud may also have lack of sexual interest, leading the breeder to believe that the bitch is not ready despite her showing interest. There is the common notion amongst many breeders that some males have the distinct ability to determine exactly when a bitch is in peak heat (at her most fertile) and will only mate her in that time and not "waste" his time by mating her on times not in peak heat. Whilst there may be truth to the observation that studs may show increased sexual interest in bitches as they approach the fertile period, it should not be relied on too much. Dogs with good libido may show very keen interest in any bitch which is in season irrespective of how close she is to the fertile period in her cycle. Dogs may even show interest in bitches which are not in season and have a vaginal discharge related to vaginitis or other vaginal pathology. On the other hand, dogs which lack libido may also confuse the breeder. These dogs may fail to show adequate interest in any bitch for more than 2-3 consecutive days or at times not show any interest in an "in season" bitch at all.

5.17.2. Methods used by veterinary surgeons and breeders to determine optimal breeding time

a) Use of the outward signs

Outward signs of heat such as vaginal swelling which starts to recede, change in colour of the vaginal discharge from serosanguinous to straw coloured at the onset of standing heat and intensity of the vaginal and tail reflex, may all act as clues that the bitch is in heat and receptive. It will, however, not indicate that the bitch is in the fertilization period. This method is no more helpful than evaluating the response of the stud to the bitch.

b) Physical changes during heat

Physical changes occur in the vagina during heat. Vaginal slime, pH, viscosity of the vaginal slime, electrical conductivity of vaginal slime and glucose content change during heat. Some companies market devices that measure these changes. Studies have shown that all these have limited clinical usefulness and that they have poor correlation with hormonal events.

c) Use of vaginal cytology

This involves making a smear of the vaginal epithelium and evaluating the cell types. Because there is poor correlation between onset of cytologic oestrus and ovulation it is concluded that cytology is not useful in breeding management to determine the optimal mating period. Vaginal cytology may be useful in confirming that the bitch is in oestrus in cases of bitches exhibiting silent heat or suboestrus. This is characterised by bitches exhibiting vaginal cornification with few or no outward or behavioural signs of oestrus. Vaginal cytology is, however, very useful for determining the onset of cytologic dioestrus (D1). D1 is clinically significant as it occurs 6 days after ovulation with little variation. D1 may also be of use in narrowing down the expected whelping date. This usually occurs ± 57 days from D1. However, D1 only has retrospective value and is therefore of no use in optimising the timing of breeding in the bitch.

d) Use of vaginoscopy

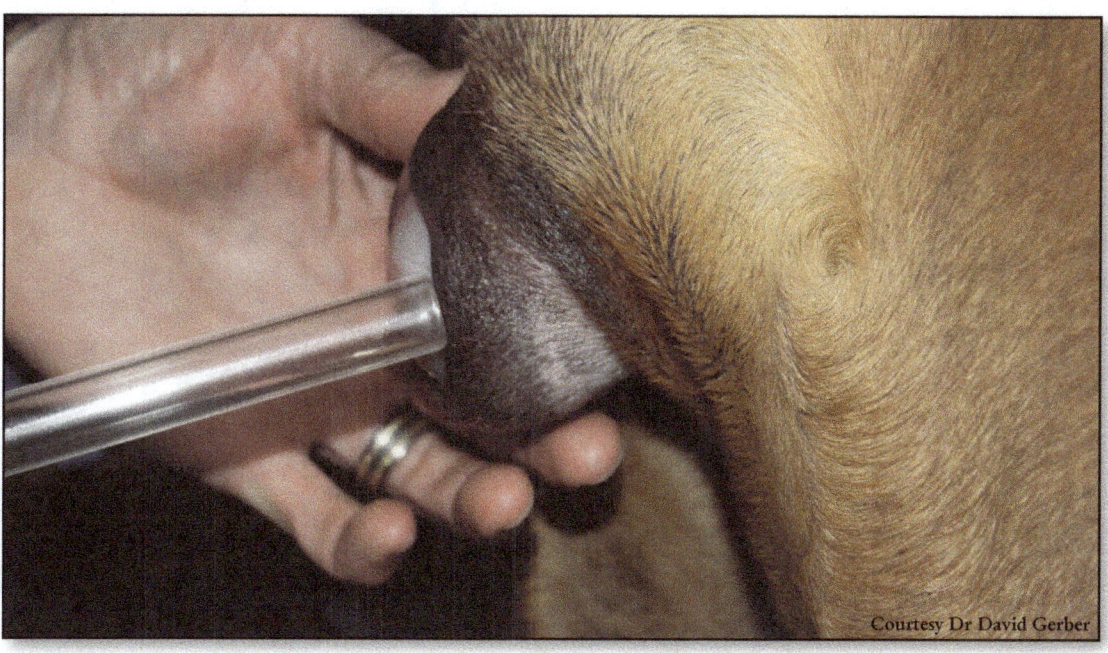

Courtesy Dr David Gerber

Vaginoscopy

This involves inserting a vaginoscope (speculum) into the vagina and evaluating the appearance of the vaginal mucosa. Using vaginoscopy, the veterinary surgeon may identify the first sign of angularity of the vaginal folds, which more or less coincides with the time of ovulation. It is, however, not considered accurate enough for timing ovulation with frozen semen inseminations. Despite this, the main advantage of vaginoscopy is that it allows the veterinary surgeon to identify the stage when the bitch allows matings, but has oedematous folds and could not have ovulated yet. This may considerably reduce the length of time between first breeding and fertilization period and is even more useful in bitches with exceptionally long cycles. For the experienced operator, vaginoscopy is a useful tool for timing breeding. It is very useful for breeders wanting to take their bitch to a stud which is either far away or when there is restricted access to the stud. This method is also valuable for timing fresh or chilled semen inseminations. Of all the "non-laboratory methods", this is the most useful and accurate. It offers the operator the very best real-time information. It is also useful in cases where the breeder has no idea how long the bitch has been in heat for or when a bitch is not available for daily examinations. A series of vaginoscopic examinations however, gives more accurate predictions of the crucial events ahead and therefore daily examinations whilst monitoring the heat cycle, is ideal.

e) Use of hormone assays

Hormone assay remains the most accurate predictor of ovulation time in bitches. The two hormones measured are usually luteinising hormone (LH) and progesterone. These hormones may be measured using commercial assay kits or laboratory quantitative assays. The kits are usually semi quantitative assays, meaning they indicate the presence of the hormone but do not accurately measure hormone concentrations. They therefore only narrow down the time of ovulation and thus for accurate results, quantitative results for progesterone are preferred. Not all hormone kits available to the breeder are the same. Some have limited value and others are totally inaccurate and considered useless. LH measurement by quantitative assay is not practical as few laboratories have the test available. There is a semi-quantitative LH test kit available which, in the opinion of the author, shows promise and warrants further investigation and validation. However, the short duration of the LH peak necessitates daily or even twice daily sampling and confirmation with progesterone assays. Therefore, LH assays are less practical than progesterone assays. Measurement of progesterone by quantitative assays, such as radioimmunoassay (RIA), chemiluminescent immune-assay (CLIA) and enzyme-linked immunosorbent assay (ELISA) is generally accepted to be more accurate. RIA is the gold standard.

Progesterone concentrations have been adequately correlated with key events in the canine oestrous cycle and can be used to determine optimum time for breeding (fertilization period). Progesterone concentrations may be used in two ways, each with its advantages and disadvantages. The first would be to use progesterone to determine the first day on which there is a rise in the pre-ovulatory progesterone. In determining this day, it is recommended that the progesterone be repeated at least once after the first rise to ensure that the rise is sustained and steep. It is advised that vaginoscopy be used to guide the veterinary surgeon in the timing of blood sampling. The aim is to take samples on the days when the progesterone concentration increases sharply on two consecutive days with the former being the day of first rise in progesterone. Key events are then timed from this day. The advantage of this method is that it has prospective value in that it gives the veterinary surgeon prior notice of the optimum breeding time. The second is using absolute progesterone concentration values. Using absolute values, the veterinary surgeon can stage the cycle and confirm that ovulation has occurred. Hormonal assays are the method of choice where the most accurate results are required. It is therefore the method of choice in timing inseminations with frozen semen, chilled semen or poor quality semen. Although hormonal assays are currently the best method available, thorough investigations by various reproductive scientists have led them to speculate that there is a margin of error of approximately one day using hormonal assays. For the veterinary surgeon performing assisted reproductive techniques this information is important. It explains to them and the breeder why when using compromised semen, two inseminations with a 24 hour interval achieves better results than when only one insemination is performed. It makes sense that if the error was zero, that only one perfectly timed insemination should be sufficient. Work is in progress to achieve that goal. Progesterone concentrations may also be used to monitor progress of pregnancy, investigate abnormal cycles and confirm presence of ovarian tissue in apparently sterilised bitches.

The drawbacks to hormonal assays include the considerable costs associated with the kits, laboratory assays, need for daily monitoring, access to a suitable laboratory and the time delay in obtaining results. Some breeders may also object to the daily blood sampling for up to a week or longer.

5.18. Breeding protocols for optimum fertility

The information in the previous section has to be translated into practical and useful protocols to breeding bitches. The time in between one breeding to the next in the same heat period, is referred to as the breeding interval. This breeding interval is mainly dependent on the longevity, quality and sperm numbers of the semen used in the breeding. Assuming the bitch is fertile, the factors which determine the success of breeding are fertility of the semen used and timing of breeding. Both the fertility of the semen and timing method used, influences the ideal breeding interval and number of breedings used. Because access to male, method of breeding and fertility of sperm used, may all vary depending on circumstances, various breeding protocols to optimise fertility may be used.

In planning breedings by means of natural matings, it is important to have prior knowledge of accessibility to the stud. Unfortunately these studs may frequently be "booked" for several bitches at around the same time. Owners of bitches whom have their mind set on a particular desired stud present the bitch for matings to this stud based on his availability rather than upon information gathered by ovulation timing. For this reason it is vital that the veterinary surgeon assisting the breeder, advise them to have a second choice stud (plan B).

5.18.1. Natural mating with unlimited access to a stud dog; without heat timing

This is the most common breeding protocol. A fertile stud dog is a dog which consistently impregnates fertile bitches which are bred during the fertile period, and which result in normal sized litters. Generally a good stud dog, under ideal circumstances, should attain a pregnancy rate of 80% and above. Their semen evaluation will reveal good motility, good morphology and adequate numbers. If the only means of assessing the optimal time for breeding is behaviour and vulvar discharge, the breeder has no choice but to breed a bitch on the first or second day of standing heat and every second day thereafter, until the bitch refuses to mate. This mating protocol is wasteful in terms of stud dog management because it is possible that the stud dog will perform numerous unnecessary matings using this protocol. Although wasteful, this method is better than the counting method explained earlier.

5.18.2. Natural mating using one stud dog on two bitches, alternating matings, without heat timing

It often happens that the same stud needs to mate two bitches simultaneously. As will be discussed later in 10.10, healthy studs can easily manage this. Each bitch is mated every alternate day for the entire period that the bitches remain receptive. Provided the stud dog has good fertility, his ejaculate should be able to maintain a sizable sperm population in the reproductive tract of each bitch, to ensure fertilization. Again, this mating protocol is also frustrating for the stud dog owner because it is likely that the stud dog will have to perform numerous unnecessary matings.

5.18.3. Natural mating with limited access to a stud dog (2-3 matings)

A breeder should seek veterinary assistance to monitor the bitch's cycle if the number of matings are restricted. Vaginoscopy and vaginal cytology are accurate enough to determine the period when matings will be fertile. From the time that this period begins until the end is narrowed down to 5 or 6 days or so. Given that a fertile stud dog's semen remains fertile in the genital tract of the bitch for at least 2-3 days, alternate day matings for 2-3 days should ensure that viable sperm are available to impregnate the bitch's eggs, at the correct time. If a veterinary surgeon is competent in vaginoscopy and vaginal cytology, the number of matings can be reduced to two, with good results.

5.18.4. Natural mating with access limited to a single mating

If access to the stud dog is limited to a single mating, accurate timing is required. This can be achieved by performing a progesterone assay. A bitch may be bred when progesterone exceeds 16 nmol/l to about 30 nmol/l (may vary somewhat depending on laboratory). This corresponds more or less with 6 days after the progesterone levels first started to rise above basal levels. Alternatively excellent results, almost equivalent to those obtained using hormonal assays, can be achieved by vaginoscopy This is because the semen which is used under these circumstances is fresh and uncompromised and it can last for at least 2-3 days with ease in the female urogenital tract, which allows for only one mating. This is the only circumstance under which a single breeding is likely to have consistently good results.

5.18.5. Breeding using compromised semen

Compromised semen may be fresh semen from a stud with poor quality semen, chilled semen or frozen semen. Ideally, in all these cases, the breeder should opt for blood progesterone assays in order to optimise the time of breeding. It is important to realise that when semen is suspected or known to be of poor quality, two successive breedings, 24 hours apart from each other, render better results than a single breeding. This is because, the margin of error in determining the time of ovulation, even when using blood assays, may be out by a day or so. Therefore, the second breeding is likely to boost already diminished sperm numbers and because compromised semen is suspected to have severely diminished longevity (in the order of hours rather than a day or three).

a) Fresh semen of poor quality

Fresh semen is considered compromised when either one or a combination of the following are present; inadequate number of sperm, poor motility or an abnormally high percentage of sperm defects. Pregnancy rates are poor when using this semen. Two breedings are recommended on consecutive days timed using progesterone assays. Depending on the extent of semen compromise and sperm count, the pregnancy rates may be vastly improved if the method of breeding is artificial insemination by intra uterine semen deposition. In fact, in cases where the semen contains a critically low number of normal sperm, intra uterine insemination may be the only means by which this semen may have a realistic chance to impregnate a bitch. Two inseminations 24 hours apart are advised.

b) Chilled semen

Chilled semen is considered compromised because the cooling process decreases its vitality, quality and longevity. Two inseminations are recommended on consecutive days, timed using progesterone assays. The semen may be deposited intra-vaginally or intra-uterine. If the semen is of poor quality to start off with, the breeder should strongly consider not using this method of breeding. When using semen of good quality and good chilling media, good results may be expected.

c) Frozen semen

Frozen semen is considered compromised because the freezing and thawing process severely decreases its vitality and longevity. Two inseminations are recommended on consecutive days timed using progesterone assays. The semen must be deposited intra-uterine. To achieve good results, only semen of adequate quality should be considered by breeders.

5.19. Examination for breeding soundness

A breeding soundness examination for a bitch may be requested, prior to sale or purchase, or as part of an infertility examination in a breeding colony. Some owners of studs insist on a breeding soundness examination as it may help protect the stud dog's reputation by preventing unnecessary breeding failures. They may also be concerned about the safety of the stud dog if a natural breeding is chosen. What follows is a list of possible examinations the breeder and their veterinary surgeon may consider as part of the breeding soundness examination. Again, the extent of the examination may be dictated by what the breeder is prepared to spend, breeding history of the bitch and the value of the dogs involved. Geographic location influences the type of examinations advised. Therefore these matters should be discussed with veterinary surgeons experienced in the subject. No complete generic list can be compiled for breeders around the world. In some areas it may be considered negligent not to test for diseases such as Lyme disease, Brucellosis or heartworm while in other areas it would be a waste of time and money.

5.19.1. Pre-breeding bacterial cultures

Pre-breeding vaginal swabs are often collected to establish whether the bitch harbours a genital infection. These examinations are best completed before the bitch is about to cycle or at the very beginning of her cycle. Although it is true that overt genital infections would be easily identified with clinical signs of a vaginitis or uterine infection, subclinical, low-grade infections would not. These swabs may reveal the presence of bacteria which may be implicated in a genital infection in the bitch and will also indicate which antibiotic is likely to be most effective in its treatment.

It is important that the swabbing technique is such that it avoids contaminants from faecal origin or from the skin. Both the bitch's vagina and the dog's penis have similar normal populations of bacteria which can potentially cause uterine infections. Careful interpretation of such routine examinations is required as it may be difficult to distinguish normal populations from potential pathogens. Results from swabs should therefore be interpreted in conjunction with result from clinical examinations as well as white blood cell counts. Many bitches which do not harbour an infection and do not require treatment are treated with antibiotics because of misinterpretation of culture results. When these breeders then achieve pregnancies with treated bitches, they erroneously deduce that this practice works well. Therefore the practice routine treatment of bitches based on swab results in the absence confirmed infection or predisposing factors may be questioned.

5.19.2. White cell count
The white blood cell count reveals whether the body is fighting an infection or not. If the white blood cell count in a bitch is elevated, it warrants further examination. Elevated white blood cell counts may reveal the presence of an infection which would otherwise remain undetected. Uterine infections are not the only cause of elevated white blood cell counts in cycling brood bitches but they should nevertheless be excluded. Low-grade bacterial infections of the uterus make it an unfavourable environment for conception and maintenance of pregnancy and white blood cell counts are helpful in their detection.

5.19.3. Ultrasonography of uterus and ovaries
Ultrasonography of the uterus and ovaries may reveal abnormalities such as neoplasia, infection and or cystic changes. The skill of the operator, as well as resolution of the ultrasound machine used, may all influence the accuracy of the ultrasonography findings. Ultrasonography is an easy and non-invasive examination to perform and should form part of any breeding soundness examination in bitches.

5.19.4. Thyroid function
Thyroid hormone must be present at adequate levels in all dogs to support normal function and reproduction. True hypothyroid bitches are easy to recognise and diagnose. Dogs which have marginally low values and poor reproductive performance may be problematic. This is because it might be difficult to ascertain whether the low thyroid levels are a primary condition or secondary to some other condition. The decision whether a bitch should receive thyroid hormone replacement therapy should be based upon not only laboratory results but also on clinical indicators of hypothyroidism and absence of concomitant disease. Hypothyroidism as cause of reproductive failure may be over-diagnosed by some veterinary surgeons. This may prompt some breeders to seek a second opinion. However, hormone replacement therapy for bitches which need it, may help re-establish reproductive capacity in these bitches.

5.19.5. Brucellosis
Brucellosis is comprehensively discussed in 12.3. It is vital that breeding bitches taken to outside studs be tested for brucellosis to prevent either transmission of this devastating disease or accusations thereof. The tests may be performed twice per year or soon before breeding to a stud. Generally in countries where this disease occurs, results obtained within the last 6 months are considered recent if the dog in quest is known to reside within a Brucella-free colony. Brucella testing should form part of any pre-purchase breeding soundness examination within the preceding month or so. Generally, in countries where Brucellosis is absent, testing of imported dogs is mandatory.

5.20. Oestrus induction and oestrus synchronization
Oestrus induction is the scientific term used for bringing a bitch into heat. Clearly this could be used to bring two bitches into heat simultaneously, thereby synchronising their heat cycles. This may be of interest to the breeder when breeding opportunities have been missed or bitches have failed to conceive. It can also be used as treatment of bitches which do not cycle (anoestrus). Oestrus induction is easy and frequently employed in farm animals where it is used to synchronise cycles for various reasons. Before embryo transfer and other new developments and technologies can be applied in the dog, reliable and easy induction of fertile oestrus must be possible.

Many different attempts at finding a way to effectively and safely induce fertile oestrus in the bitch have been made with poor results. None of these methods have found their way into everyday practice. This is because they have failed to induce fertile oestrus in many cases, are not risk free and have serious limitations as to how much time is really gained by inducing the oestrus. In many of the protocols, success was only attained when the protocol was applied to bitches very close to the time (20-40 days) that the bitch was about to cycle naturally. An ideal oestrus induction protocol does not yet exist.

Oestrus induction should however be considered in bitches suffering from confirmed anoestrus.

5.21. Superovulation of the bitch

This topic is discussed as some breeders have knowledge or experience with farming practices where superovulation is applied in other species.

Superovulation refers to the induction of more ovulations than would normally be the case under natural conditions in a normal heat cycle. In many species, including the cow, ewe and human, this is commonplace. Although this has been attempted in both natural occurring oestrus cycles as well as induced oestrus cycles in the dog, the success rate has been very poor.

5.22. Fertility drugs

As is evident from the experience with superovulation and oestrus induction, the bitch has a heat cycle which is difficult to manipulate and poorly responsive to exogenous hormones when compared to other species. There are no wonder-drugs available for use in the bitch. Some breeders hold the view that exogenous administration of hormones may act as "fertility drugs" by increasing conception rates and litter sizes. Many breeders use hormones at the time of breeding that are reputed to enhance ovulation. These drugs only have a place in bitches which fail to ovulate, in other bitches they are either useless or cause harm. Numerous nutritional supplements, herbal and homeopathic remedies are reputed to "boost" fertility, but scientific evidence of their efficacy is scant.

Chapter 5 Reproduction in the Bitch

Chapter 6

Pregnancy

Pregnancy is defined as that period during which fertilised eggs develop into embryos and later into foetuses in the bitch's womb (uterus) until birthing takes place.

6.1. Prevention of pregnancy

6.1.1. The pharmacological control of the heat cycle

Drugs called progestins were commonly used to postpone or prevent the bitch from coming into heat. These drugs are available in tablet form and injectable formulations. Their use can no longer be recommended because of serious side effects such as pyometra, permanent infertility and diabetes. Breeders whom wish to skip a heat and want to breed at a later stage are strongly advised to use drugs which are safe. Gonadotrophin releasing hormone (GNRH) analogues are such drugs. In countries where safe medication is not available, it is best not to use any drug to suppress or postpone heat. It is best to kennel these bitches and keep them away from the stud.

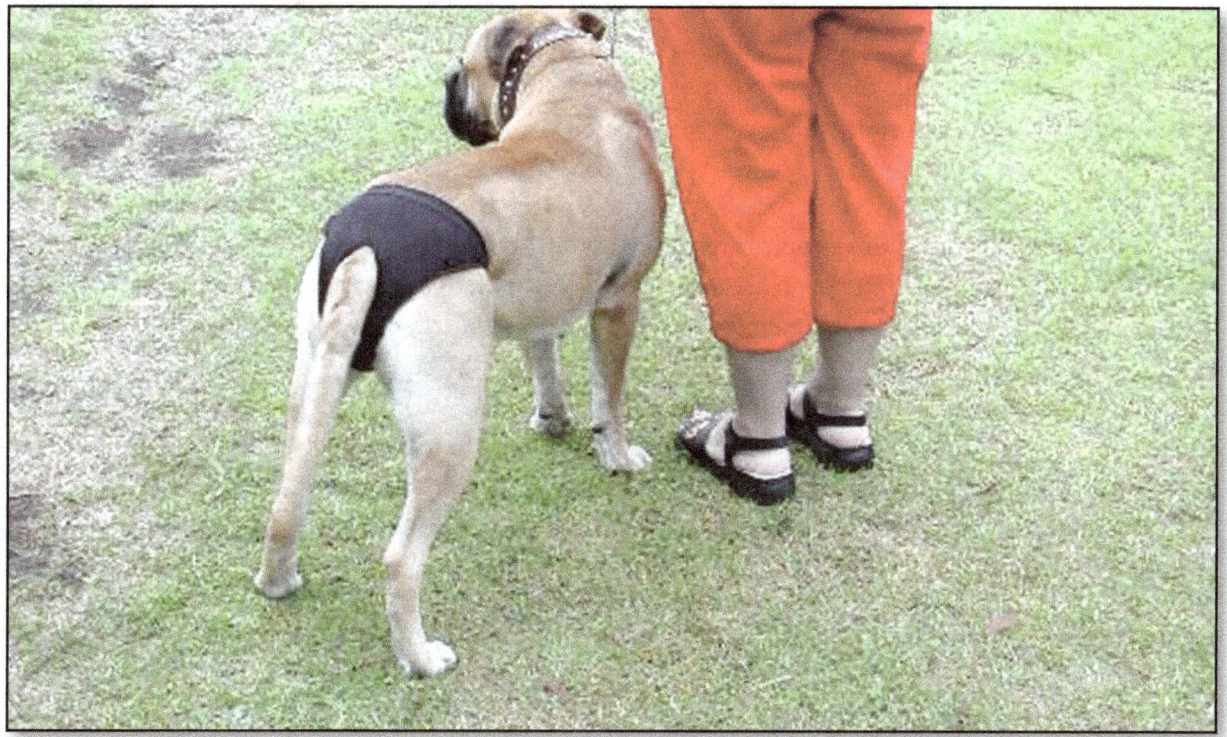
Mechanical prevention of mating as is often practised in countries where routine sterilisation is prohibited by law

6.1.2. Surgical control of reproduction in bitches

Breeders do sterilize individuals in their breeding colony from time to time for various reasons. It is necessary that breeders acquaint themselves with the advantages and disadvantages of sterilisation because new puppy owners might request a recommendation from them. Sterilisation by surgical removal of the ovaries and uterus is known as ovariohysterectomy or spaying, and is the best way to prevent pregnancy in bitches. The surgery can be performed in the conventional way through surgical incision of the abdominal wall or indirectly via endoscopy. Sterilization by tying off the fallopian tubes, as it is performed in woman, makes no sense because the bitch might still cycle, bleed and attract male dogs or develop uterine disease. Some surgeons prefer to remove the ovaries only (ovariectomy), especially in pubertal bitches because it is less invasive and achieves the same goal. In time, ovariectomy is likely to gain popularity as will early spaying. In some countries the sterilization of dogs is prohibited and it is only allowed if there is a medical reason for it.

a) Age of sterilization

Early-age neutering in this text is defined as the neutering of puppies at 6-7 weeks of age, but before 4 months of age, rather than the conventional age of 6 months or older. Early age neutering is becoming increasingly popular all over the world. This increase in popularity results from accumulated information regarding the safety of the procedure and the lack of long-term adverse side effects. As veterinary surgeons become more comfortable and familiar with the procedure, they are likely to encourage more clients to consider early-age neutering. Puppies which are neutered at an early age have a shorter recovery period as opposed to those neutered at a more traditional age. Mortality and morbidity rates are also reported to be lower. It has been categorically proven that the prepubertal spaying of bitches reduces the incidence of mammary neoplasia to almost zero.

Traditionally, female dogs and cats are neutered at approximately 6 months of age and male dogs and cats at approximately 6 to 9 months of age. Enforced sterilization in animal shelters has been the main driving force behind early sterilization. This stems from the fact that new owners of adopted pets seldom fulfil the terms of adoption and fail to present the pet for sterilization. Some breeders insist on puppy sterilization before the puppy is sold, to enforce breeding restrictions.

Some breeders may still have questions regarding early sterilization. There is no increased risk of infectious disease provided the puppies are vaccinated on schedule and are not exposed to a virulent virus at the time of sterilization. It is advisable to postpone sterilisation until 1 week after the completion of the vaccination regimen if non-exposure to an infectious virus cannot be guaranteed.

Many breeders and veterinary surgeons may still believe that early sterilization of puppies affects their growth but several research studies have refuted this. Obesity can occur in both neutered and intact animals as it is influenced by factors such as diet, calorie intake and activity levels. Obesity is more likely in spayed bitches and neutered males irrespective of whether the surgery was performed at an early age or not.

Dogs neutered at traditional ages can develop urinary incontinence within days of the surgery or several years later. Oestrogen-responsive urinary incontinence can occur in up to 4% of bitches which are spayed at the conventional age. To date, there is no evidence that suggests that the incidence of urinary sphincter incompetence which leads to urinary incontinence is higher in bitches which were spayed at an earlier age.

The anaesthesia of very young puppies requires extra care to prevent hypoglycaemia and hypothermia. The use of modern and safe anaesthetic agents is imperative. If these principles are observed, there is no increased risk of surgical or anaesthetic complications.

In conclusion; there is no conclusive evidence that the early sterilization of young bitches holds any increased risk other than the normal risks associated with sterilization at a conventional age. A bitch should be sterilised as soon as possible or as soon as it is decided not to breed with her anymore.

b) The effects of spaying on the behaviour of dogs
Breeders often show and work their dogs in various arenas and therefore they may be concerned about effects of sterilization on behaviour. It is important to realise that breed and sex differences have an effect on the manifestation of behaviour changes following sterilization. The effects are difficult to measure due to the non-objective parameters within which the effects are measured. It is therefore not surprising that there is no clear consensus on what the real effects are. The effects that have been studied include: stranger directed aggression, owner-directed aggression, dog-directed aggression, trainability, excitability and the effect on the energy levels of a dog. The results of the study suggest that spayed females tend to be slightly more aggressive or assertive toward their owners and strangers than intact females. Both males and bitches have slightly reduced energy levels and drive following neutering. This is perhaps the main reason why breeders are reluctant to sterilise dogs that they are competing with.

The advantages of sterilization on both the dog's long term health and behaviour far outweigh the disadvantages and should be considered by owners of pet dogs.

c) Resistance to sterilizing bitches
In addition to the health benefits, sterilization brings about other benefits too: spayed bitches do not attract males, are less likely to fight or cause fights, do not roam in search of a breeding partner, and the nuisance factor of on heat vaginal bleeding is brought to an end. Despite the benefits, many dog owners are still hesitant to neuter their dogs. Breeders should advise their puppy buyers to sterilise their dogs. Unconvinced owners should however discuss the matter of sterilisation with their veterinary surgeon in order to make an informed decision.

There are a host of studies on-going with regards to possible adverse effects of sterilising dogs. These studies indicate that there may be a slight increase in certain cancers (osteosarcoma, lymphoma and haemangiosarcoma) as well as increases in incidence of skeletal disorders such as cranial cruciate ligament rupture and HD. More adverse effects are likely to emerge as more extensive epidemiological studies are completed. It is important to note that these adverse effects are in many cases affected by breed, age of sterilization and sex. Finally it is important for breeders and veterinary surgeons to interpret the results of such studies with circumspection. For instance it would be wrong to interpret the results as saying that sterilization causes cancer, a slight increase in a specific cancer in a specific breed may be a more appropriate interpretation. Whilst one cannot argue with the veracity of these studies, both benefits and adverse effects must be evaluated in the decision making process. Mammary cancers are less likely in sterilised bitches not to mention uterine infections which will lead to sterilisation in most bitches anyway or even death.

With regards to sterilisation of pet dogs, the advantages of sterilization on both the dog's long term health and behaviour, far outweigh the disadvantages in most instances and most breeds.

6.2. Fertilization

Fertilization in the dog occurs in the fallopian tubes. It involves the fusing of the male gamete (sperm) with the female gamete (egg or ovum) which then results in the development of an embryo. The canine ovum first has to mature following ovulation and this may take approximately 48 hours. Fertilisation is thought to occur on one day in some bitches and on two subsequent days in others. This extension in time for fertilisation to complete may be because not all eggs may have been ovulated within 24 hours and fertilisation also takes a number of hours to complete. Despite this small time delay, ovulation and fertilisation should be considered a synchronised affair. This means that all puppies in one litter will be of similar age (24 hours difference maximum). Fertilisation occurs during the last 4 days of cytological oestrus for any bitch (Usually last 4 days before bitch is off heat).

6.3. Early development in the womb

Following fertilisation the fertilized egg develops into an embryo which is transported from the fallopian tubes to the uterus and moves freely. The embryos then space themselves equally throughout the length of both uterine horns. They then implant (attach and connect with uterine wall) on day 13-15 following fertilisation. It is of vital importance for the breeder to realise that any stressors during this vulnerable period will result in embryonal death. This may be of importance in bitches which are transported over long distances to and from a stud for mating. If the bitch has to travel long distances following a visit to the stud, it is advised that the breeder do so within the 3-7 days following the last mating. If the breeder is unable due to circumstances to do so, they should consider leaving the bitch at the premises of the stud or nearby kennel and delay transport back home approximately 22 days after the last mating. Other stressors besides transport are; withholding food, dehydration, exposure to extreme temperatures, extreme exercise and social integration into a group with more dominant individuals. If the bitch happens to fall ill during this crucial period, embryonal death and thus failure to conceive may also occur.

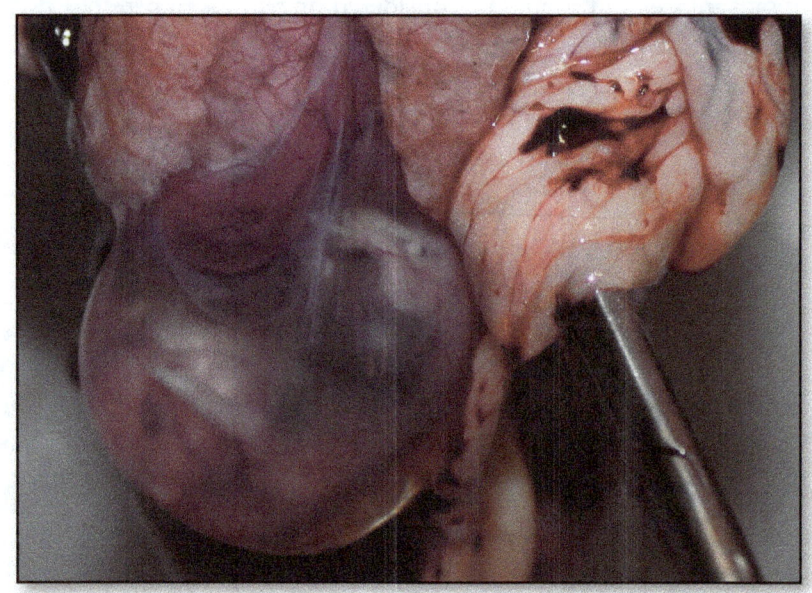
Early canine embryo

Diseases which cause a fever for a couple of days, at the time of implantation of the embryos, are particularly likely to cause embryonal death. Complicated infectious tracheobronchitis, more commonly known as kennel cough, is a frequent culprit in this regard. A mild bout of kennel cough in a bitch is however unlikely to cause embryonal death. It is of vital importance that the breeder always alerts their veterinary surgeon to the possibility of pregnancy. This is of particular importance during embryonal development as this is the most vulnerable stage of pregnancy. This should then alert the veterinary surgeon to avoid drugs which are unsafe.

Following implantation the pregnancy is less fragile but certainly not free of threat. At this stage, loss of pregnancy will result in resorption. This involves the death of the foetus, enzymatic liquefaction of the foetus, its membranes and placenta and finally resorption of all the fluids and debris. Resorption does not necessarily lead to any vaginal discharge or evidence of pregnancy loss. Indeed, the breeder might not know that the bitch had ever conceived. Many breeders however will insist that they are able to accurately either visually or intuitively assess pregnancy from about 3-4 weeks following mating. The author's experience does not confirm this. This is important because breeders may request the veterinary surgeon to examine a bitch which allegedly had resorbed. The veterinary surgeon may then erroneously investigate causes of resorption whereas other causes of infertility should be investigated because the bitch was indeed never pregnant. After day 35, the embryo develops into what is then known as the foetus. The period of the foetus (foetal development) is the time during which typical puppy features appear and rapid growth occurs. After about day 35 of gestation, the loss of pregnancy will result in abortion. Abortion differs from resorption in that fluids, foetus and membranes will be expelled from the vagina (vaginal discharge).

6.4. Sex ratios

Nature seemingly results in a very close to 50:50 sex ratio offspring born from most mammals. That is if the sample size measured, is large enough. Most breeders will be familiar with the frustration of having puppies for sale but not the "correct" sex. The question often arises whether it is possible to alter the sex ratios in a litter of puppies.

The sex of the mammalian offspring is determined by whether a Y-chromosome bearing (male sperm) fertilised the egg or not and whether the survival rate of the female embryo (XX) and male embryo (XY) are similar. Given that there are as many male as female sperm in an ejaculate, the statistical outcome dictates that for the most part a sex ratio of very close to 50:50 can be expected.

This is however not true in all cases in other species. Well documented sex ratio deviations from the normal 50:50 spread exist in nature. Most examples are in polygynous (from the word polygamy) species. The latter is a species in which males have multiple partners. In these species, the Trivers-Willard hypothesis states that evolutionary theory predicts that mothers in different stages of condition could adjust the birth sex ratio of their offspring in relation to future reproductive benefits. The Cape buffalo is an example of one of many herbivore species where climatic conditions and food availability can influence sex ratios. In the latter species the cows will produce more female offspring during droughts when food is scarce. All the mechanisms and environmental cues by which shifts in sex ratios are achieved, are not known but glucose levels appear to play a role.

Dog breeders also have their own "anecdotal recipes" of how to sway the sex ratios (mostly unproven). The notion in the breeders mind that they may be correct in assuming that this indeed is possible in dogs, is strengthened by the fact that many gynaecologists also have their own "trusted methods they advise" to woman patients to increase likelihood of boy or girl (mostly unproven). At the end of the day, in any advice one gives concerning the outcome, one has a 50% chance of being correct. There are breeders whom claim that bitches on premises where there are no resident males, produce litters with sex ratios altered in favour of male offspring. Whether this may be triggered by mechanism of lack of pheromone stimulation is speculation (if indeed true). It would make sense that nature would gear towards male offspring if males were in demand. The latter all remains speculation though and no scientifically proven reliable recipes exist in carnivores to alter sex ratios in one or another direction. However the practice of using sex sorted sperm is an established practice in many other species. It is now possible to preselect or predetermine the sex of offspring prior to conception in those species. It is a highly desired technological tool for assisted female breeding programs specifically for milk production, and in males, for meat production in cattle. The technology uses modified flow cytometric instrumentation for sorting X- and Y-bearing sperm and is about 90% accurate. This technique is however expensive and fertility of sexed sperm is lower than unsexed ones. To date this technology has not permeated clinical practice and is not used in domestic dogs to alter sex ratios in litters. This technology may become both less expensive and improved in time to come and attract future attention by the dog breeder fraternity.

It has however been proven that in the dog, in litters from carrier males mated to carrier bitches, the presence of one or more cryptorchid puppies in a litter, is associated with a shift in the sex ratio in favour of male offspring. In addition, an increased litter size in comparison with litters from non-carrier parents was reported. It is fair to speculate that this is another example of the way "Mother Nature" tries to compensate for the cryptorchid genes.

6.5. Diagnosis of pregnancy

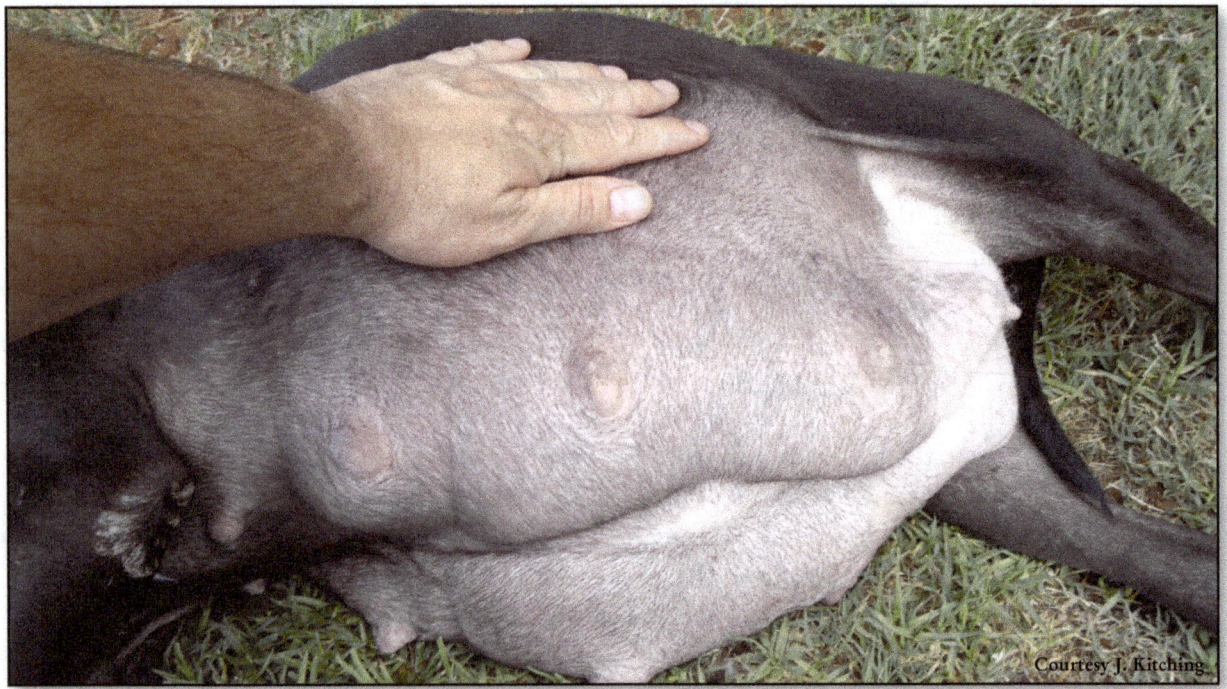

Bitch in advanced pregnancy and the breeder has huge expectations of a large litter. The size of the abdomen however may be deceptive and not be an accurate indication of litter size.

Because bitches often show pseudo pregnancy with resultant mammary gland enlargement and even lactation (milk production) as well as apparent increased abdominal size, there are no reliable external indicators that a bitch might be pregnant. Palpation is a useful tool only in the period of Day 18-28 but should rather be left in skilled hands. Excessive external pressure on the early foetus may cause damage. It may be difficult, if not impossible, to palpate a mid-trimester pregnancy in a bitch. Bitches with a barrel shaped abdomen, with a very muscular abdominal wall or nervous disposition are impossible to palpate. It is the author's opinion that palpation has serious limitations in many dogs and is therefore not always reliable.

Chapter 6 Pregnancy

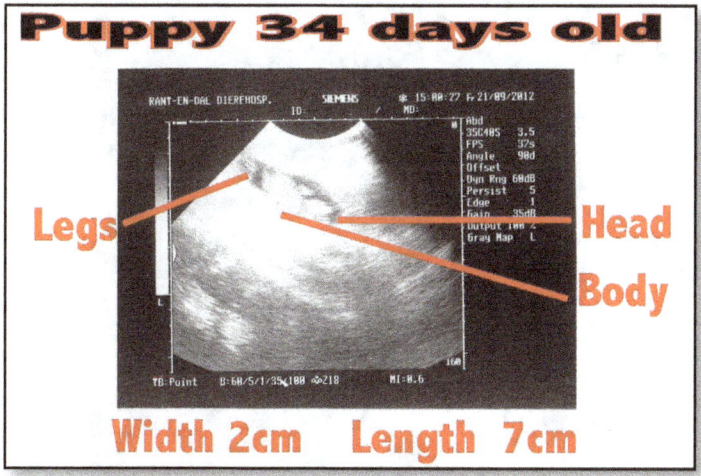
Sonogram of early pregnancy

Ultrasound scanning is a safe and accurate way to diagnose pregnancy. Note that the hair should preferably be clipped to ensure good contact of the ultrasound probe with the skin. Early pregnancy may be confirmed from day 18 (with only the best ultrasound equipment). Ultrasound is very useful to accurately diagnose pregnancy from days 24 onwards. It can however not be used to determine litter size accurately, especially with large litters.

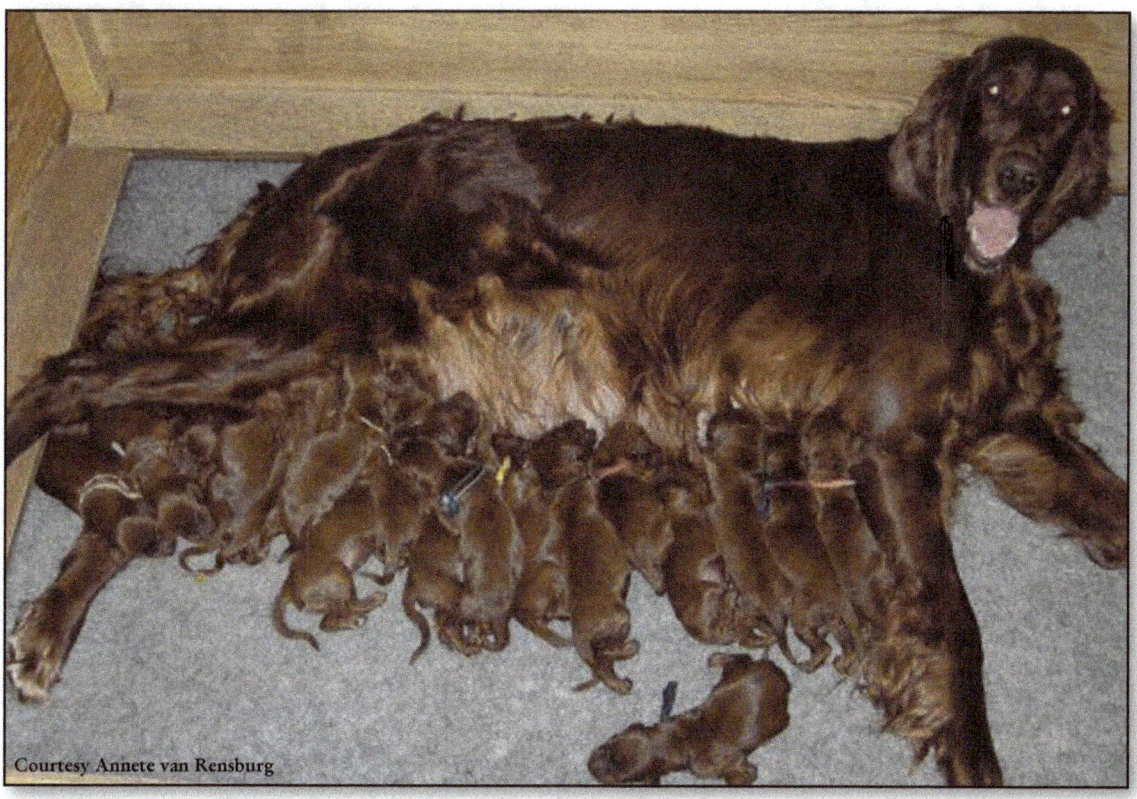
Very large litter

It also allows one to diagnose total or partial loss of a litter due to death of embryos or foetuses. It is also useful in pre-labour evaluation to confirm whether foetuses are alive or not and to pick up other gross foetal or uterine problems. There is a reliable blood test kit available that detects the hormone relaxin but this is only effective from day 32 onwards and gives no other information on the pregnancy.

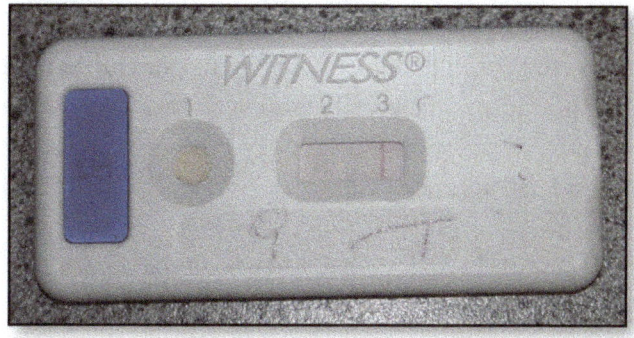
Relaxin pregnancy test

Chapter 6 Pregnancy

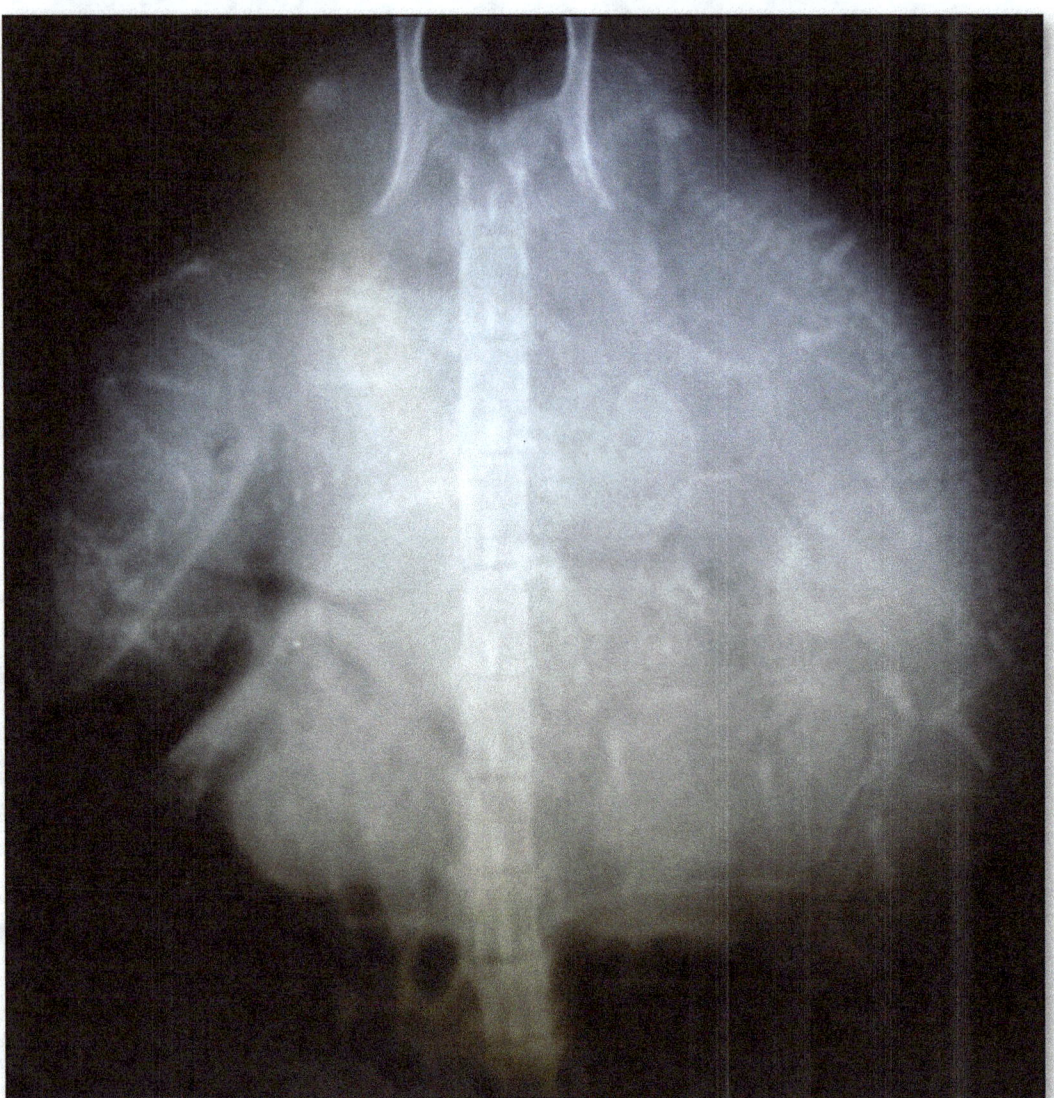

Radiograph of abdomen of bitch with large litter. Radiographs are often used to count puppies but undercounts are sometimes encountered using this diagnostic modality

It is possible to diagnose pregnancy using radiographs. This is possible during the last 3 weeks of pregnancy with excellent radiographic equipment only. Radiographs are particularly valuable in the last 7 days of pregnancy because it is then possible to count the number of foetuses accurately. This method is however not fool proof as undercounts are possible, especially in large bitches.

Knowledge of accurate count of litter size may be very useful for the breeder as it gives them an accurate assessment of how many puppies they must still wait for to be born during the whelping process. It takes the guessing out of whether this bitch has completed the birth process or not! Radiographs and ultrasound may be very helpful in confirming whether a bitch is carrying a singleton. Some companies market Doppler devices that the breeder themselves can use to diagnose pregnancy but these are not considered accurate at all.

The size of the abdomen close to term may not be an accurate assessment of the litter size. Some bitches appear huge with small litters whilst some bitches which appear small may deliver a very large litter. Breeders are often disappointed by the true litter size based on their estimation of size of abdomen.

6.6. Phantom pregnancy (pseudopregnancy)

Pseudopregnancy is also known as pseudocyesis, false pregnancy or phantom pregnancy and refers to a state following heat where a bitch appears to be pregnant whilst in fact she is not. Both mated bitches and non-mated bitches can become pseudopregnant. Pseudopregnancy in the bitch is possible because the hormonal events following heat are almost identical in pregnant and non-pregnant bitches. False pregnancy can be very misleading and convince breeders that when failing to produce puppies, the bitch may have lost its litter through resorption or abortion!

False pregnancy is characterised by apparent enlargement of the abdomen, mammary gland enlargement, milk production and finally nesting behaviour. It is not necessary to treat pseudopregnancy as it will usually resolve spontaneously within 1-3 weeks. Spaying can be considered, but in certain bitches it prolongs pseudo pregnancy. There are a number of drugs, each with their own adverse side-effects, which can be used to resolve pseudo pregnancy. Pseudopregnancy may be displayed by as much as 50% of bitches following heat and should be considered a normal phenomenon in bitches following a cycle. In the dog, pseudopregnancy may be an evolutionary adaptation to survival of the fittest. This is because in wild dogs and wolves, lower ranking bitches that were not allowed to mate by dominant ones (alpha bitches), will frequently show pseudopregnancy, start lactating and indeed help nurse the suckling puppies of the dominant bitch. Pseudopregnancy is also believed to have evolutionary advantages in the wild dog, because it made it possible for other females in the group to produce milk and take over the nursing of the puppies if something befalls the mother.

Nature's ability to synchronize heat cycles also plays a role. Because of the dormitory effect, most bitches within the pack will, in time, synchronise their heat cycles, making available bitches that are hormonally primed to start lactating, even if they are not pregnant. There are other mechanisms, beside pseudo pregnancy, which can trigger milk production in a non-pregnant bitch. Bitches with very strong mothering instincts are known to start lactating in the presence of nursing puppies. It is speculated that the audio-visual and olfactory stimuli offered to a bitch by nursing puppies trigger neuroendocrine events which result in lactation. This phenomenon has even been observed in sterilised bitches, and in rare cases, the stimulus even prompts the nursing of offspring of another species, e.g. rabbits or cats.

6.7. Parentage testing

Parentage testing is possible to categorically include or exclude individuals as parents/siblings to the tested individual/s. Cost of these tests is decreasing as it becomes more commonplace to perform them. Parentage testing has typically been employed to confirm parentage in cases of suspected mismatings or to resolve disputes regarding alleged parentage. It may be used to confirm parentage when frozen semen was used provided a sample or profile on the donor is available. It can positively confirm identity of imported breeding stock. It can confirm parentage of puppies in cases of multi-sire breedings. It may also be used when a natural mating was performed on a bitch which had already been inseminated with semen from another sire and certify identity of the sire when using artificial insemination. Parentage testing is performed by DNA analysis of microsatellite markers. It was established that when ≥ 15 microsatellite markers were used, accuracy in excess of 99% was achieved. This type of technology may also assist in confirming breed heritage, and identifying frequently used sires. Work is in progress to improve these techniques and increase their accuracy.

6.8. Gestation length

The duration of pregnancy is also known as gestation length. In the bitch this can vary depending on which event in the cycle is determined as the starting point or chronological landmark. If the starting point is the point at which the progesterone increases for the first time, then the gestation length is estimated to be 65 days. If ovulation is considered the starting point, the estimated gestation length is 63 days. If fertilisation is the starting point, the estimated gestation length is 61 days. Lastly if the end of the cycle (first day of dioestrus) is used as the starting point, the gestation length is 57 days. In most cases, breeders have no information about abovementioned events. They only have at their disposal breeding dates which they use as their point of reference. Therefore, breeders have adopted 63-65 days as the correct gestation length in the bitch. This is because of the observation that many bitches whelp 63-65 days after the first mating. This interval is however very variable ranging from 55-71 days. This is the reason why many bitches are erroneously considered overdue in the eyes of the breeder. Some of these bitches are then presented to the veterinary surgeon with clients insisting on intervention by caesarean section. Conceding to this request may lead to delivery of non-viable premature puppies as well of increased risk of uterine haemorrhage following surgery. These complications accentuate the need for the breeder to, with assistance of their veterinary surgeon; establish a protocol designed to predict whelping dates in their bitches. Even the best methods to predict whelping dates are likely to vary by at least one day on either side of the predicted date. With regards to factors which may influence gestational length, it is fair to speculate that the difference in gestation length between breeds is either non-existent or negligible and that litter size probable does have a small influence with large litters having slightly shorter gestation (perhaps less than 1 day). The only exception is the bitch carrying only one puppy (singleton pregnancy), see 9.1.2. Parity and age has no effect on duration of pregnancy.

6.9. Prediction of whelping date

It is necessary for breeders to know what the whelping date (parturition date or due date) is. In breeds which usually do not have whelping problems, it is less important but still convenient to know. The information is used to move bitches to their whelping quarters, to change the diet and feeding regime and to plan the breeder's whereabouts around the due date to ensure that supervision is possible. Bitches which usually have whelping problems require a more accurate prediction of the whelping date because these bitches might be destined for delivery by caesarean section and would therefore have to be presented to a veterinary surgeon at the correct time. A breeder can estimate the due date, but with the assistance of a veterinary surgeon, a more accurate date can be established.

6.9.1. Whelping date relative to breeding dates

As mentioned before, most bitches whelp between 62 to 64 days after the first or the only mating, however, the interval can be as short as 55 days, and as long as 71 days. This variation is brought about by the long fertile life span of canine sperm inside the female genital system and the long, yet variable, duration of behavioural oestrus. The variation, that can be as long as 14 days, can throw the breeder's determination of the due date out of kilter to the detriment of proper parturition management. The sole use of breeding dates to determine due dates does not provide dates with adequate accuracy. Despite this, many breeders report that the method of counting 63 days from the first mating frequently provides them with an accurate due date. Some count 61 days from the last mating and report that it works well. These methods can provide an acceptable approximation of the due date for those bitches which have heat cycles of average lengths, but the lack of accuracy is problematic if things go wrong and veterinary intervention is required; timeous intervention is essential to prevent serious complications.

6.9.2. Whelping date relative to decline in rectal temperature before labour

Rectal temperature can drop shortly before the due date. The drop in rectal temperature has some value but it was found that a variance in rectal temperature exists between different individuals to the extent that it cannot be used as the sole criterion to predict the time of parturition. Some bitches do not demonstrate a detectable pre-partum drop in rectal temperature, even if they are monitored three times per day. Preparturient temperature drop can give important clues, but it is not accurate or reliable enough to use as the sole criterion to accurately predict the time of parturition; neither does it indicate foetal maturity so that intervention, by parturition induction or caesarean section, can be performed safely.

6.9.3. Whelping date relative to behavioural signs of impending labour

Breeders, by virtue of the fact that they frequently observe bitches which are about to whelp, claim that they can "spot" a bitch in pending labour. They say that they can detect that the abdomen has changed shape or, in breeder's jargon, "the abdomen has dropped". This kind of observation is not reliable because it is difficult to spot if the litter is small, and not all bitches necessarily "drop" before they go into labour. Behavioural signs of impending parturition are either inconsistently displayed by bitches or is inconsistently observed by the person who is witnessing pending labour. The time interval between the first display of behaviour and labour is also variable; for instance: nesting behaviour, bouts of panting, milk production and the release of the cervical mucus plug (characterised by white grey mucus discharge from vagina) have been observed up to 7 days prior to the due date.

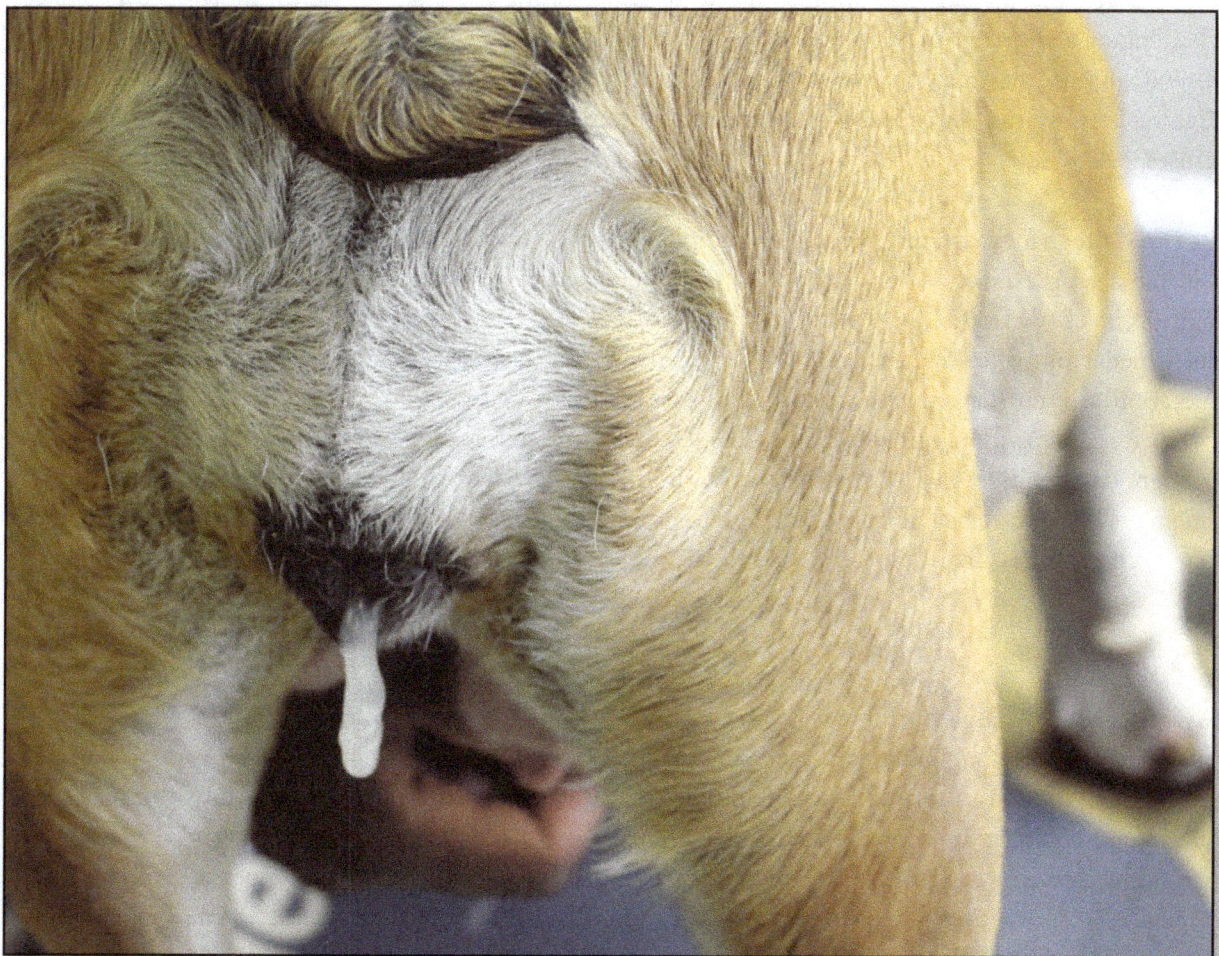

Greyish white mucous vaginal discharge is frequently evident during the last week of pregnancy

6.9.4. Whelping date relative to veterinary observations made during heat

The breeder's veterinary surgeon can assist the breeder to time ovulation more accurately by measuring either progesterone concentrations, or luteinising hormone (LH) levels, or by determining cytologic dioestrus (D1) through vaginal cytology. The results of these measurements provide a reasonably accurate estimate of the parturition date. Generally, onset of dioestrus occurs 8 days after ovulation and parturition is expected after 57 ± 1 days. In a study involving a large number of whelpings, parturition was established to be 57 ± 2.8 days from the first day of cytologic dioestrus. Measuring progesterone concentrations also provides accurate information with which the partition date can be determined.

6.10. Complications of pregnancy

6.10.1. Loss of pregnancy

Loss of pregnancy can only be a consideration if the breeder is sure that the bitch was pregnant, in the first place. It is difficult to determine an incidence of early loss of pregnancy (resorption) because it is impossible to diagnose pregnancy at the time when resorption would occur, consequently, it is impossible to distinguish between fertilisation failure, early embryonal death or uterine insufficiency. Loss of pregnancy at a later stage often goes unnoticed because bitches usually eat the aborted foetuses and clean vulvar discharges. Abortion should only be investigated if there is sufficient evidence that the bitch was indeed pregnant. Evidence should be sought by performing a relaxin test or an ultrasound, or by searching for expelled aborted foetuses. Establishing the exact cause of abortion can be very challenging. Abortion may be due to: foetal defects, illness in the dam, uterine insufficiency, hypoluteodism (insufficient progesterone to maintain pregnancy), nonspecific infections, specific infections, Canine herpesvirus, *Brucella canis*, trauma, drug interaction during pregnancy and some other obscure causes.

In early pregnancy around the time of implantation (second to third week) stress and any disease causing a febrile reaction for a sustained time may lead to resorption. After about 30 days abortion will occur characterised by the expulsion of foetuses and foetal membranes. It is very important for the breeder to realise that in advanced pregnancy (last trimester), the bitch is haemodynamically and metabolically challenged. As a result, a disease that is usually mild, may become a life threatening condition in heavily pregnant bitches. The lesson that breeders need to take home is that a seemingly innocuous condition such as mild enteritis, should be viewed with much more seriousness in heavily pregnant bitches. A heavily pregnant bitch is more likely to die of an affliction than a non-pregnant bitch which suffers from the same affliction.

6.10.2. Vaginal discharges during pregnancy

Any vaginal discharge during pregnancy, besides a scant mucosal discharge (greyish white to ivory coloured cervical slime), is considered abnormal. A bloody, green or black discharge usually indicates a detachment of one or more placentas from the uterine wall and often precedes foetal death and abortion. It also indicates that the cervix is no longer closed because it allowed uterine content to escape and so an ascending infection is possible. In late pregnancy (last week or so), cervical incompetence might cause a vaginal discharge, but it is rare. It is thought that the cervix dilates somewhat and that a partial placental release of the foetus closest to the cervical opening occurs. This and other causes of vaginal discharges should be investigated without delay, because it is an indication that the pregnancy is in peril.

6.10.3. Torsion of the uterus

This is a very rare condition referring to the twisting of one or both of the uterine horns. It is usually seen in late pregnancy. The bitch may present with signs of abdominal pain and this is a medical emergency which requires immediate veterinary intervention which may include either sterilization or removal of one horn. In cases where the one uterine horn is removed it should be removed with its ovary and the pregnancy should be very closely monitored and considered a high risk pregnancy with caesarean section as a likely method of delivery.

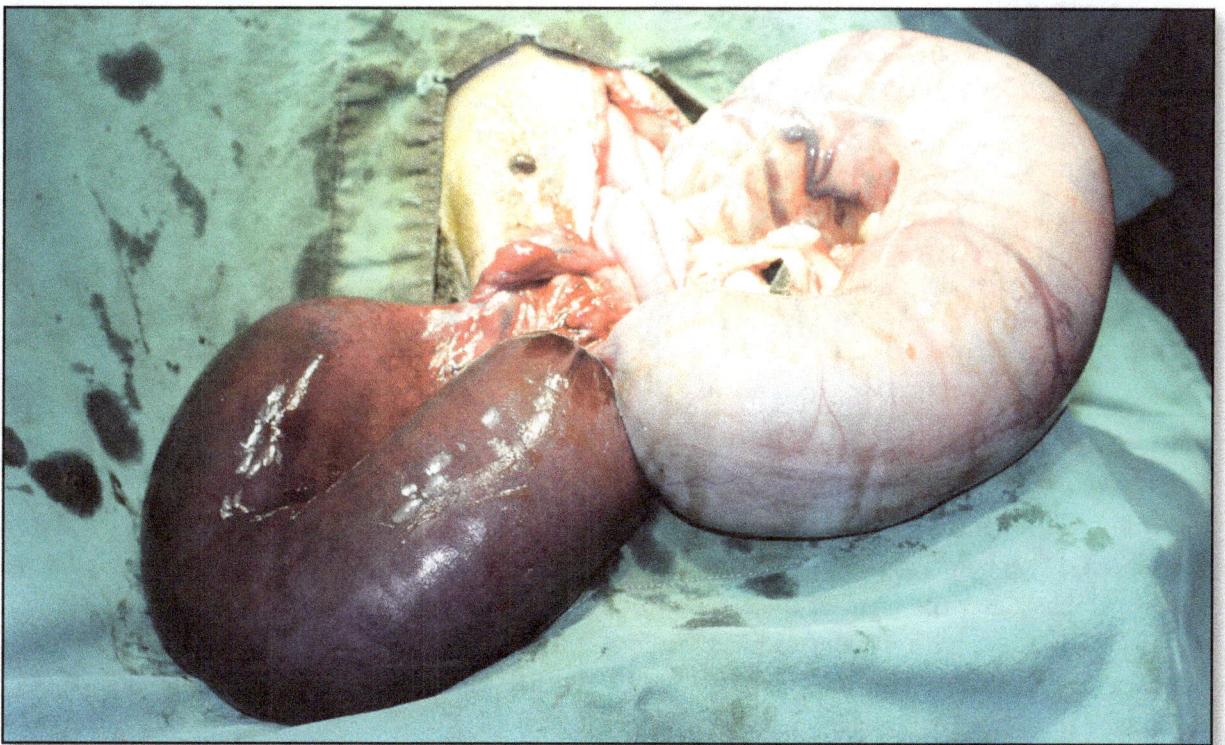

Uterine torsion

6.10.4. Pregnancy associated oedema (swelling) of hind legs and surrounding areas

In rare instances, some bitches in the last two weeks of pregnancy may show marked swelling of their hind legs and the ventral abdominal subcutaneous tissues (under-belly). It is more common in large breeds which are heavily pregnant with large litters. It is speculated that this swelling occurs because of the heavy gravid uterus partially obstructing the venous blood from the hind quarters. This swelling can appear very alarming but is usually inconsequential and subsides within a day or so following delivery of the litter. As there may be more sinister causes of oedema in this region, it may be safer to have the bitch examined if this is noticed.

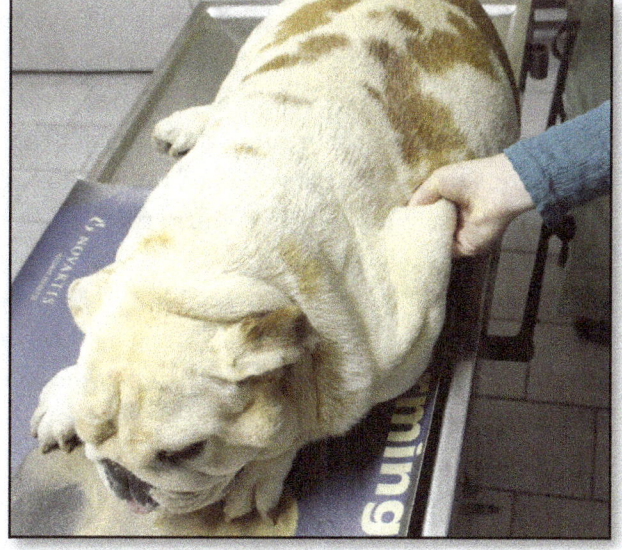

Pregnancy associated ventral oedema

This swelling should not be confused with swelling of the vulva which may occur in some bitches in the last week prior to whelping. This is a perfectly normal phenomenon and the extent of which may vary from negligible to very pronounced.

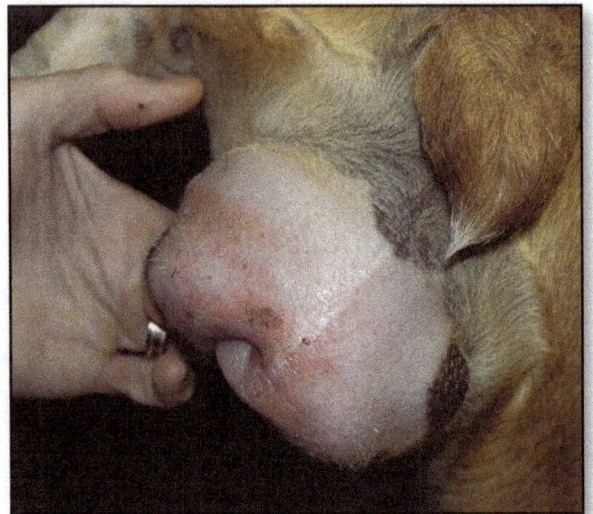
Pregnancy associated vaginal and perineal swelling

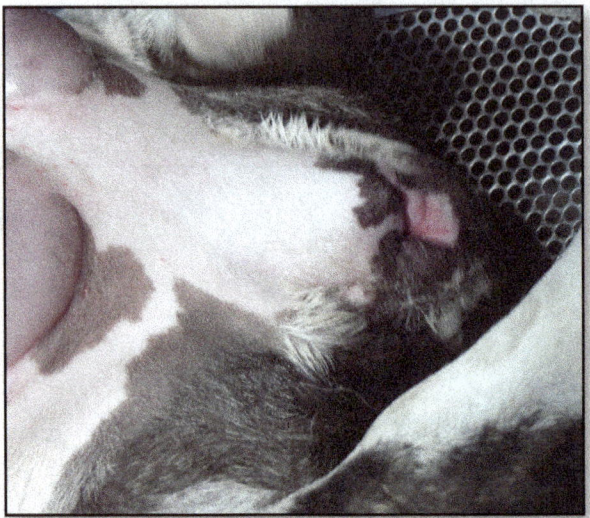
Dramatic pregnancy associated vaginal and perineal swelling

6.10.5. Retained placentas (afterbirths)

Placentas will normally be expelled simultaneously with the expulsion of the foetuses or within a short period thereafter; sometimes even hours thereafter. If placentas remain in the uterus for 12 hours or longer after the birth of the last puppy, they are deemed to be retained placentas. A bitch will usually present with a green to black discharge. It can develop into severe uterine infection if the placentas are retained for longer than a day. If retained placentas are suspected, the bitch should be presented for veterinary examination and confirmation. Treatment normally involves antibiotics and ecbolics (drugs which cause the womb to contract so as to expel its contents); seldom surgery.

6.10.6. Retained foetus

Inability to whelp all the foetuses will result in retention of a foetus. This may be a sequel to dystocia. Generally bitches which have not delivered all the puppies in the uterus will not settle down and continue to hyperventilate. In some cases however, a puppy may be retained and the bitch will act perfectly normal leaving the breeder to erroneously believe that all is well and whelping is complete. Bitches with retained foetuses will then later (usually within 24 hours or so) fall desperately ill and can die. Immediate medical or surgical delivery of the retained puppies is indicated. Some breeders wish to present a bitch which is presumed to have completed whelping for routine veterinary examination "post whelp examination" to confirm that all is well.

6.10.7. Uterine infections after whelping

Uterine infections are common after whelping. They occur when bacteria ascend into the uterus via the open cervix within the first week after whelping. If the bitch has poor uterine tone, has retained placentas or has suffered from dystocia, the likelihood of a uterus infection is increased. Bitches which whelp in unhygienic conditions, wet muddy environments, are in poor nutritional condition or have other underlying conditions may be predisposed to uterus infections. Blood, afterbirth and debris from whelping may accumulate on the hind quarters of bitches and these may act as an ideal growth medium for bacteria to cause uterine infections. Long haired breeds should therefore be trimmed before whelping and washed with antiseptic soap.

Transferring bitches some time before the whelping date to clean, dry, temperature controlled whelping quarters may all aid in reducing uterine infections and neonatal losses.

Bitches with a post-partum uterine infection will present a high fever, anorexic, neglect of puppies and reduced/no milk production. These bitches may also have a smelly vaginal discharge. Uterine infections after whelping may be a medical emergency which requires intensive fluid and antibiotic therapy and in exceptional cases may require ovariohysterectomy.

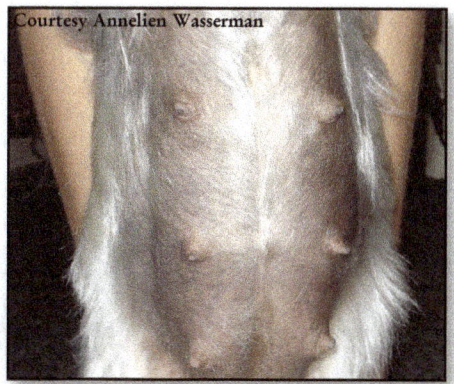

Trimming of long haired breeds prior to whelp

6.10.8. Post-whelping "blues"

After whelping, bitches may suffer from a low grade fever for a day or two, have a poor appetite and suffer from general malaise. Some breeders refer to this as post-whelping "blues". It occurs so frequently that it is considered normal by many breeders. This mild "condition" lasts for a day or two and doesn't affect the puppies or milk production negatively. If however, the condition persists for longer than 2-3 days, the bitch will lose weight and suffer from poor milk production with consequent demise of the puppies. The cause remains unclear but is speculated to be associated with low grade inflammation of the uterus after the whelp.

Stimulating appetite by making food more attractive is a good principle in order to keep up with caloric requirements of the bitch at this critical stage. The most important is to make sure that this condition is not confused with more serious post whelping complications.

6.10.9. Continued haemorrhaging after whelping

Bitches might bleed for a couple of hours after natural whelping and it normally subsides to a few scant drops, over the next 3 to 4 days. Bleeding which continues and does not reduce in quantity after the first week of whelping is abnormal. Abnormal haemorrhage is normally associated with anaemia but other illnesses can also be the cause. Bitches which have had a caesarean section are more prone to develop serious uterine haemorrhaging. This condition requires immediate veterinary attention.

A less serious cause of post whelping haemorrhage is subinvolution of the placental sites. This is when the placental sites keep on bleeding because, for some unknown reason, they do not heal. The only symptom is a continued (sometimes for longer than 6 weeks) bloody vaginal discharge. The puppies are unaffected by this condition. Although this condition occurs in bitches of any age, younger bitches appear to be more susceptible. Fortunately this condition is unlikely to return at the next pregnancy. There is no known treatment and the condition spontaneously resolves within a month or two, but in some instances it continues, on and off, until the bitches' next season.

6.10.10. Uterine rupture

Uterine rupture is an uncommon complication of pregnancy. It can occur spontaneously during dystocia, or it can inadvertently be induced through the administration of ecbolics (drugs which induce uterine contractility). It occurs in all bitches whether they previously had a caesarean section or not but the latter are more prone. Due to the rupture a foetus might land up in the abdominal cavity. If this happens immediate surgical intervention may be required to save the bitch.

6.10.11. Uterine or vaginal prolapse

Both are very uncommon complications of pregnancy. It usually occurs soon after natural or assisted whelping and is characterised by fleshy, bloody protrusion from the vagina. Veterinary attendance is required immediately. As an interim intervention, the breeder can protect the fleshy protrusion with gauze soaked in a bactericidal ointment on the way to the veterinary facility.

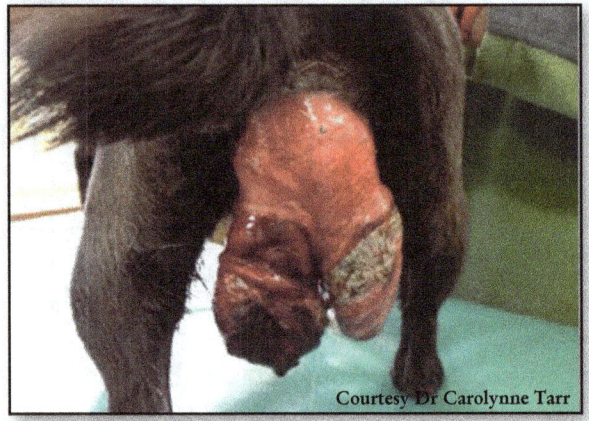

Uterine prolapse

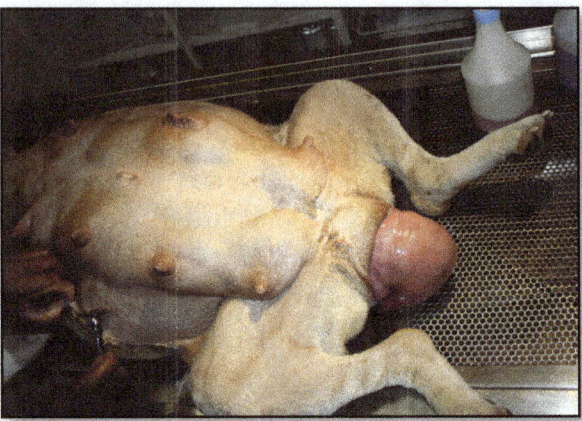

Vaginal prolapse during pregnancy

6.10.12. Post whelp hair loss

Some bitches may suffer from outspoken bilateral symmetrical hair loss after whelping and lactation. There may be a general loss of condition and coat but the hair loss is most outspoken on the flanks of the bitch. This condition is ignored unless it does not resolve and starts to improve within 6 weeks of weaning the puppies. Some breeders report similar, yet less severe, loss of coat condition and hair loss following heat.

6.11. Safety of drugs during pregnancy

Knowledge about drug treatment in pregnancy is not satisfying at all. It is recommended to avoid any drug administration to pregnant bitches unless absolutely necessary. The effect in one species is not a reliable indicator of what the effect may or may not be in another. The mere fact is however that pregnant bitches may need to be medicated with a variety of drugs for various reasons. Breeders should therefore make sure that their veterinary surgeon is prescribing safe drugs to their bitches during pregnancy and should always inform their veterinary surgeon that a bitch might be pregnant or is soon to be mated before any treatment is administered. Non-steroidal anti-inflammatory agents are singled out as culprits because they are increasingly used perioperatively because of their analgesic properties in all types of surgery. No anti-inflammatory agents have been approved for use in pregnant bitches and their use may be associated with loss of pregnancy, foetal abnormalities, prolonging or delaying the whelping process and renal impairment in nursing puppies.

It is best that bitches be current on vaccinations prior to breeding so that there is no need to vaccinate them other than herpesvirus. If however vaccination is due, there are safe vaccines registered for use during pregnancy.

6.12. Pregnancy termination

Breeders might want to terminate a pregnancy because of an accidental mismatch mating, also termed mésalliance or mismating. The injection of oestrogen as the "day after" injection might work but it is not recommended. A real risk of pyometra, extension of the heat cycle, and occasional failure to terminate pregnancy exists. Sterilization may be the best option if the bitch is not destined for breeding. If further breeding is intended, the breeder's veterinary surgeon might opt to terminate the pregnancy by using various drug options which are registered in their country. There are drug options which can terminate a pregnancy from essentially the first week up to close to labour. It is best to terminate pregnancy as early as possible. Early pregnancy termination has a higher success rate and a lower complication rate.

6.13. Labour induction in the bitch

An idealised labour induction protocol would be one that induces whelping, with a consistent predictable time frame between administrations of induction agent and whelping, with acceptable whelping times, without affecting lactation and that is safe. Breeders wishing to embark on such reproductive interventions should do so only in association with veterinary surgeons or reproductive specialists who are familiar with ovulation timing methods and the use of labour induction protocols. In practical terms its use in clinical practice is limited to the instances where ovulation time is accurately determined and the whelping date is known. The main disadvantage may be when the labour induction causes an extended whelping process with possible puppy losses. Another disadvantage of labour induction is that not much is usually gained because the bitch needs to be supervised throughout the entire labour process. It is advised that this supervision occurs at the veterinary facility (whelping centre) where progress and ultrasonographic monitoring of foetal heartbeats is possible and emergency surgical intervention can take place.

Chapter 6 Pregnancy

Chapter 7

Mammary Glands and Lactation

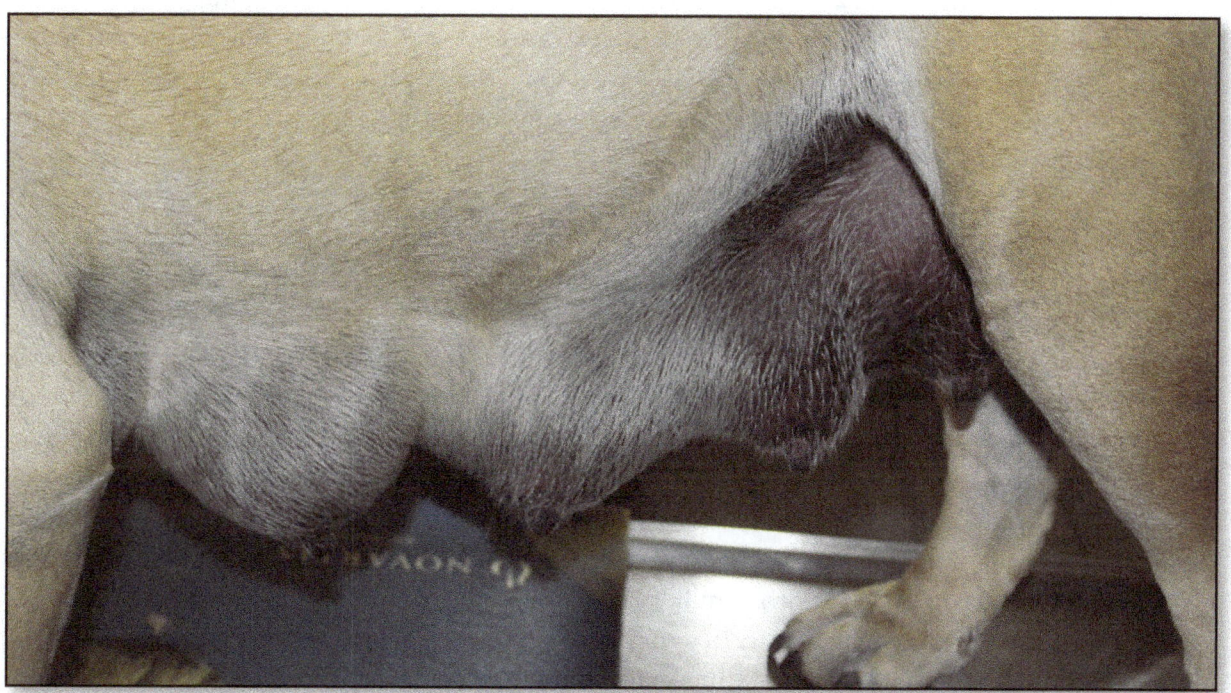

Bitch with obviously advanced mammary gland development

Depending on its size, a dog has 4-6 mammary glands on each side of the midline, therefore, 8-12 in total. Mammary gland enlargement starts at about mid-pregnancy and by the last trimester they are obviously enlarged. Breeders should note that mammary gland development and lactation is not limited to pregnancy, it can also occur in pseudo-pregnancy, as explained in section 6.6.

7.1. Uptake of colostrum by puppies

Colostrum is the first milk present in the mammary glands following delivery of the puppies and is present for the first 2-3 days. It is more viscous (thicker) than regular milk and appears slightly yellow.

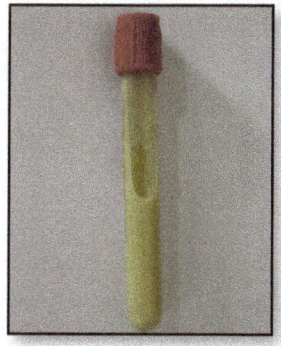

Tube filled with colostrum to be frozen in the colostrum bank for future use

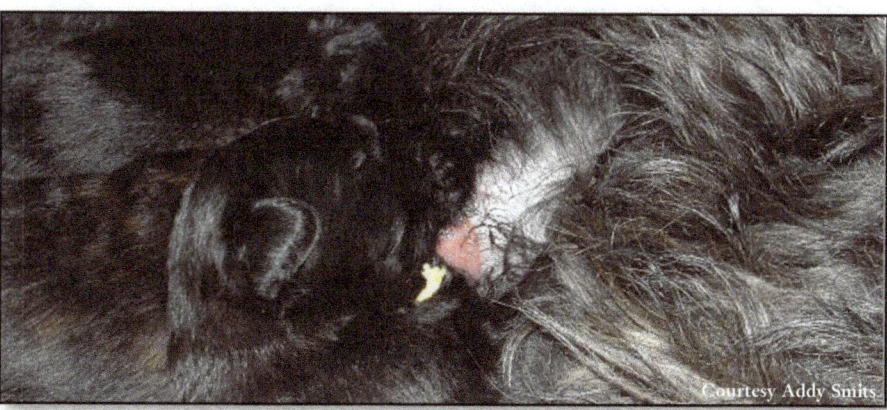

Yellow colostrum showing as puppy sucks

Chapter 7 Mammary Glands and Lactation

Colostrum is rich in immunoglobulins (antibodies). These maternally derived antibodies (MDA) are vital to the puppies' survival in that it provides the immunological defences immediately after birth for 6-9 weeks or so and protects the puppies against infections. This transfer of immunity from dam to puppy is termed passive transfer of immunity via the colostrum. Many mammals depend on transfer of colostral immunity. In the dog $\geq$ 90% of antibodies have to be consumed via the colostrum within the first 24 hours of life. This 24 hour deadline for colostrum ingestion is very important in dogs. This is because during the first 24 hours the puppies' intestines are highly permeable to antibodies allowing them into circulation immediately. After 24 hours these "gaps" close and the intestinal cells lining the intestinal tract become impermeable to intact antibodies and they would be digested as any other protein would.

In contrast, in humans, the vast majority of antibodies are transferred through the placenta to the baby and hence milk or colostrum consumption is not that important to them. It may at first impression appear that placental transfer of antibodies is a more sound method and nature has "failed" the canine species in electing colostral transfer instead of transplacental transfer. However, it may be speculated that colostral antibody transfer is an evolutionary adaptation in polytocous species not to waste unnecessary resources on the weak. For instance, if there were weak or stillborn puppies, they would not "waste" their mothers very valuable resource.

Colostral transfer of immunoglobulins has important implications for puppies. Puppies from bitches which suffer from agalactia (poor or no milk production) may require supplementation using milk replacers. Although the bitch might start lactating some time later, the puppies will by then be beyond the age where they can absorb the vitally important antibodies. For this reason it might be beneficial to establish a colostrum bank. This involves milking a bitch for colostrum and freezing it in small tubes. The amount of colostrum which each puppy requires is estimated to be the same as what they can drink in a single meal (stomach capacity), which is approximately 2-3% of bodyweight. If puppies weigh approximately 400 gram they would require around 12 ml colostrum each; a single meal is sufficient. Colostrum can be kept frozen in a household freezer for up to 12 months. Breeders could collaborate to collectively keep a colostrum bank going for everyone's use and convenience. Bitches of giant breeds are the best donors of colostrum because they are much easier to milk than toy breeds. Colostrum donors should be fully vaccinated and this should include vaccination against herpes virus. If colostrum isn't available, the serum of an adult dog, as source of protective antibodies, can be administered orally to the puppies within the first 24 hours after birth The serum should be dosed at 4 ml/100 gram bodyweight. A veterinary surgeon can prepare the serum by collecting blood (in a sterile tube) from the dam or any other adult dog. The blood is allowed to clot and is spun down in a centrifuge. The clear liquid fraction is the serum. Again, after 24 hours this serum would be useless in achieving maternally derived immunity. Theoretically, the serum should be effective in transferring antibodies to the puppy if it were administered intravenously even if the 24 hour period had lapsed. Serum, as a source of antibodies, is not nearly as efficient as colostrum and should only be considered if colostrum is not available at all.

Although puppies can only absorb antibodies in the colostrum for the first 24 hours, milk containing antibody is not entirely useless after the 24 hour period. This is because the antibodies present in the milk will have some local immunological effect in the intestine, before they are digested. This is beneficial in digestive upsets during the first few days of life. For this reason some intestinal remedies contain colostrum derived antibodies, albeit heterologous colostrum (from another species e.g. Cow). It is good to have frozen colostrum at hand to treat puppies which develop diarrhoea in the first few weeks of life.

The extent of protection which the puppies derive from the dam warrants discussion. The quantities and types of antibodies which are present within the milk are directly proportional to the levels of antibodies present in the mother. It therefore follows that puppies which start out with higher levels of colostrum derived antibodies in their system will remain protected for a longer period than those which do not. It is obvious that puppies can only receive antibodies against diseases which the dams' themselves were exposed to or vaccinated against. For instance, a puppy can only be expected to acquire immunity from its dam against the herpesvirus or against canine parvovirus enteritis if the bitch was adequately vaccinated against these diseases or if the bitch naturally acquired them and recovered, with the resultant acquisition of protective levels of antibodies. The implication is that antibodies in colostrum can have local geographic relevance. This is because not all areas have the same bugs and consequently it may be speculated that not all colostrum may therefore be equally effective. However, any colostrum from dogs administered to puppies is far better than none.

In cases where puppies did not receive colostrum within the first 24 hours of life and if alternative sources of colostrum were not available, consideration must be given to vaccinate the puppies at an earlier age (3 weeks) than the accepted norm. Colostrum-deprived puppies have a poorer chance of survival; besides being susceptible to parvovirus, distemper and other diseases, which they can be vaccinated against, they are even more susceptible to bacterial infections. Although not ideal, it is possible to raise puppies which were colostrum deprived.

7.2. Lactation and agalactia (poor or no milk production)

Breast milk is superior to all milk substitutes because it possesses highly digestible nutritional constituents and immunologic properties which cannot be mimicked by the very best milk replacers. Maintaining normal lactation in the bitch following whelping should therefore be a priority. It is cheaper, less labour intensive and associated with fewer complications if the bitch raises puppies than if breeders do it. In most cases "mother nature" does a better job than we do. Optimal nutrition of the lactating bitch is far more economical than spending money on milk replacers. Also, hand rearing of puppies may be associated with many complications and should be avoided as far as possible.

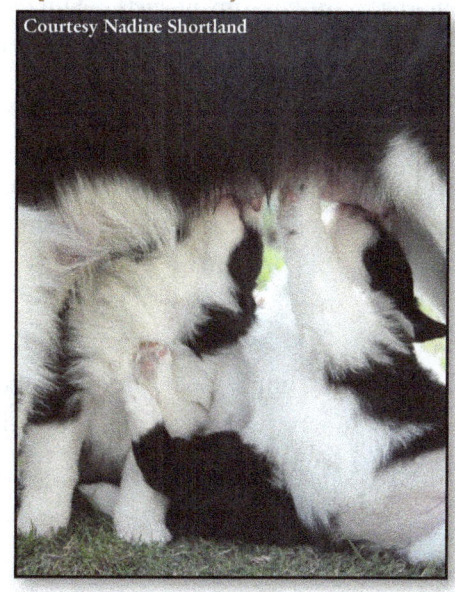

Puppy suckling strongly

Insufficient milk production is known as agalactia. It is not easy to assess whether a bitch has sufficient milk. The mere presence of a drop of milk on the teat when it is squeezed does not necessarily mean that the bitch is producing enough milk. If the puppies suckle vigorously and they gain weight, then the bitch's milk production is adequate; if not the bitch most probably, suffers from agalactia. The time before milk appears in the teats can vary from bitch to bitch. Some bitches might have milk as early as a week or more before whelping, whereas others only start producing milk shortly after whelping. Heavily pregnant bitches appear to be particularly prone to suffer from temporary agalactia, around late pregnancy and soon after birth. It is presumed that the weight of the gravid uterus exerts pressure on large blood vessels, partially occluding them, which in turn impairs the blood supply to the mammary glands. It corrects itself within the first day after delivery of the puppies but it can unfortunately lead to starvation and or colostrum deprivation during the critical first 24 hours.

Most bitches will have a reduced appetite in the last few days before whelping and others will have blatant anorexia for a few days after whelping. If these bitches are not in a good condition or are unable to mobilise energy from body reserves, poor milk production will result. It might be a good idea to add appetisers to the ration to induce consumption so that a caloric deficiency with resultant poor milk production is prevented. Post whelp diseases such as uterine infections, mastitis, and other conditions can also bring about anorexia and consequently, agalactia. It is speculated that poor milk production is genetically linked because poor milk production seems to be a recurring problem in certain bitches. It is very important to investigate the possible causes of agalactia as soon as possible because interruptions exceeding 48 hours might halt milk production altogether or cause insufficient milk production for the remainder of the lactation. If lactation is interrupted for less than 48 hours due to illness, the chances are good that it will resume normally after recovery.

The phenothiazine group of tranquilisers can be administered to stimulate the hormone prolactin, which in turn stimulates milk production. In addition, it is known to have a calming effect on the bitch so that normal maternal behaviour can set in. These tranquilisers are beneficial when stress and nervous behaviour is the cause of agalactia. Other drugs are also frequently used to enhance or stimulate milk production. Optimal nutrition is of crucial importance and the reader is referred to section 4.6 where optimal nutrition and its positive effect on milk production is discussed. Breeders should exercise extreme caution before tranquilisers are administered. The breeder must be a hundred percent sure that whelping is complete because these tranquilisers can halt the whelping process before the bitch has delivered all the puppies. Breeders report that bitches which have had a caesarean section seem more likely to suffer from agalactia. The use of medication to improve milk production or to sedate bitches although indicated in many cases, should always be used in consultation with a veterinary surgeon.

7.3. Galactostasis

Galactostasis refers to stasis of milk in the mammary glands; the glands enlarge and become warm and painful. This is a rare condition and usually occurs in bitches which produce more milk than their puppies can consume. It also befalls bitches which lose their litters shortly after whelping or after the puppies are weaned. Some breeders are very concerned when galactostasis sets in and promptly treat the mammary glands with hot/cold compression and a gentle massage. If no further milk production is required, simply reduce food intake for a day or two and the problem will usually resolve itself. In some countries specific drugs are available to halt milk production. Galactostasis if not resolved, can progress into mastitis.

7.4. Mastitis

Each mammary gland of the bitch has one teat or nipple. The nipple has 8-20 individual openings through which the milk may escape to the outside. Mastitis refers to an infection of the mammary gland usually during lactation. One, more or rarely all mammary glands may be involved. Initially the mammary gland is inflamed, swells, is painful to touch and the milk becomes more viscous and discolours from white to yellow or even brown.

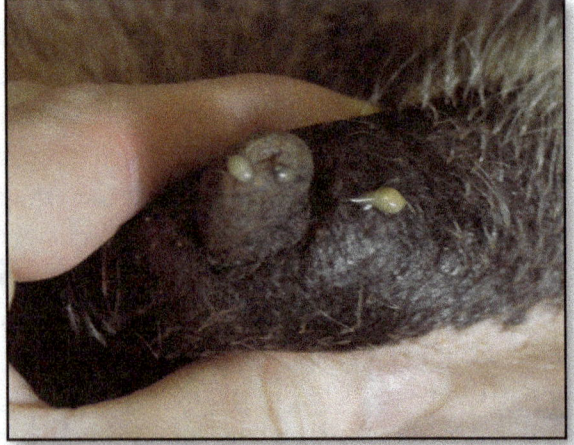

Gentle massage of the mammary gland reveals puss at the teat opening of a mammary gland with mastitis

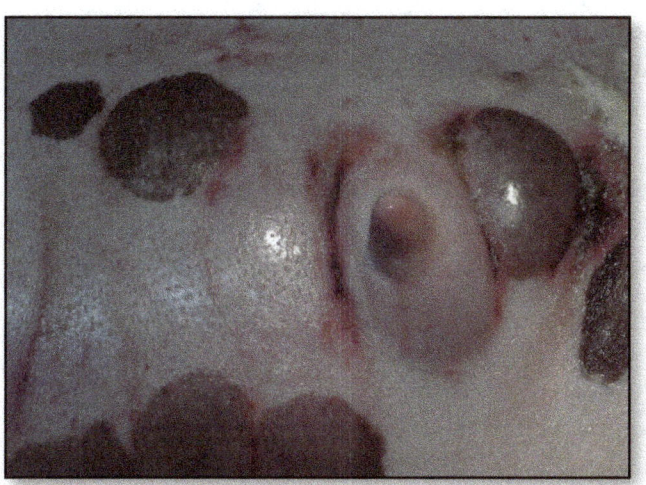
Fissured mammary glands

The bitch will frequently not allow suckling from that teat. Usually a day later the affected mammary gland swells even more. Bitches suffering from mastitis develop a fever, become anorexic and her puppies may become restless and cry. Untreated bitches may become desperately ill from septicaemia (blood poisoning) and may even die. Mastitis may occur at any stage of lactation but is more likely to occur in the first two weeks.

Mastitis is caused by bacteria which enter the teat openings and ascend into the mammary gland or get there via the blood and causes infection. This accentuates the need for a clean and hygienic whelping area because unhygienic conditions increase the incidence of both mastitis and uterine infections. Nevertheless, despite the best efforts, some bitches will still develop mastitis. Some bitches have very taut skin and when abdominal distension and mammary gland engorgement stretches the skin, a fissure can occur. This is very common in certain breeds. These fissures become infected and serve as a source of bacteria which feed the development of mastitis. Bitches which are kept on rough abrasive surfaces might have dry and fissured teats which are prone to infection. If this is the case, teats should be treated with creams which have moisturising and antibacterial properties. Sometimes puppies damage the teats and mammary glands with their sharp nails, if this happens, the breeder must take steps to blunt them.

Treatment involves the use of antibiotics. Drainage of the gland might be required if it becomes abscessed. The draining of a mammary gland abscess can leave a huge open wound but this usually heals very quickly. A very important consideration in the treatment of mastitis is what to do with the puppies? If the puppies are 3 weeks or older; it might be the safest to wean the puppies early (See section 13.4.3). If early weaning is not possible or the puppies are younger than 3 weeks, the puppies should be allowed to continue suckling on the dam, even if she has mastitis. However, the breeder must first check whether the dam displays aggressive behaviour towards the puppies due to pain when they suckle. The choice of antibiotic must be safe for both puppies and dam. Non-steroidal anti-inflammatory agents must be used with caution in lactating bitches and must be used for a limited period, not exceeding 2-3 days. If the puppies start showing signs of illness because of toxic milk syndrome, they should be removed from the dam and hand reared.

7.5. Milk fever (eclampsia)

Milk fever is also known as eclampsia, puerperal tetany or hypocalcaemia. The underlying cause is inadequate free calcium ion concentrations in the blood. This usually occurs when bitches which are good milk producers have large litters. A large litter consumes more milk; the greater consumption of milk translates into a greater loss of calcium for the bitch. These bitches are unable to replace the calcium; neither through the diet nor from their bone reserves. The inadequate intake of dietary calcium plays a key role in the manifestation of milk fever. Bitches can develop milk fever even if they are on an adequate diet but inferior diets can predispose them. Bitches which have both a poor ability to rapidly mobilize calcium from bone and also with large lactational demands are at increased risk to develop milk fever.

Chapter 7 Mammary Glands and Lactation

Genetic factors are thought to play a role in susceptibility because mostly bitches in the small breed category develop milk fever; however, almost all breeds are affected. Oral calcium supplementation during pregnancy is not helpful in the prevention of milk fever; to the contrary, many actually think that it is a contributing factor. However, calcium supplementation during the time of peak milk production might aid the prevention of milk fever, especially in those bitches which developed milk fever during previous lactations. Calcium supplementation may also help prevent the recurrence of milk fever during the same lactation. The importance of Vitamin D in conjunction with calcium supplementation was discussed in section 4.15.1 and 4.15.2.

Milk fever commonly presents at around 2-3 weeks after whelping and usually coincides with peak milk production. It occasionally occurs in late pregnancy or around the time of labour. Bitches which suffer from milk fever hyperventilate excessively, salivate, have muscle tremors, show stiffness, are unable to walk and develop a very high fever. The onset can be sudden and there is a rapid progression into seizures, coma and ultimately death. Eclampsia is a medical emergency and requires prompt treatment with intravenous calcium solutions, correction of acidosis (abnormal increase in blood acidity) and attention to the glucose demand of the bitch. Recovery is usually quick and dramatic. Breeders must discuss possible preventative protocols with the attending veterinary surgeon to prevent recurrence. The causes which led to the development of the eclampsia in the first place, still exist at the time of discharge from the veterinary clinic following treatment and the condition is likely to recur when the bitch resumes nursing.

Puppies which are 20 days or older are able to start eating themselves and it might be a good idea to wean the puppies early. If the puppies are younger than 20 days, the breeder can opt to hand rear them using milk replacers. If hand rearing is employed, the puppies need to be isolated from the bitch. This is because an awareness of their presence can continue the stimulation of milk production and a recurrence of the condition. If the puppies cannot be removed from the bitch because hand rearing, for whatever reason, is impossible; the breeder, assisted by a veterinary surgeon, must establish a preventative protocol to minimize the possibility of recurrence. In these cases the bitch will require daily subcutaneous injections of calcium until the puppies are able to eat by themselves. Breeders must understand that a bitch which developed milk fever during lactation might do so again when she next lactates, even if attempts are made to prevent it through oral calcium supplementation.

Chapter 8

Whelping

8.1. Signs of impending labour

It is useful to know what the signs of impending labour are. It is even more useful to know which signs represent normal progress and which do not. The application of this knowledge is complicated by the fact that the signs of impending labour that are exhibited vary considerably from bitch to bitch. Prudent breeders do not rely on a single sign to alert them but rather look at a combination of signals. The interval between the first signs of impending labour and actual labour also varies. For instance, lactation can start as long as 2 weeks before labour, or as early as a few hours before birth, and in exceptional cases, even after birth. The interval between the onset of lactation and parturition is often only one day in primigravida bitches (maiden bitches) and a few days in multipara bitches (bitches which have whelped before).

A decrease in body temperature usually occurs from 2-12 hours before the onset of second stage labour. Many breeders use this decrease in body temperature as a warning signal of impending labour. Unfortunately, it is not standard in all bitches and it is, therefore, not reliable if it is the only warning signal that a breeder uses. At best, it should only be used as a guideline because a drop in temperature can occur days before labour or it might not drop at all.

The mucus plug is the thick slime which seals the cervix and prevents ascent of bacteria into the uterus during pregnancy. This plug usually dissolves towards the end of pregnancy and is visible as a slimy vaginal discharge. This discharge becomes visible around 3 weeks before labour but also just a few minutes before or not at all; and so, the visibility of a discharge on its own is not a reliable warning signal of impending labour.

Most bitches will become partially or completely anorectic (stop eating), restless, seclude themselves and show nesting behaviour (scratch and dig) a few days before labour. The onset of behaviour and also which behaviour is exhibited varies from bitch to bitch. Some bitches will eat up to a few hours before labour although restlessness and nesting behaviour started a week or longer, before the due date.

The "drop" in the bitch's abdomen refers to the relaxation of the abdominal muscles, the pelvic muscles and the vulva, in the last few days prior to labour. Although subjective, it appears to give the abdomen a sagging shape. This subjective perception should not be used as the only warning signal of impending labour.

What follows is a summary of the different stages of labour and how long they normally last.

8.1.1. First stage

The signs of first stage labour, namely excitement, restlessness, panting, seclusion, nesting and sometimes vomition, typically start 12-24 hours prior to whelping. During this stage the uterus contractions become stronger and more frequent and the cervix dilates completely and the first membranes appear.

Chapter 8 Whelping

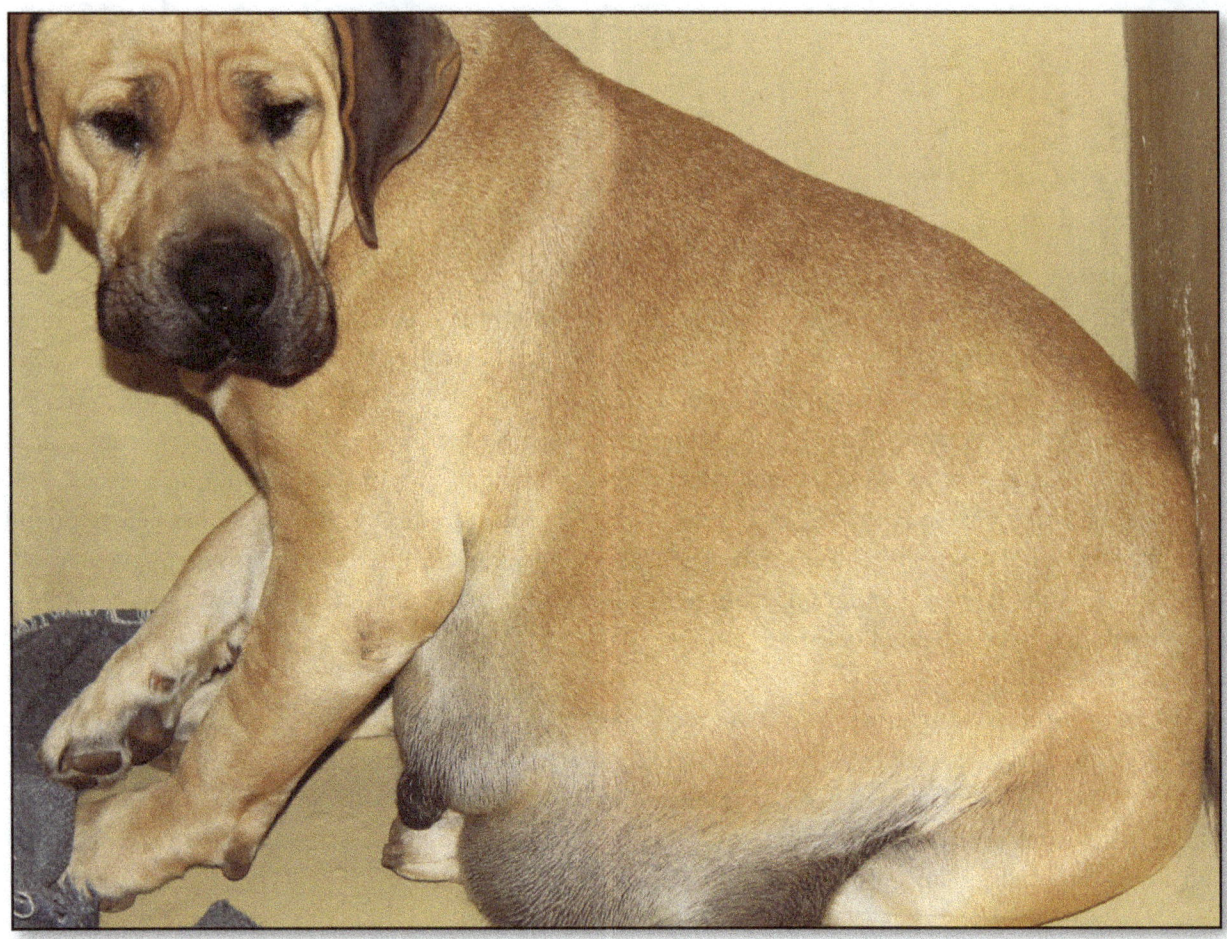
Bitch appearing uncomfortable and constantly looking at her flanks during first stage of labour

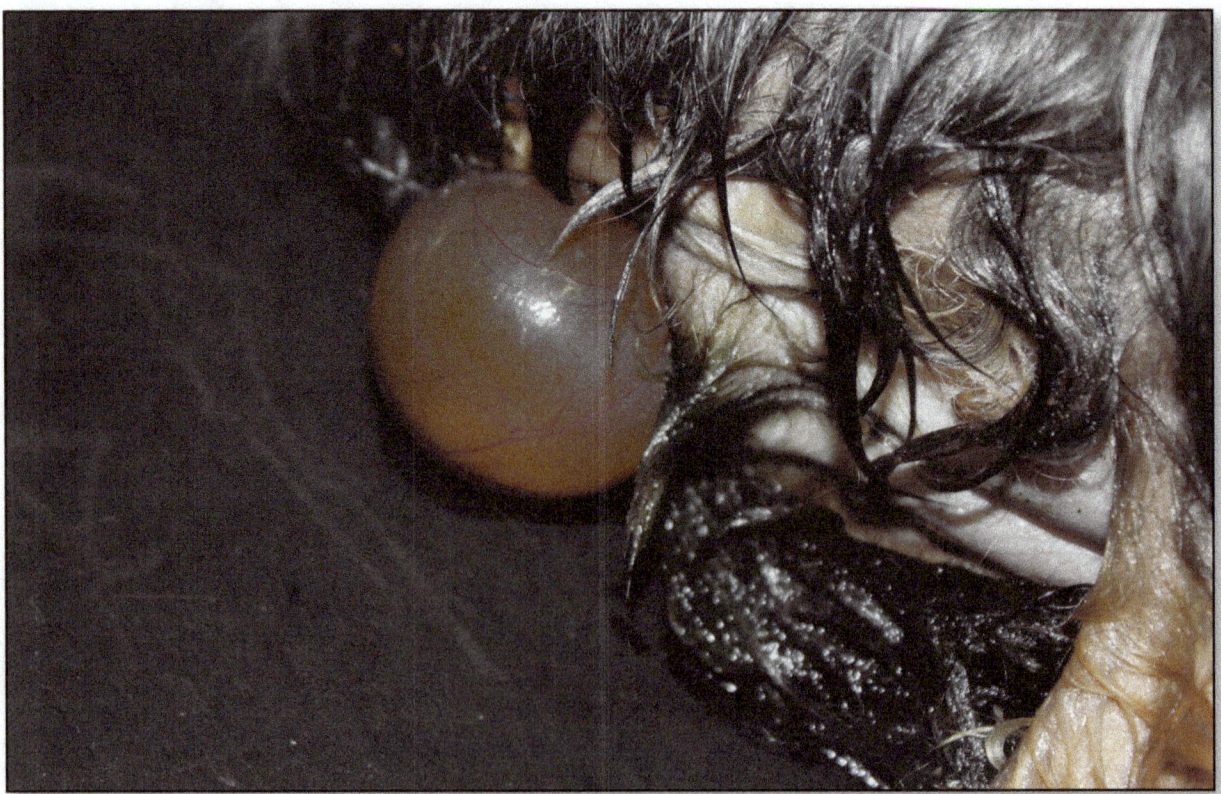
Membranes appearing during first stage of labour

Chapter 8 Whelping

8.1.2. Second stage

During this stage the bitch starts contracting her abdominal muscles which the breeder can see as straining or pushing. This is the stage during which the foetuses are expelled. During this stage the puppy is pushed into the birth canal. The breeder will at first see the membranous sack filled with fluid part the vulva. The fluid may be cloudy coloured water or have a green tinge. It is not necessary for the breeder to intervene at this stage as long as there is progress. The fluid filled membranes path

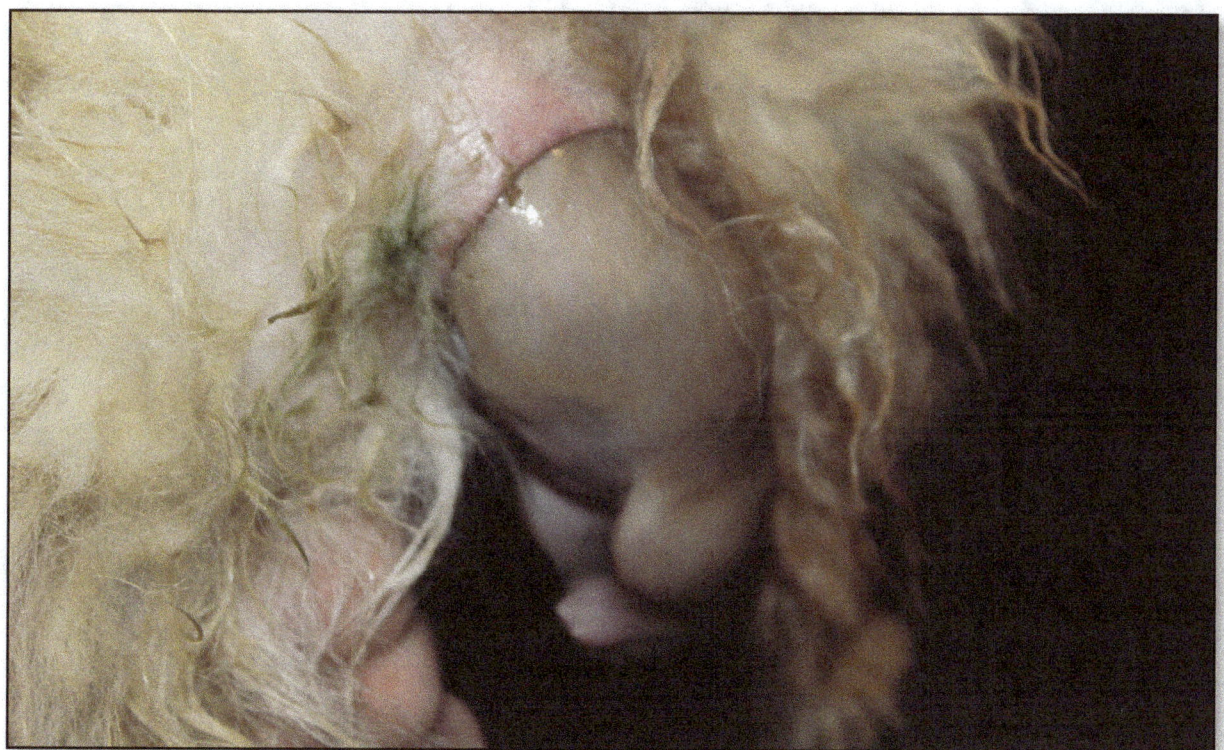
Puppy apears in birth canal and protruding from vagina

the way for the birth process by dilating the cervix and birth canal by mechanical action and making the surfaces of the birth canal slippery. Sometimes the membranes break inside the birth canal and a gush of water is expelled from the vagina. In other cases the puppy is born with all its membranes intact (inside the sack).

The bitch should immediately turn around and break the membranes to allow the puppy to start breathing. If the bitch fails to do this the breeder should do it for her and wipe the puppy dry with a clean towel. The sack consists of two layers which should both be torn. Puppies may be born feet first, head first or with their hind quarters first. All are normal.

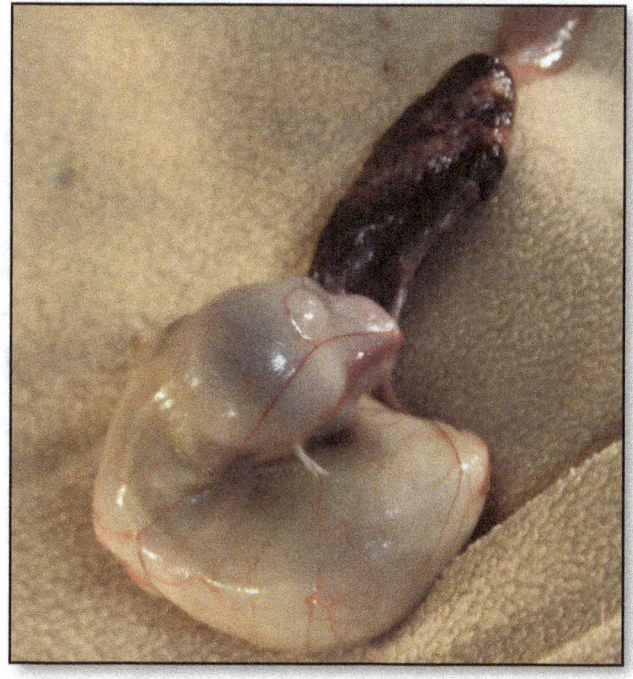
Puppy in membranes

Chapter 8 Whelping

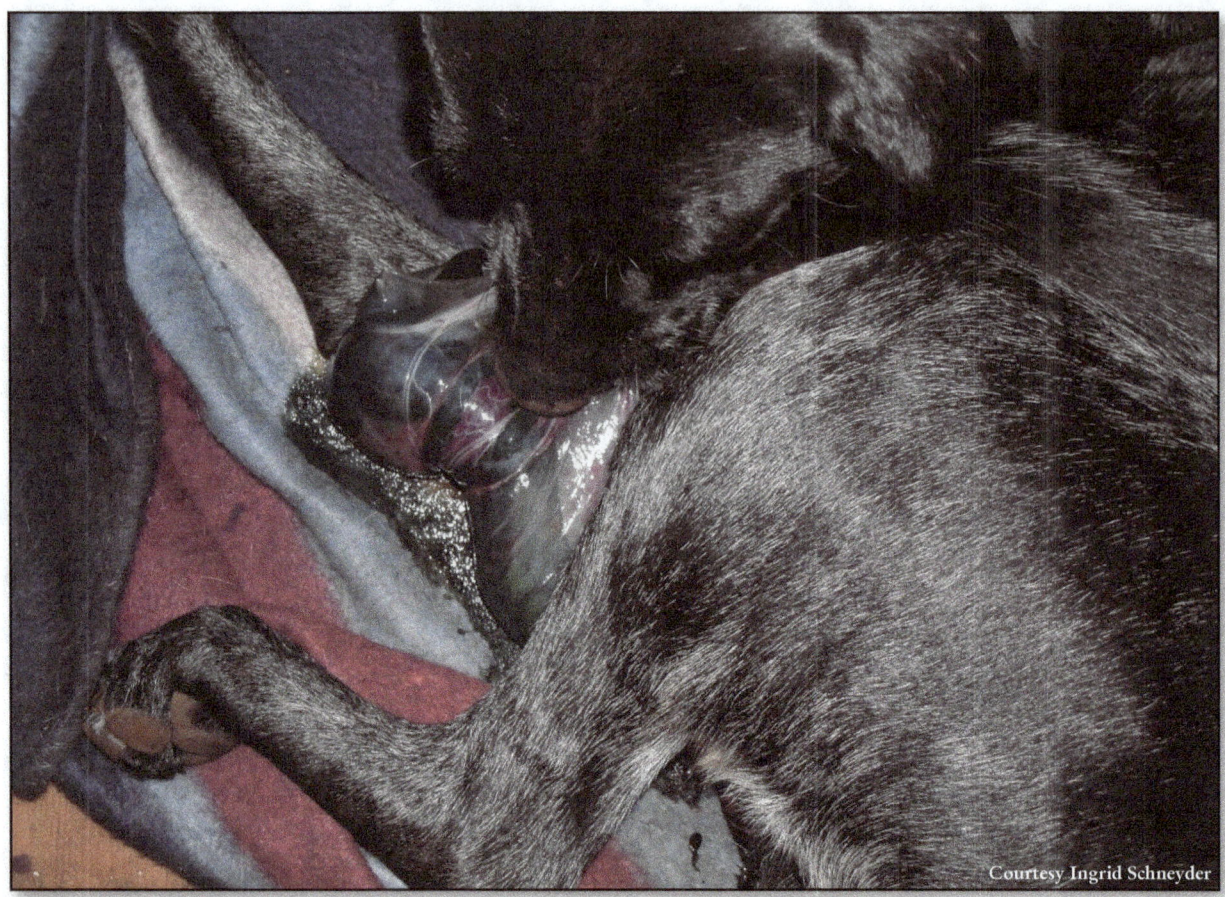

Puppy born within sack and placenta around it clearly visible

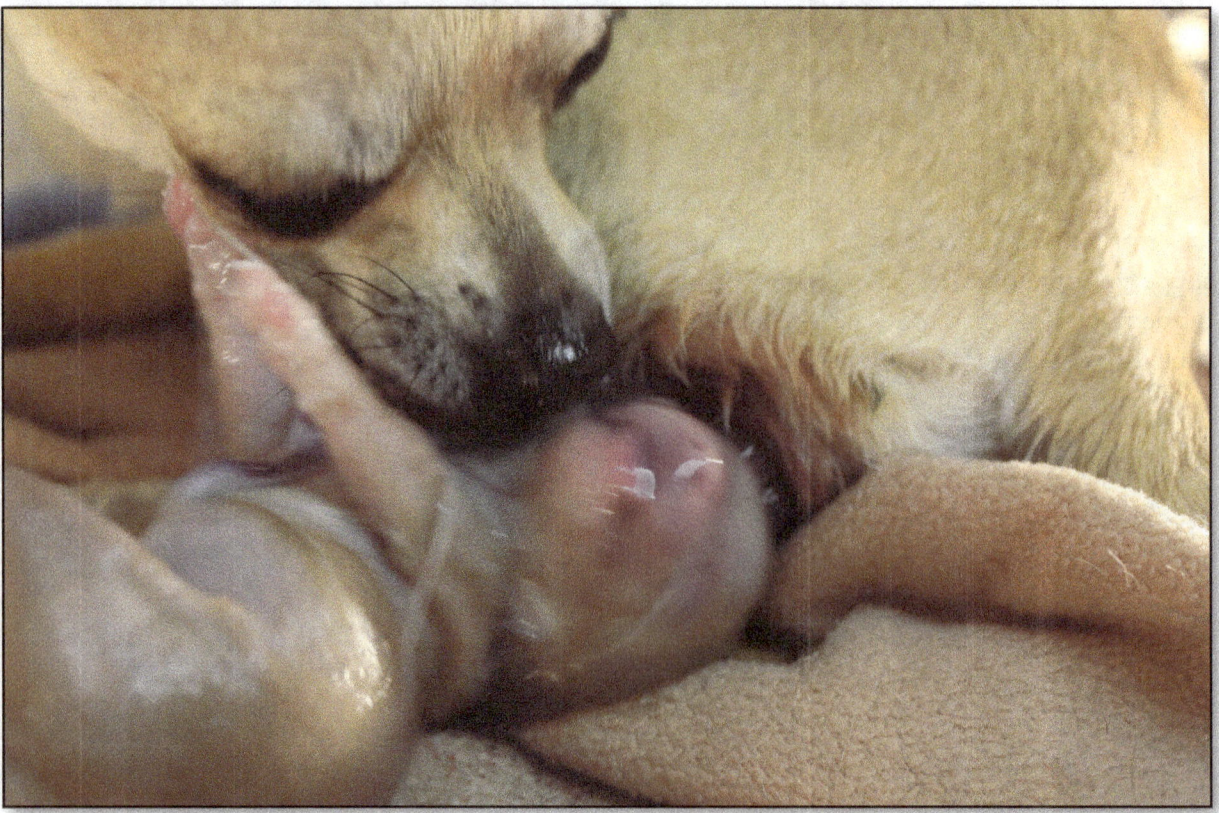

Bitch starts chewing membranses off puppy immediately after birth

This stage may last up to 24 hours depending on litter size but averages 4-8 hours. The birth of the first puppy may take as long as one hour after the onset of straining whereas the duration of straining prior to the birth of subsequent puppies is seldom longer than 15 minutes. Unproductive, uninterrupted straining for longer than 20-30 minutes indicate labour difficulties. The interval between subsequent puppies is very variable and may be as long as 4 hours. Intervals of 24 hours and longer have been recorded resulting in delivery of live puppies, but this is highly unusual and risky. Usually, interpup intervals are shorter than one hour. It is important to monitor the bitch during these intervals. Intervals longer than 2 hours become suspect but are not too harmful if the bitch is resting during this time. This resting period may be confusing to breeders as they may not know whether the bitch has completed the whelp or not. Extended inter-puppy intervals associated with long periods of straining is cause for concern. The third stage of labour follows the birth of each puppy. The placenta of each neonate is usually released within 5-15 minutes after birth. Sometimes two puppies may be born before both placentas are released simultaneously.

8.2. Management of the whelping bitch

The management of a whelping bitch starts with the preparation of the whelping quarters. It further involves the transferral of the bitch to the whelping quarters, observation of the whelping process and it ends after the last puppy is born and all puppies suckle. This can be a very tough time for the breeder because the whelping process places restrictions on the breeder's time and movements at that time. If the breeder only has mating dates to work on, they will be unsure of when to expect labour. Consequently breeders will waste a lot of time looking out for signs of impending labour, which might even be a week or two away. Breeders often suffer from sleep deprivation during this time, particularly if circumstances dictate additional feeds or the hand rearing of puppies. For this reason, it is strongly advised that breeders seek veterinary assistance to predict the whelping dates more accurately. This could shorten the period of increased vigilance to around 3-5 days.

About 10 days before the expected due date the bitch should be placed in the whelping area (whelping quarters). This allows her to adapt and settle down in her new environment. It is better to transfer the bitch to the whelping quarters earlier rather than later in order to ensure that she does not "surprise" the breeder and whelp in less than ideal conditions, before she is transferred.

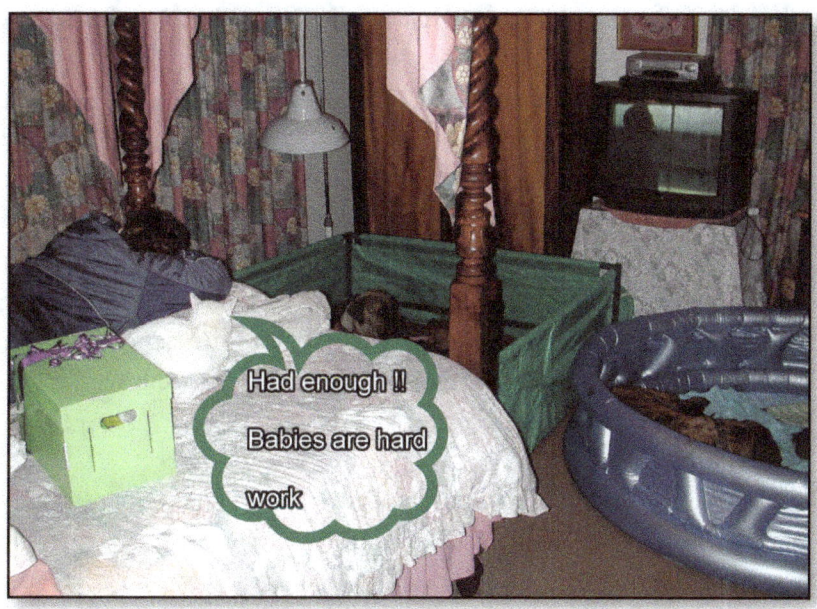

8.2.1. The whelping quarters

In nature, pregnant bitches will withdraw from the pack and retreat to a warm cosy well-padded den well in advance of the due date. This is exactly what a breeder tries to simulate when a bitch is transferred to a whelping quarter. There are a number of reasons why transfer to a whelping quarter is important. It signals the time when a "whelping trim" needs to be performed on bitches with long hair. This involves a hygienic trim around the perineum (the region of the abdomen surrounding the urogenital and anal openings) as well as around the mammary glands and nipples, to facilitate access. All bitches, irrespective of breed, should be washed with antiseptic soap. A separate whelping quarter isolates the bitch from the general dog population preventing provocation of anxiety and the possibility of other dogs interfering with the neonates.

Pregnant and lactating bitches have different nutritional needs and should be fed in accordance with the guidelines given in 4.6.

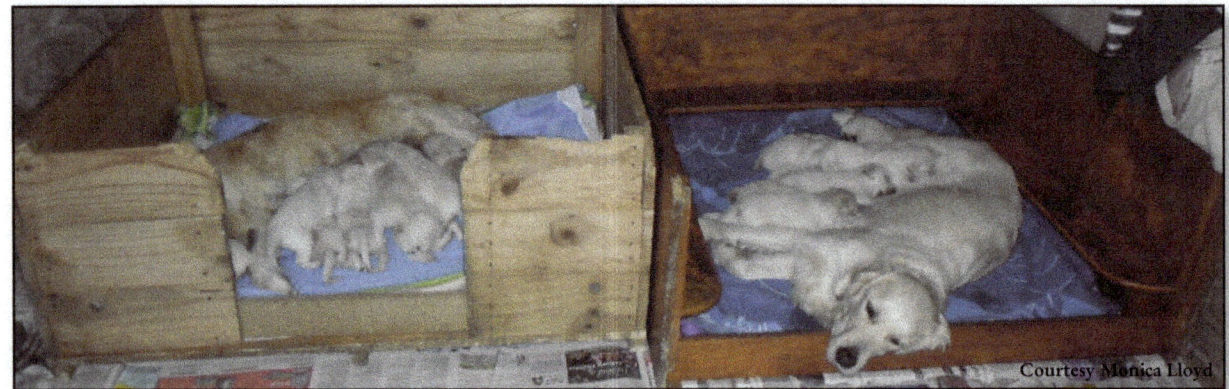

Although some breeders may manage to keep two lactating bitches with puppies together in the same room without incident, many regard this as too risky

Some breeders might have the luxury of a dedicated whelping room with all the necessary paraphernalia and others even have custom built whelping kennels. For many breeders however, the whelping quarters is a make shift "maternity ward" in the kitchen, garage, shed, any utility room or even their own bedroom. One might work as well as the other, provided it meets the minimum requirements, i.e. it should be a space that is dry and clean, providing shelter against inclement weather.

The bitch should have access to a whelping box. The dimensions of this box will depend on the size of the dog. It should be large enough to accommodate her lying down in a fully stretched out position, with still enough space around her for the litter. The sides of the box must be high enough to prevent puppies of around 3-4 week old from escaping. A protective side rail which prevents the bitch from lying directly against the box's side panels helps prevent clumsy bitches from crushing their puppies against the side of the whelping box. Bedding material, i.e. blankets, carpets and so on should be kept clean and the breeder must ensure that the puppies cannot be trapped underneath it and suffocate. Care should be taken if food or water bowls are placed inside the whelping box to prevent puppies from drowning in them.

Because neonates do not have the ability to thermo regulate, the whelping quarters should be warm. The ideal ambient temperature should be around 22-27°C, from a few days before the due date and maintaining it for the first 2 weeks of lactation; where-after it can be allowed to drop by a few

Chapter 8 Whelping

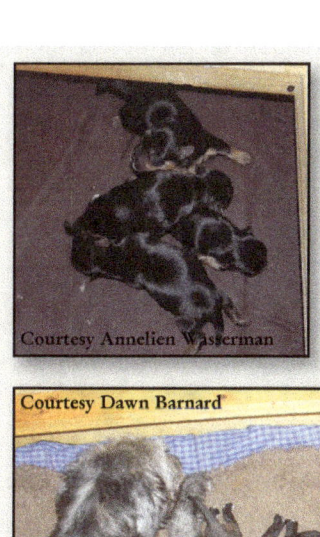
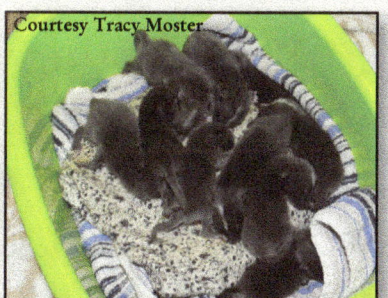
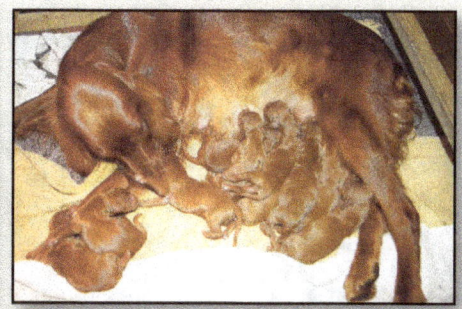
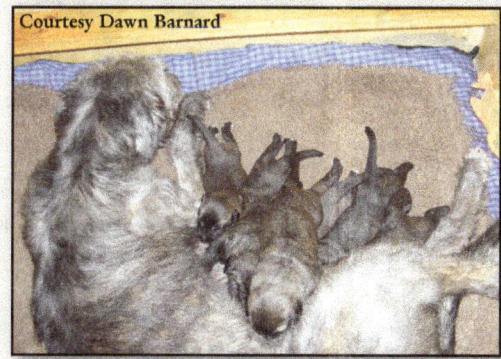
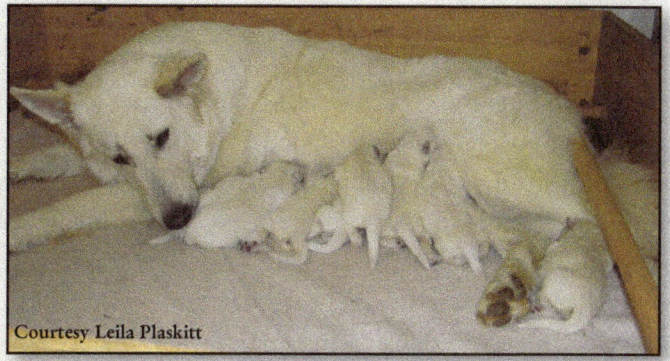
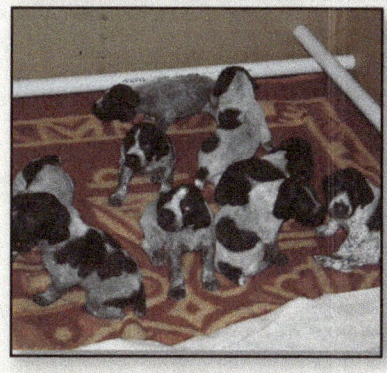
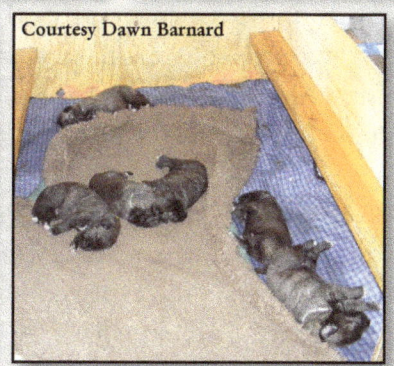
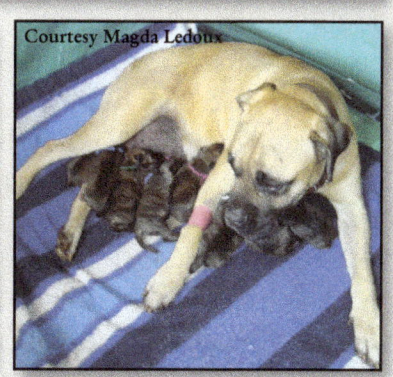
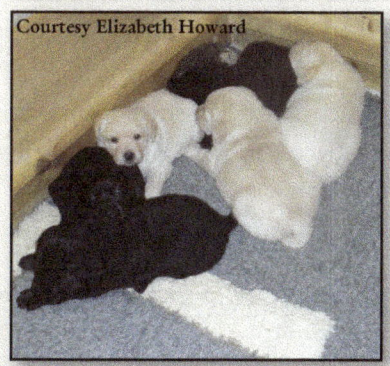
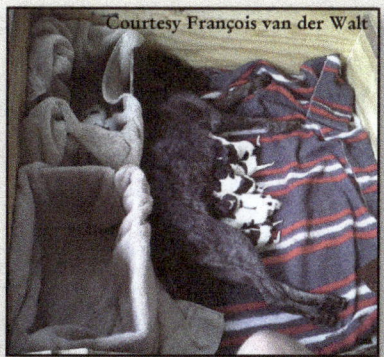
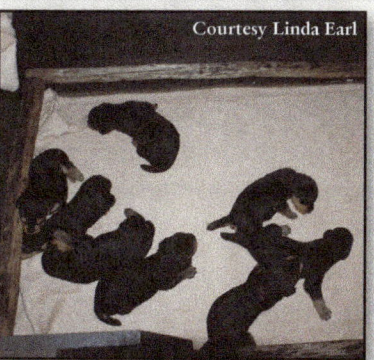
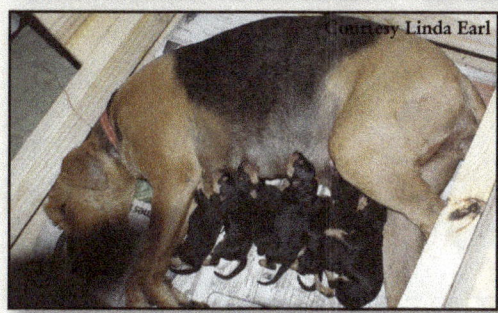
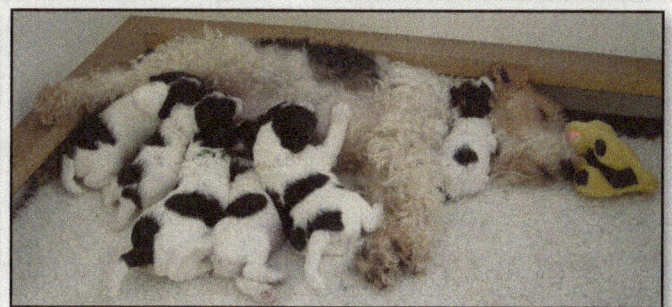

Whelping boxes may vary from very simple to profesionally made and complex structures

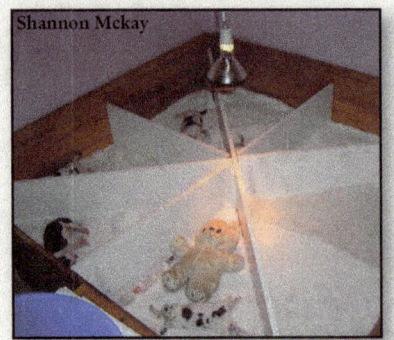
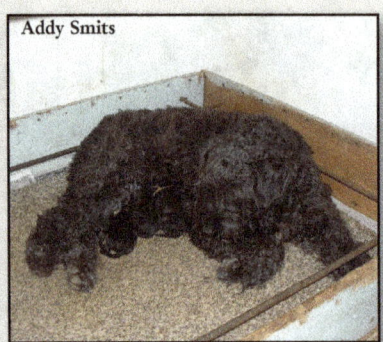
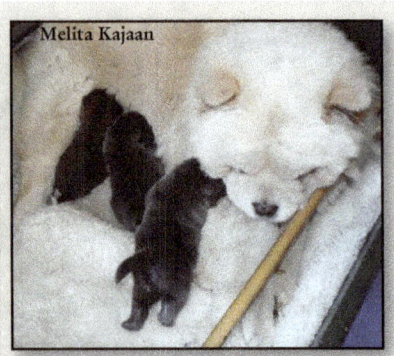

degrees. Temperature can be artificially controlled by placing heating devices in the whelping box. Care must be taken to place them in such a way that thermal or electrical trauma is not possible. In very cold countries, if whelping quarters are outside, breeders attempt to conserve heat by keeping vents and windows closed. In doing so, care must be taken not to compromise proper ventilation. Good mothers will be able to maintain their puppy's temperature in cold climates if the whelping quarters are outside, provided the quarters are well-constructed, have a proper whelping box and are padded with adequate insulating material and blankets. Nonetheless, this is not ideal because extreme cold spells cannot be predicted. It is also inconvenient to properly supervise outdoors. Ideally, the whelping quarters should be indoors where proper lighting, temperature control, adequate ventilation and clean surfaces are easily organised. Also, the breeder should have easy access to the whelping quarters to monitor the entire whelping process.

8.2.2. Observation of the whelping process

The breeder should look for the signs of impending labour as described in section 8.1. The breeder should, ever so often, look in on the bitch around the expected whelping time. Some breeders place audio monitoring equipment in the whelping quarters so that they can hear the "sounds of whelping" (panting, moaning, whining, scratching). Others install cameras to enable remote visual monitoring of the bitch. Many keep the whelping bitch in their bedroom for direct monitoring purposes whilst some even sleep in the bitch's whelping quarters. In stark contrast to this, some breeders elect not to supervise at all. This is because they feel that the bitch should not be disturbed when she is whelping. It is true that some bitches do not need any assistance, however, most breeders will soon learn that maximum puppy survival requires a hands-on approach.

Puppies are born either with their foetal membranes intact or ruptured with the umbilical cord usually still attached. The bitch ruptures the membranes immediately after birth and nibbles through the umbilical cord and thereafter she licks the puppy dry. A good dam will attend to the puppy and attempt to gather it close to her abdomen. If the bitch does not remove the foetal membranes immediately, the breeder has to remove it manually. This has to be done within minutes after parturition to avoid suffocation. It is good practice to disinfect the umbilicus and to tie it off, using umbilical tape or string.

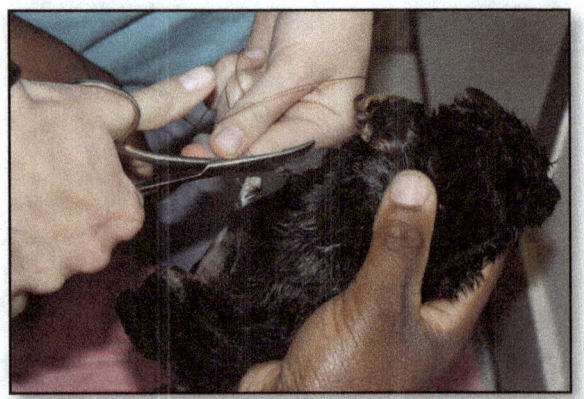

Umbilicus is tied off with catgut in this instance immediately after delivery by caesarean section

Some breeders take the puppies away from the bitch as they are born, to prevent her from injuring the puppies during the whelping process. Others prefer to leave the puppies with the bitch, especially if she is aware of their presence and concerned for their welfare. Most breeders will temporarily remove the puppies until the whelping process is complete, especially if they are medium or large breed dogs. Even with the best mothers, some degree of neglect will be evident during the birth of a large litter.

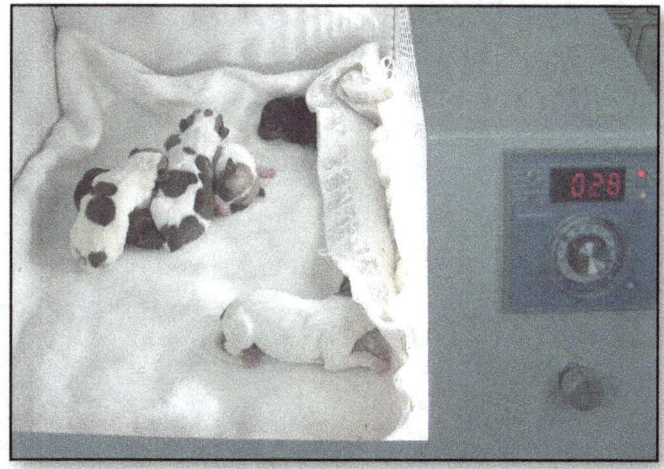
Dedicated puppy incubator with accurate temperature controls

If the puppies are removed from the bitch, they should be transferred to a warm and insulated container. The containers which breeders use vary from a simple box with some towels in it to an advanced incubator with temperature and humidity control. Puppies will do well in any of the containers, provided they are kept warm (35°C). Sometimes the "puppy box" is left in sight of the bitch, and sometimes it is placed out of sight; whatever action is taken usually depends on how the bitch reacts to it. Crying puppies can disturb a bitch and delay the whelping process if she constantly attempts to attend to those which are already born, whilst other bitches are not bothered at all. Breeders must be warned that during the early stages of whelping a bitch might behave aggressively towards them. It is quite possible that an otherwise loving bitch suddenly becomes vicious upon the delivery of the first puppy; she might even bite to resist interference with the new-born puppy.

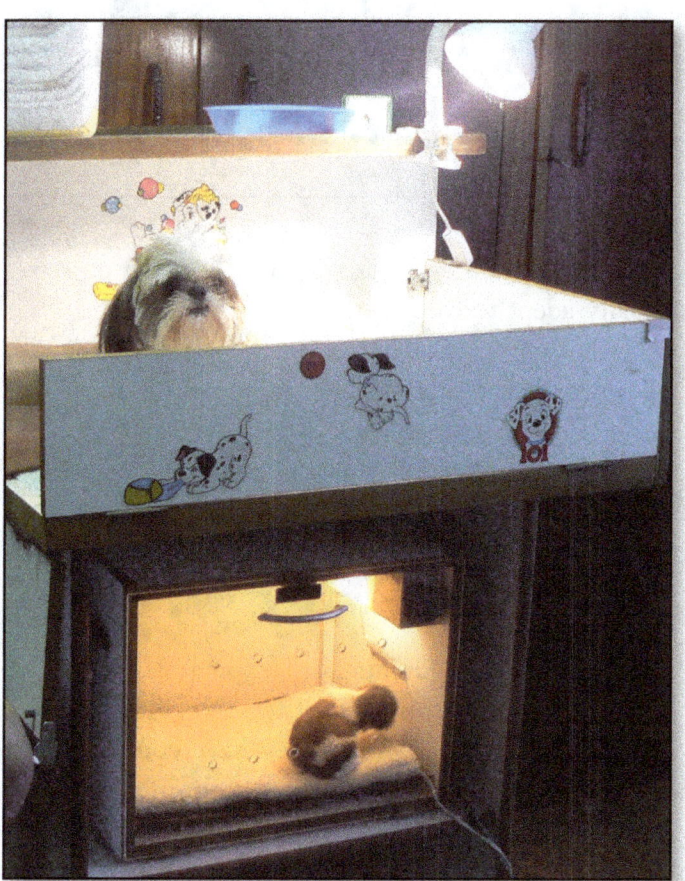
Example of home-made incubator using lamps as heat source

Soon after delivery of the puppies, the placentas will be expelled and most bitches will consume them. This is a natural phenomenon and is probably an evolutionary adaptation; firstly to conserve calories and secondly to remove blood which might attract unnecessary attention to her vulnerable state and the new-borns. Some breeders remove the placentas themselves and are motivated to do so either through revulsion or nausea or both. Some bitches vomit up the placentas, either during the whelping process or soon after, which unfortunately serves to heighten breeder revulsion.

Chapter 8 Whelping

Signs which should alert breeders to the fact that the whelping process is not progressing normally are described in the section on dystocia in 8.3.1. As a general rule most bitches will settle down and stop hyperventilating within minutes of the delivery of the last puppy. Some breeders choose to seek veterinary confirmation that labour is complete. Prior knowledge of the litter size is helpful in this regard. Supervision of the whelping process is complete when the puppies are all suckling and ingesting colostrum, which is the most important meal of their lives.

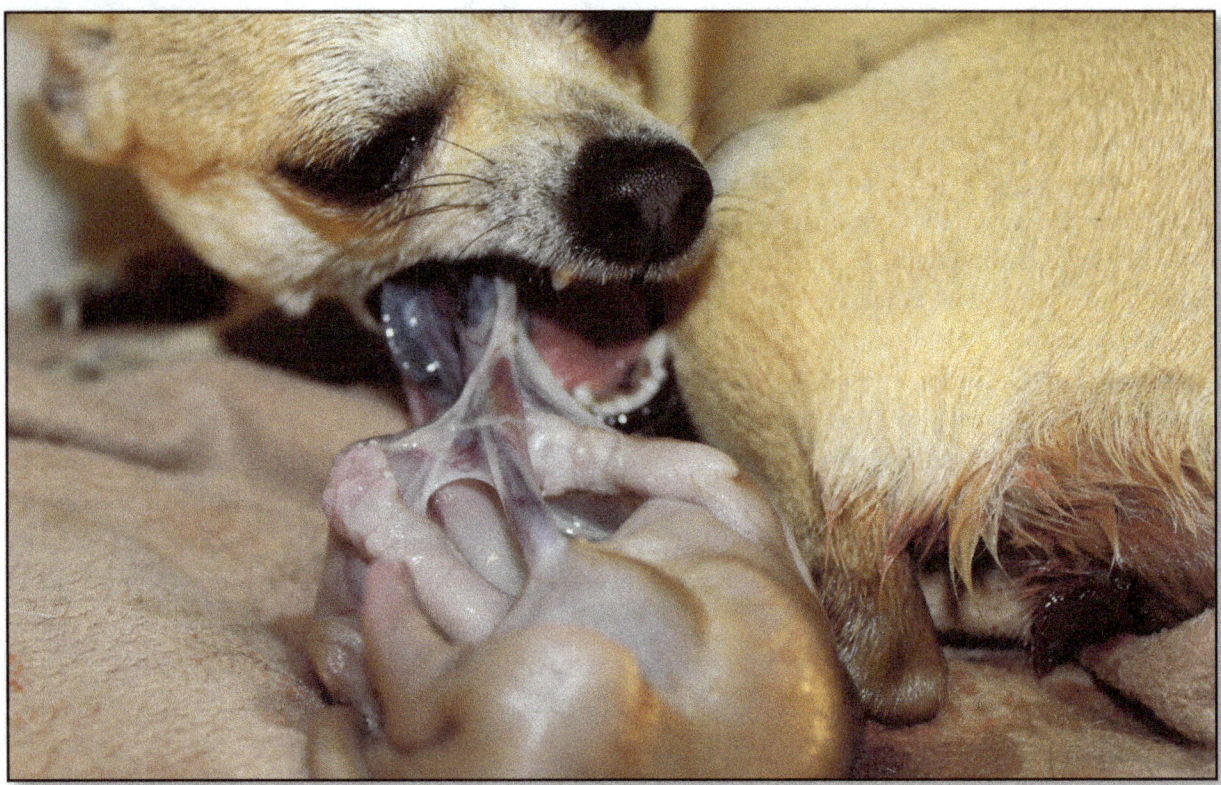

Bitch consumes placenta

Early on in the whelping process the breeder will be able to evaluate whether the bitch possesses good maternal instincts. Not all bitches are equally adept to care for and nurse the puppies. Poor mothering skills, are: "over mothering", clumsy behaviour, neglect, or the worst case scenario, aggressive behaviour towards the puppies. Bitches which over-mother their puppies do so by licking the neonates excessively. They can lick off the skin on their abdomens or even cause evisceration by opening the umbilicus. Incessant nibbling can result in the loss of extremities, evisceration, or biting the umbilical cord off too near to the abdominal wall, which can result in fatal haemorrhage. This type of behaviour is often instigated by the puppy's cries and over mothering is the bitch's response to it.

Clumsy bitches might unintentionally harm their puppies by squashing or stepping on them. This type of behaviour is mostly exhibited during labour and serves as a signal to remove the puppies from the whelping box. Most bitches will become more cautious once they have completed the whelping process and have settled down. The bitch produces the hormone oxytocin in response to the puppy's stimulation (suckling) of the nipples. This hormone not only stimulates milk let-down to ease suckling, but it is also believed to strengthen maternal instincts and behaviour to aid in the bitch's bonding with her litter. A tranquiliser can be prescribed at a low dosage to calm nervous bitches which fail to settle down after the birth of the last puppy. Some of these drugs will also increase milk production.

Infanticide refers to the killing of puppies by the dam. It is usually encountered in bitches which are particularly nervous after labour, or it happens in response to the puppies incessant crying. Bitches which commit infanticide may also kill other bitch's puppies. Bitches who are poor mothers are likely to display this behaviour in subsequent litters. Bitches will often eat a stillborn puppy or one which dies soon after birth. This is known as cannibalism and it is normal behaviour in all wild carnivores.

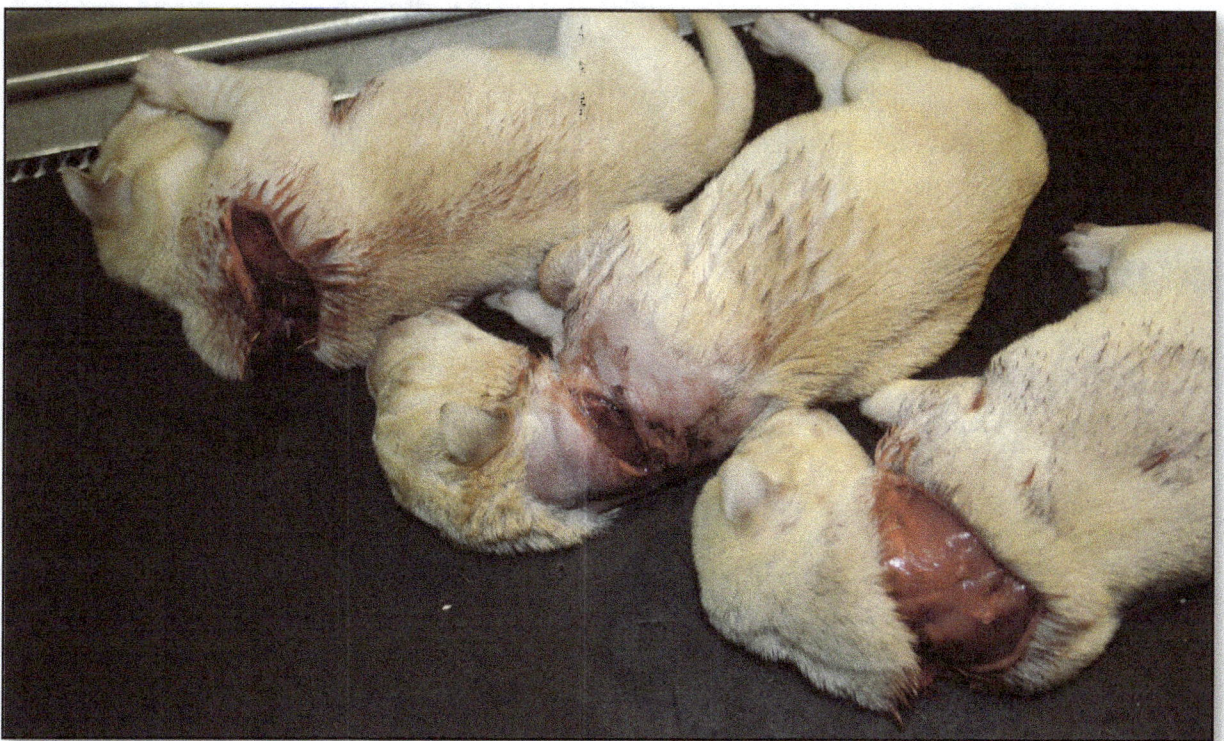

Infanticide, in this image the dam had killed her entire litter in stereotypical fashion by biting the back of their necks

A bitch will sometimes selectively neglect an individual puppy. In many instances it is the smallest or weakest puppy but there are exceptions to this rule. It is suggested that bitch's have an instinctive ability to identify a puppy with a defect and consequently neglect it. Although it is true that most of these puppies die, even if hand rearing is attempted, some do survive and turn out to be perfectly normal dogs. This is probably another example of evolutionary adaptation to ensure that resources are not wasted on individuals which are unlikely to survive ("survival of the fittest").

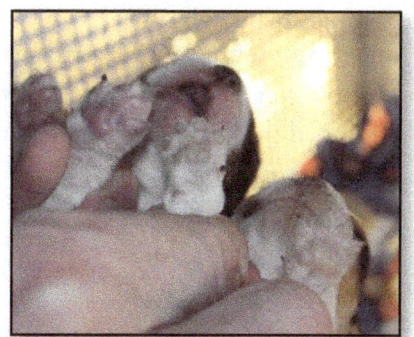

Note anaemic feet of puppy on the right

Because new-born puppies do not have an adequate blood clotting mechanism until they are at least 72 hours old, some breeders and even veterinary surgeons administer vitamin K to bolster the clotting mechanism. Most breeders do not and their puppies do not appear to have an increased risk of umbilical bleeding or haemorrhagic tendency.

8.3. Dystocia (difficulty in labour) in the bitch

A discussion of labour difficulties is necessary to help breeders understand the decision making process in the management of labour. This discussion will be especially valuable to breeders who breed with dystocia prone breeds. Although dystocia has many causes and can befall any breed, several dog breeds are associated with an increased risk for dystocia. Scientific reports have singled out the Scottish terrier, Boston terrier, Chihuahua, Dachshund, Pekingese, Yorkshire terrier, Pomeranian and the miniature Poodle; however, most small, miniature and toy breeds, as well as all brachycephalic breeds (breeds with a short, broad, and almost spherical head) are at an increased risk. Breeding for extreme miniaturisation in certain breeds has become very popular in some parts of the world because a huge demand for this oddity is displayed by puppy buyers. So called teacup-sized (pocket-sized) Yorkshire terriers, Miniature Pinschers and Chihuahuas are mostly represented in this category. Besides subfertility, dystocia is common in these breeds. To many breeders of low risk breeds, this chapter may be of little value as their breeds whelp unassisted with little supervision and no interventions. There are however exceptions and breeders are reminded that dystocia is indeed possible in every single breed.

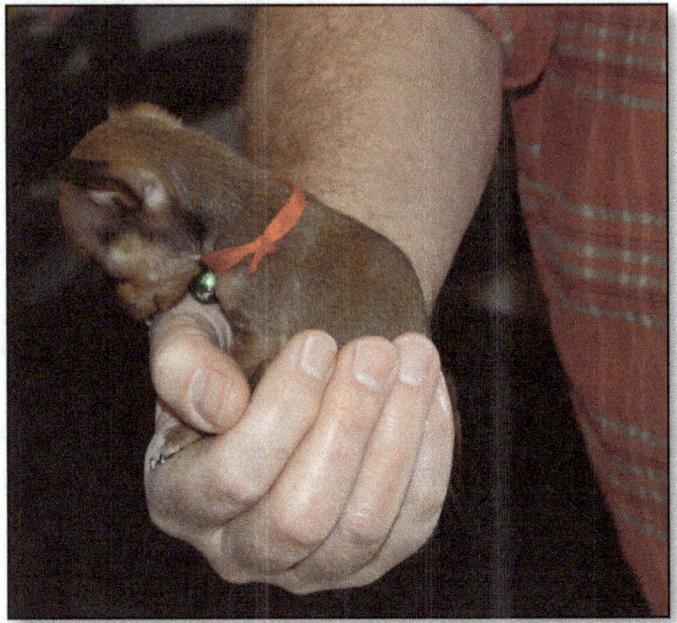

Pocket size puppy of 4 months old as an example of extreme miniaturisation

Dystocia is the inability to pass a foetus through the pelvic canal. The origin can be maternal or foetal. The most common maternal cause is uterine inertia (uterine fatigue) and it is the inability to expel a foetus from the uterus when no obstruction exists. Uterine inertia can be classified to be primary or secondary and or complete or incomplete. Complete primary uterine inertia occurs when

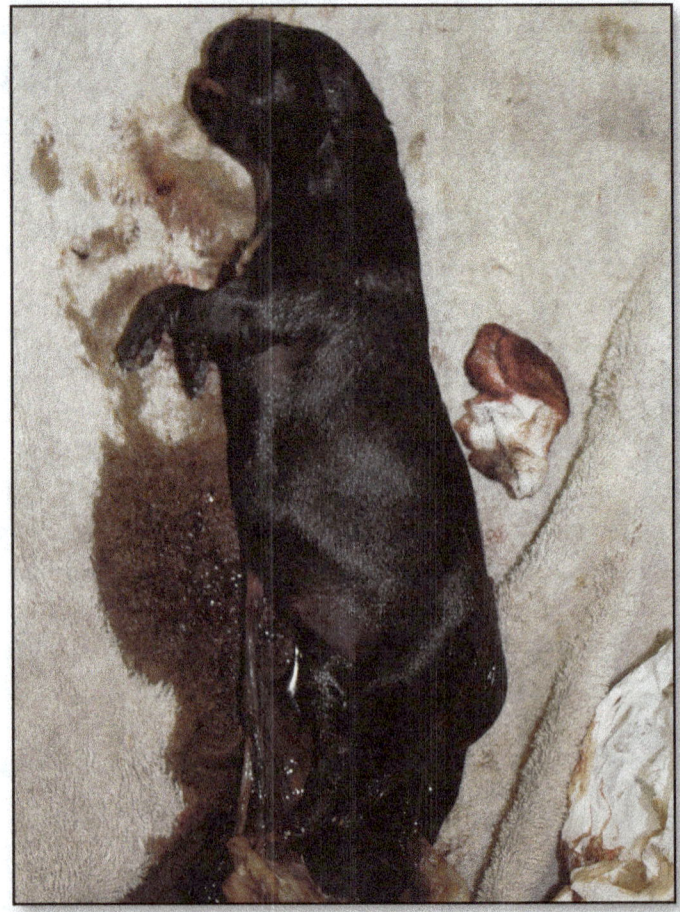

Dead puppy as result of dystocia. Note brown-black fluids surrounding puppy

labour fails to commence and no puppies are delivered. Partial primary uterine inertia is when normal labour is initiated but not all puppies are delivered. Primary uterine inertia can occur because parturition does not commence at all; it usually transpires if a bitch carries a single puppy (singleton). This can be a very frustrating form of dystocia because the bitch does not show any signs of labour, and the breeder is only alerted to the fact that something is amiss when a green or black vaginal discharge is noticed. Dystocia can also set in if the uterine wall is overstretched, as would be the case in bitches which carry large litters. Severe debilitation, obesity, senility and low blood sugar levels (particularly toy breeds) can all contribute to dystocia. Foetal anatomy and changes in the foetus' orientation account for most cases of obstructive dystocia, followed by oversized puppies. For the purposes of this text, dystocia also includes delays in the whelping process which results in poor puppy survival.

8.3.1. Deciding when to intervene

During whelping it is difficult to decide whether intervention is necessary, and more importantly, whether intervention should be medical or surgical. The decision is influenced either by the bitch's response to medical therapy, or what breed of dog it is, or what the breeder's preference is, or perhaps a combination of all three. Intervention is necessary if one or more of the following scenarios are evident:

- Stage two labour lasts more than 2 hours without progress
- More than 2 hours have elapsed between delivery of successive puppies
- The dam shows signs of illness or distress
- More than 20-30 minutes of strong abdominal contractions without delivery of a puppy
- Weak but sustained contractions for more than 2 hours without the birth of a puppy
- Green or black discharge prior to delivery of the first puppy
- Vaginal discharge (water broke) for more than 2 hours and no progress
- Stage 2 labour lasting longer than 8 hours
- Membranes or part of puppy protruding from the vagina and no progress
- Confirmed prolonged gestation

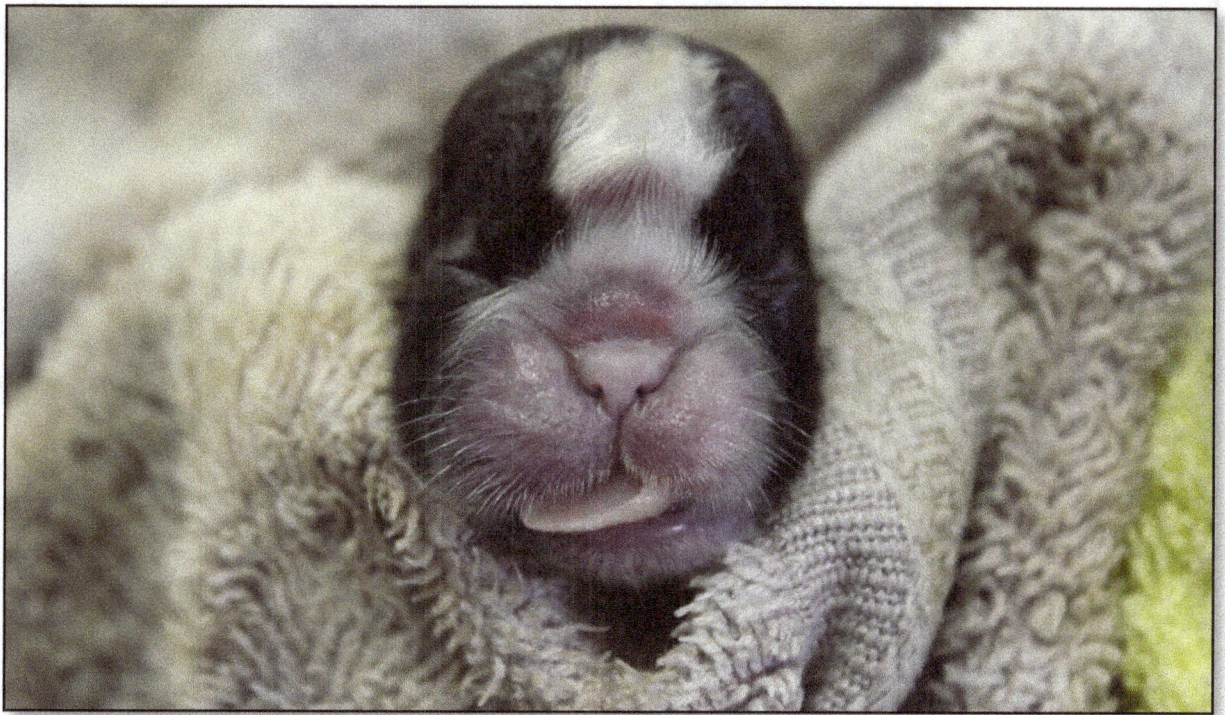

Dystocia pup, note purple colour because of constriction and oxygen defiency in birth canal

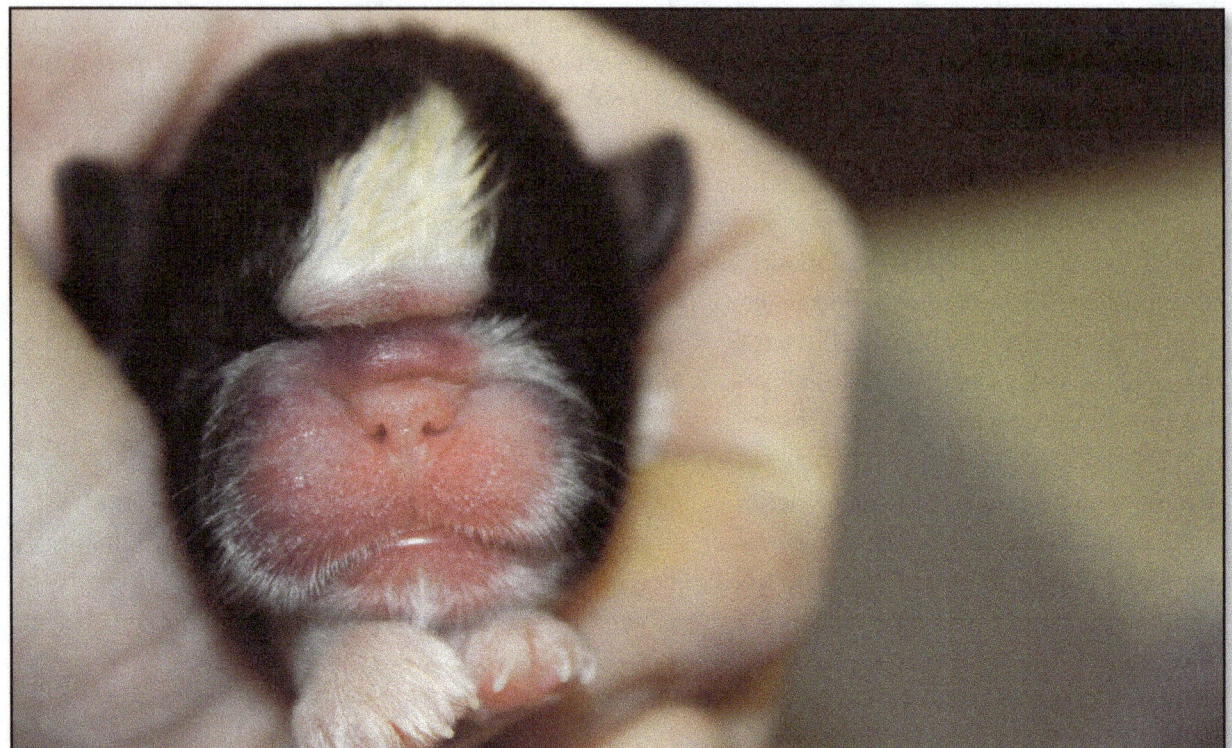
The same dystocia puppy some time later. Note improvement in colour of muzzle from purple to a more healthy pink

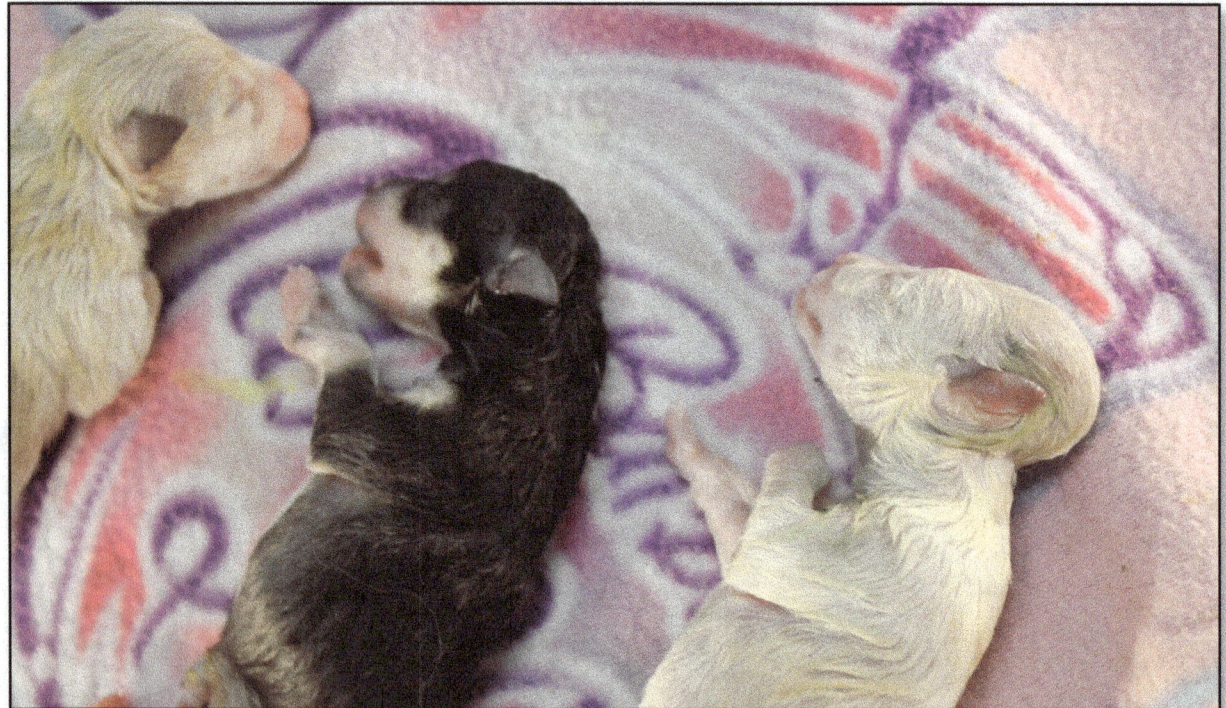
Dystocia led to distortion of puppy's head on right

A veterinary surgeon can assist in this assessment by making use of ultrasonography and or evaluation of the foetal heart rates. Heart rates of 200 beats per minute and above are considered normal; 140–160 beats/minute suggest poor viability if the puppies are not delivered within the next 2–3 hours; and foetal heart rates of less than 120 beats per minute indicate that immediate veterinary intervention is required. There are external monitoring devices available on the market which record uterine activity and foetal heart rates. Their usefulness however requires critical evaluation in controlled scientific studies because their reliability is questioned. Despite this disagreement, some breeders claim that it lowers their rate of stillbirths, and they credit these devices for the early detection of dystocia and foetal compromise. These devices do not have any predictive value and overnight monitoring of late pregnant bitches is therefore not obviated.

Medical management to relieve dystocia is indicated if the dam: is in good health and labour has not been protracted, if the cervix is dilated, if foetal size appears normal and if foetal heart rates are normal. Medical management is contraindicated if obstructive dystocia is present or if there are several foetuses in utero at the time of diagnosis, and it is confirmed that one or more of them are already compromised or dead. Medical treatment of these dystocia cases can lead to either stillborn puppies or delivery of dead puppies by later caesarean section.

8.3.2. Medical management of dystocia

Medical treatment for dystocia is indicated if there is evidence of cervical dilatation, the foetus is not oversized and the foetal heartbeat does not yet signal distress. Oxytocin, calcium gluconate, fluid therapy and glucose remain the cornerstones of medical therapy in dystocia.

8.3.3. Oxytocin and its role in dystocia

Oxytocin is the natural hormone responsible for the stimulation of myometrium (uterine muscles) during delivery and mammary myoepithelial (muscle) cells during lactation. Its release is dependent on the Ferguson-reflex, which is initiated when the foetus transports into the cervical canal. Digital stimulation of the dorsal vaginal wall might also stimulate uterine contractions. Oxytocin is probably the most common ecbolic (drug promoting uterine contractions) used (usually abused) by breeders to aid labour. Oxytocin is a drug best used in veterinary practice because if it is administered the progress of labour and foetal compromise must be monitored and this can only be done effectively, in a veterinary hospital. For this reason, Oxytocin cannot be used by breeders merely to speed up the whelping process, during normal labour. However, in the right hands and under the correct conditions, oxytocin is an effective drug to augment labour. Excessive oxytocin use is, however, counterproductive; it further compromises foetuses which had no realistic chance of being delivered normally in the first place. It is also known to cause uterine rupture in unproductive labour. A bitch which is already violently contracting does not need oxytocin treatment; in fact it will do more harm than good.

It is, however, a fact that breeders gain access to oxytocin and that they do use it during the whelping process. Breeders must not administer oxytocin if the bitch has weak contractions or none at all. Oxytocin can be repeated after 30-40 minutes if there is no evidence of an obstruction. If foetal survival is not very important, a third injection can be administered, following a rest period of one hour. If a bitch does not response to oxytocin therapy, a caesarean section may be indicated.

Oxytocin might indeed be beneficial in controlling post-partum uterine haemorrhage. Many breeders have successfully used oxytocin as a so called "clean out" injection after whelping and they claim that it helps control post whelp haemorrhaging, the induction of milk let-down, and the improvement of maternal care and prevention of post whelp uterine infections.

8.3.4. Calcium gluconate

Calcium ions must be present in all muscles before contraction can take place. In the medical management of dystocia it was found that far better results were achieved when calcium was administered together with oxytocin. The diagnosis of hypocalcaemia is not always practical but since the subcutaneous administration of therapeutic doses of calcium gluconate is safe, it can be given alongside oxytocin in most, if not all, cases of uterine inertia, provided it is done under veterinary supervision or instruction.

8.3.5. Glucose

Most bitches have normal blood glucose levels during normal labour. However, hypoglycaemia, as a cause of dystocia (primary inertia) in toy breeds, is well documented. Within these breeds, individuals which have a very low fat percentage and low muscle mass, can rapidly deplete all their glucose reserves and become hypoglycaemic. The effect of medical treatment should be the resumption of normal labour and the delivery of healthy puppies, preferably in quick succession. If this does not happen breeders are encouraged to seek veterinary intervention. In the end, the decision whether to surgically intervene or not should be based on a risk benefit assessment. The breeder and veterinary surgeon must also be in agreement that surgical intervention is the best course of action.

8.3.6. Traction on foetuses

Breeders must be warned that the manipulation of a foetus can jeopardize its survival. If the survival of the foetus is paramount, a caesarean section is the better option. A foetus should only be pulled if parts of it are visible from outside the vaginal opening. Gentle traction on the foetus is required to speed up delivery as the foetus is likely to die within minutes of appearing at the vaginal opening, if its umbilicus is constricted in the birth canal. In other cases, if just the head is protruding, the puppy may remain alive for quite some time. The use of whelping forceps is not advised and should only be used by those who are experienced and familiar with its use. It will be difficult to remove a puppy which has been stuck for a long time, without dismembering a limb or even beheading it.

Chapter 9

Caesarean Section in the Bitch

9.1. Indications for caesarean sections

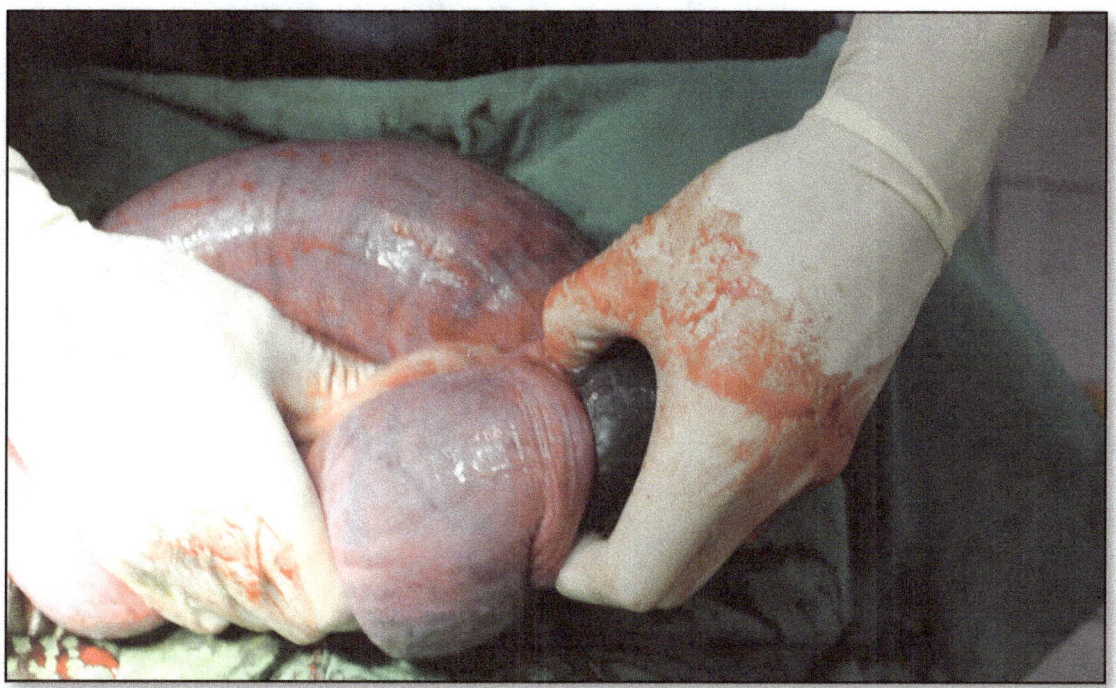
Puppy delivered by caesarean section

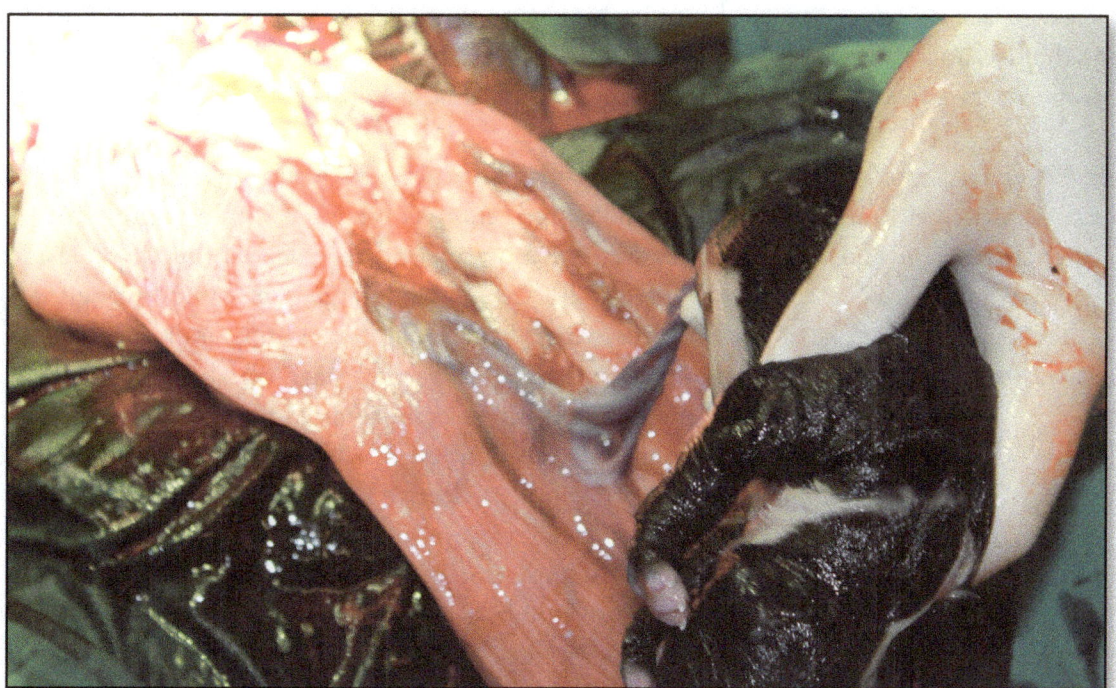
Puppy delivered by caesarean section

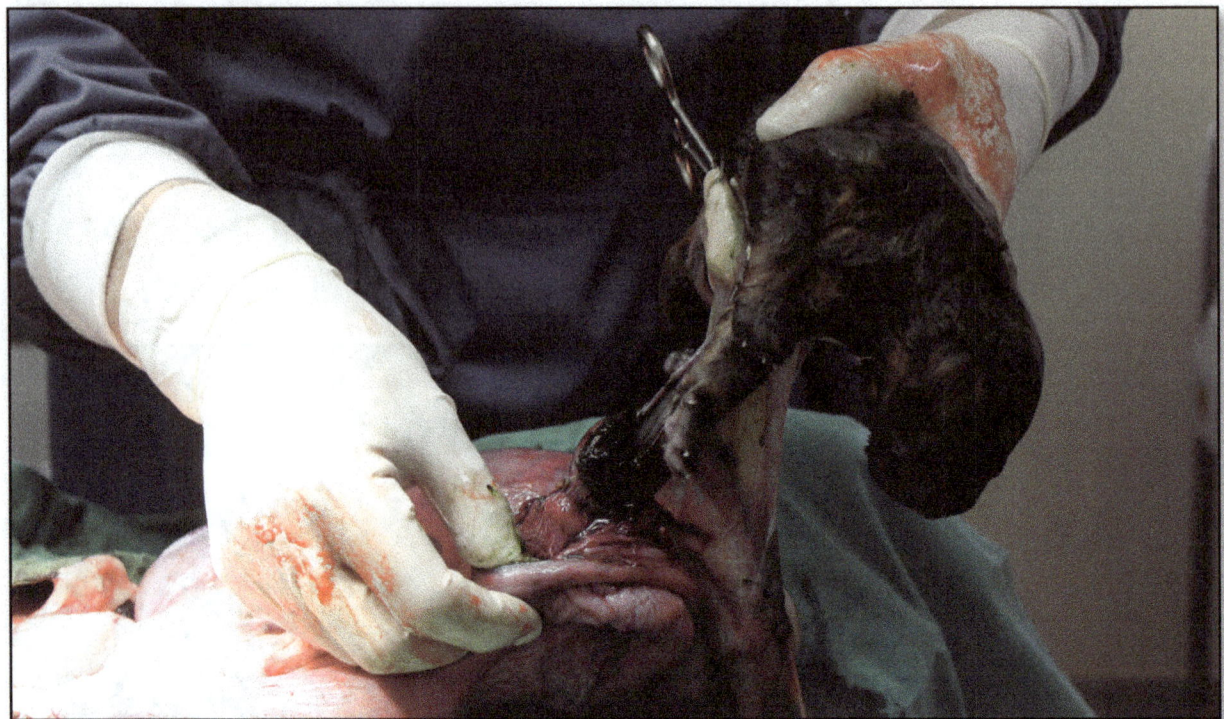
Puppy being delivered by caesarean section

9.1.1. Dystocia as indication for caesarean section

Labour difficulties related to uterine inertia that are unresponsive to medical management and foetal distress are the two main indicators for CS. Experienced dog breeders sometimes prefer CS over medical management and its potential for puppy losses. They feel that they would rather pay for a CS, whether it is indicated or not, and have live puppies than two veterinary bills; one for medical treatment and another for a CS, with a number of dead puppies in tow. Others favour a more conservative approach, in a sense, a minimalistic approach to intervention. Given a choice, these breeders will always choose medical intervention over surgical intervention. However, to a large extent, the decision whether to perform a caesarean section or not will be influenced by a bitch's whelping history as well as the breed of the dog and the circumstances at the time.

In cases where medical treatment has failed to resolve obstructive dystocia, there is no choice other than CS. In the case of uterine inertia, the decision is more complex. Considering that more than 60% of dystocia's end up with caesarean sections anyway, and that delays due to failed medical management, might lead to an increase in foetal losses, a strong argument can be made for CS at the earliest indication of dystocia, in breeds which are prone to it. Puppy mortality increases if time is wasted on ineffective medical management in the second stage of labour. Also, there are many bitches of high risk breeds, that might already have compromised foetuses in the early stages of labour. These puppies can only be rescued by timeous performance of a CS. The fact that more puppies are delivered alive when CS is performed on an elective basis rather than on an emergency basis, illustrates the point. This is an important point to consider and certainly supports performing elective CS in dystocia prone breeds and high risk pregnancies. Not all theriogenologists will agree on this but at least in the hands of the author, better results are obtained performing an early CS rather than attempting medical treatment first. This is particularly true in high risk pregnancies where prevalence of complications is likely to be higher than that of the general obstetrical population. The

English bulldog is an example of such a breed. In this breed the risk of dystocia which is detrimental to both the maternal and perinatal health is extremely high. Properly planned CS is a safe and effective treatment but, of course, not without risk. The advances that are being made to improve the accuracy and precision with which whelping dates can be predicted will likely, in the very near future enable veterinary surgeons to plan preterm caesarean sections before foetal compromise occurs.

9.1.2. Singleton pregnancies

The bitch with the singleton (carrying a single puppy) presents a serious challenge to both breeders and veterinary surgeons. This is because bitches which carry singleton litters frequently do not enter labour on the due date. They frequently go over term and the puppies die without the bitch showing any signs of labour (prolonged pregnancy). Indeed, in some cases, the breeder might not have known that the bitch was pregnant in the first place and will only suspect that something is amiss, when vaginal discharges are noticed. Singleton pregnancies in large breeds are more likely not to progress normally when compared to small breeds. The foetuses in these singleton pregnancies are not necessarily oversized.

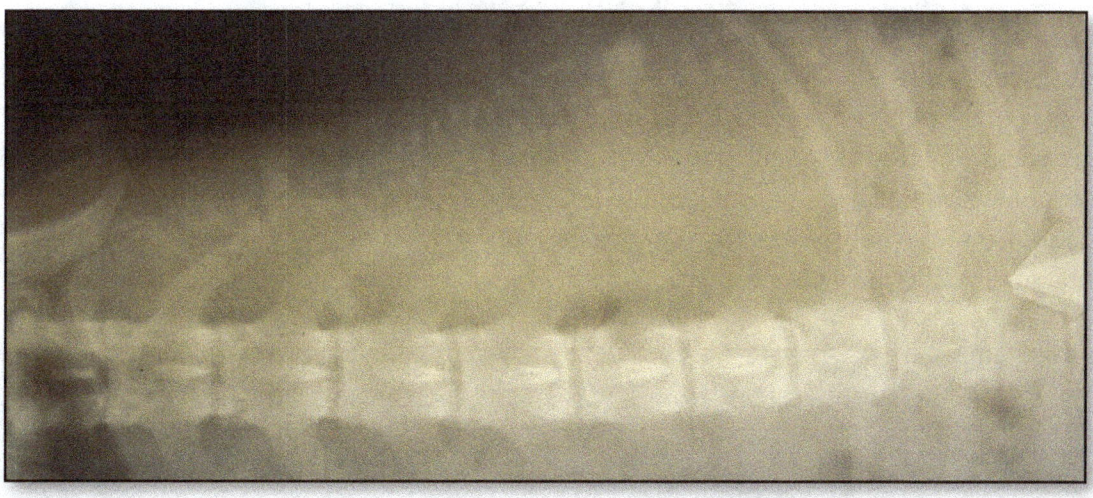

Singleton puppy

An increased gestation length is reported in bitches which carry singletons and a significantly higher incidence of whelping problems occur in large breed bitches with litters of 1 or 2 foetuses. The exact reason why certain singleton pregnancies fail to progress in a normal way and others not is unknown. It is useful to know whether a pregnancy is a singleton pregnancy or not. Singleton pregnancies are high risk pregnancies and this knowledge compels the breeder and the veterinary surgeon to be more vigilant when the whelping date draws closer.

Knowing that singleton pregnancies are high risk, breeders can decide, either to monitor the pregnancy themselves and hope for a normal birth or to monitor the bitch until she shows early signs of labour and then to present the bitch for an immediate caesarean section. Veterinary surgeons who are willing to assist breeders with the management of singleton pregnancy should only do so if they are familiar with singleton parturition management and if they have regular after hour access to the bitch, which in essence means that the bitch will have to be hospitalised. Singleton parturition management involves regular vaginoscopic examinations to look for early signs of cervical dilatation, signs of increased uterine tone, signs of discomfort, increased respiration rate and subtle abdominal contractions. If available, progesterone assay to determine progesterone concentrations may also be useful. Nevertheless, more research is required to establish the correct way to safely manage singleton pregnancies. Although skilled veterinary surgeons will save many singleton puppies, it is inevitable that some will die. This is because in many instances the bitch is not presented on time for an emergency caesarean section.

9.1.3. Prolonged pregnancy

Prolonged pregnancy can be defined as a pregnancy which goes over term without any signs of labour at term. Many pregnancies are considered to be "over term" by breeders when in actual fact, they are not. With the exception of singleton pregnancies, true prolonged pregnancies are very rare indeed. The danger exists that breeders might insist on a caesarean section because they suspect a prolonged pregnancy. If an inexperienced veterinary surgeon concedes to such a request, the delivery of non-viable premature puppies result. Prolonged pregnancy can only be diagnosed if reliable methods to time ovulation were employed. In confirmed cases, immediate caesarean section is advised.

9.2. Complications of caesarean sections

Caesarean sections are not without risk. Knowledge of the risks involved is essential in order to perform a risk-benefit assessment. The survival rate of puppies delivered by CS and those born naturally (in the absence of dystocia) are more or less the same, at around 83%. The figure is somewhat lower (75%) in brachycephalic breeds. Complications of a caesarean section normally relate to the timing of the intervention, anaesthesia and the surgery itself. Clearly, if puppies are removed long before the due date, the outcome can only be premature non-viable puppies and possibly serious haemorrhaging of the placental sites. An ill-timed CS intervention can prove deadly for both the puppies and the dam.

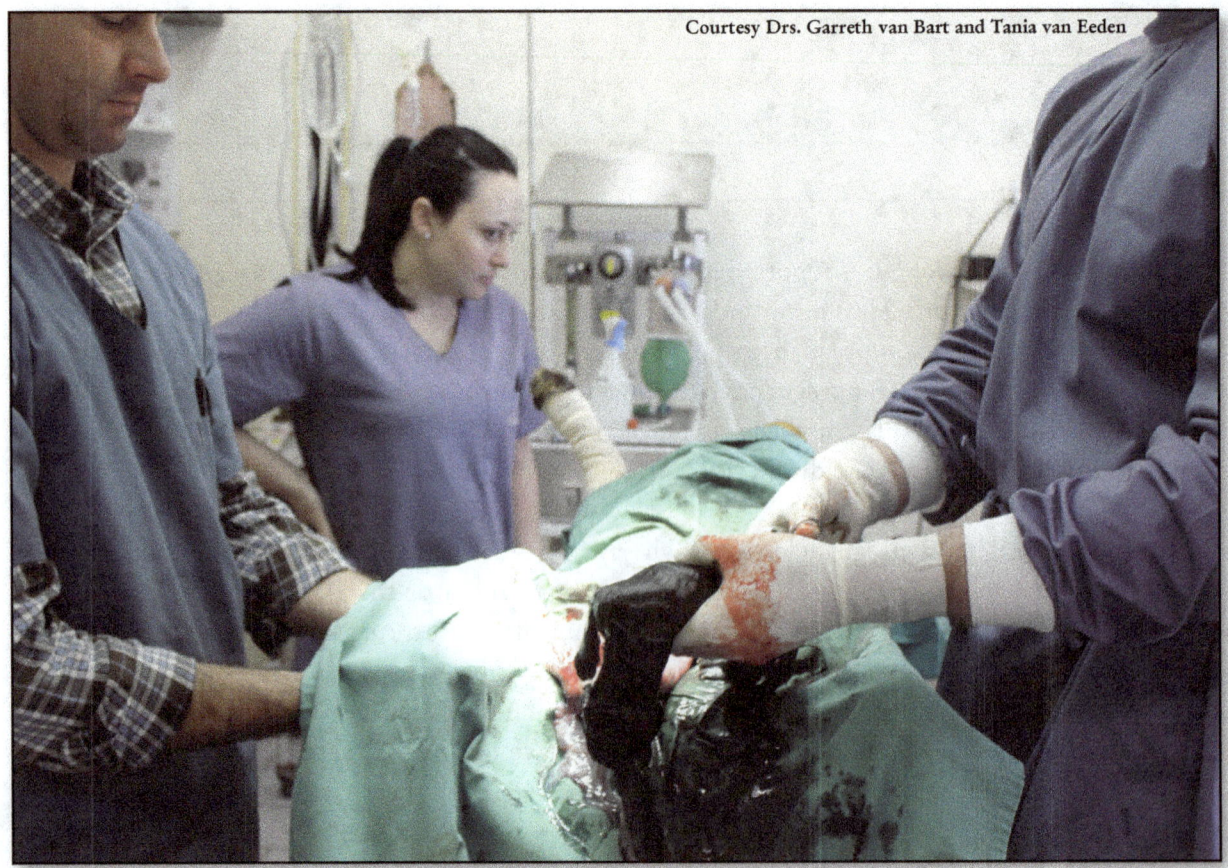

Team is required to perform a caesarean section in the bitch

Whether the placenta should be removed or not requires discussion. It is general practice in some veterinary teaching hospitals to leave the placenta and to ligate the umbilical cord. Others remove the placenta, but only if the placenta is already partially released and easily dislodged. The reason why placentas are left intact is motivated by a concern that post-operative haemorrhaging of the placental sites might occur if the placentas are removed. Some veterinary surgeons prefer to remove the placentas to avoid the risk of retained placentas and endometritis which might ensue. It is the author's experience that placentas detach easily and that haemorrhaging is not a problem when the CS is carefully timed. Leaving placentas in the author's experience leads to the development of post-operative endometritis and toxic milk syndrome in at least some cases.

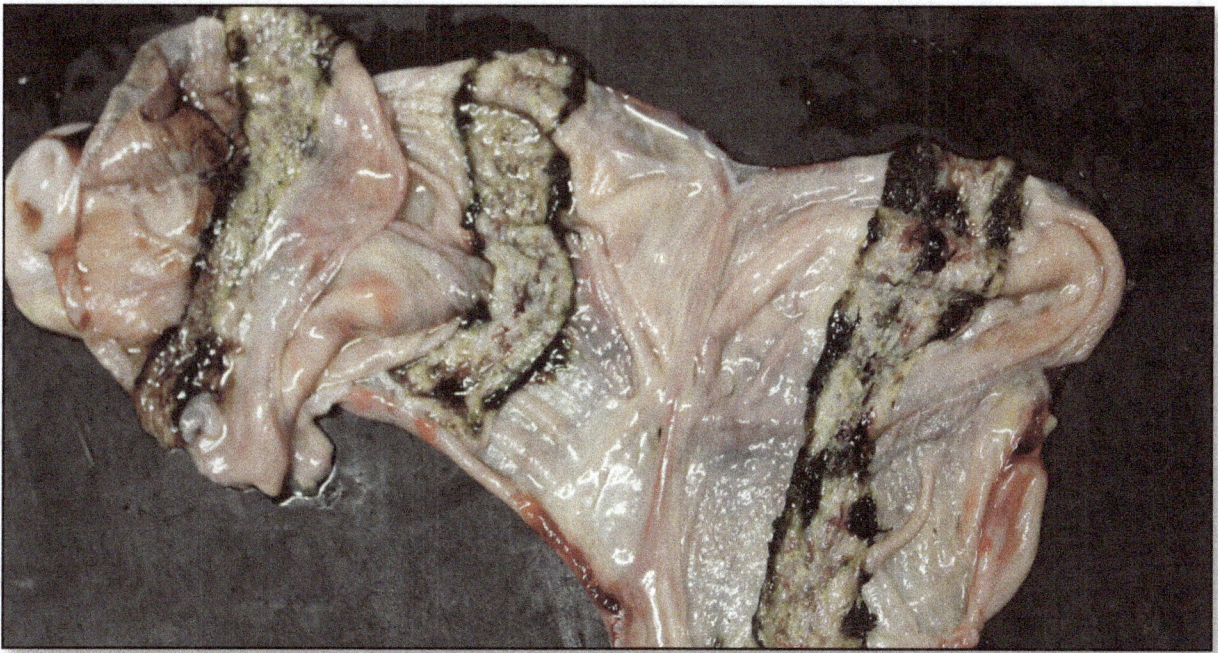

Inside of the uterus reveals three placental sites. The number of placental sites correspond with the number of foetuses (in most cases) and the placental site count may be used in cases where there is a dispute about the number of puppies delivered

With the advent of modern anaesthetic agents and its synergistic use with pain killers and sedatives, anaesthetic risk is truly minimal but not totally absent. Breeders are made aware that a veterinary hospital should, at the very least, be equipped with a gas inhalation anaesthetic machine and good monitoring equipment before caesarean sections are attempted. Haemorrhaging at the time of CS requires blood transfusions and may even require emergency spaying if it spirals out of control. Wound site infection, wound dehiscence, herniation, evisceration and bitch fatalities are also a potential threat. Up to 1% fatalities due to CS complications have been recorded. All this must be taken into consideration before a decision to do a caesarean section is taken.

Whether a bitch is spayed during the caesarean section does not appear to affect the puppy's survival or lactation. It is not known whether consecutive caesarean sections reduce the fertility of a bitch. Although a decrease in litter size is usually observed after consecutive caesarean sections, it might be due to advancing age and not necessarily the fact that consecutive caesarean sections were performed. Many bitches have undergone in excess of four caesarean sections without any adverse effects. A caesarean section increases the likelihood that a bitch will require another caesarean section in subsequent pregnancies, nevertheless it is quite possible for a bitch to whelp normally even if her previous litter was delivered by caesarean section. However, breeders should keep a close eye on such bitches during whelping. In general, experienced veterinary surgeons will be quicker to intervene surgically if there is a history of caesarean sections. This is because clinical experience shows that a delay in the whelping process is more likely to result in bitches that have had CS before and puppy fatalities are more likely in them.

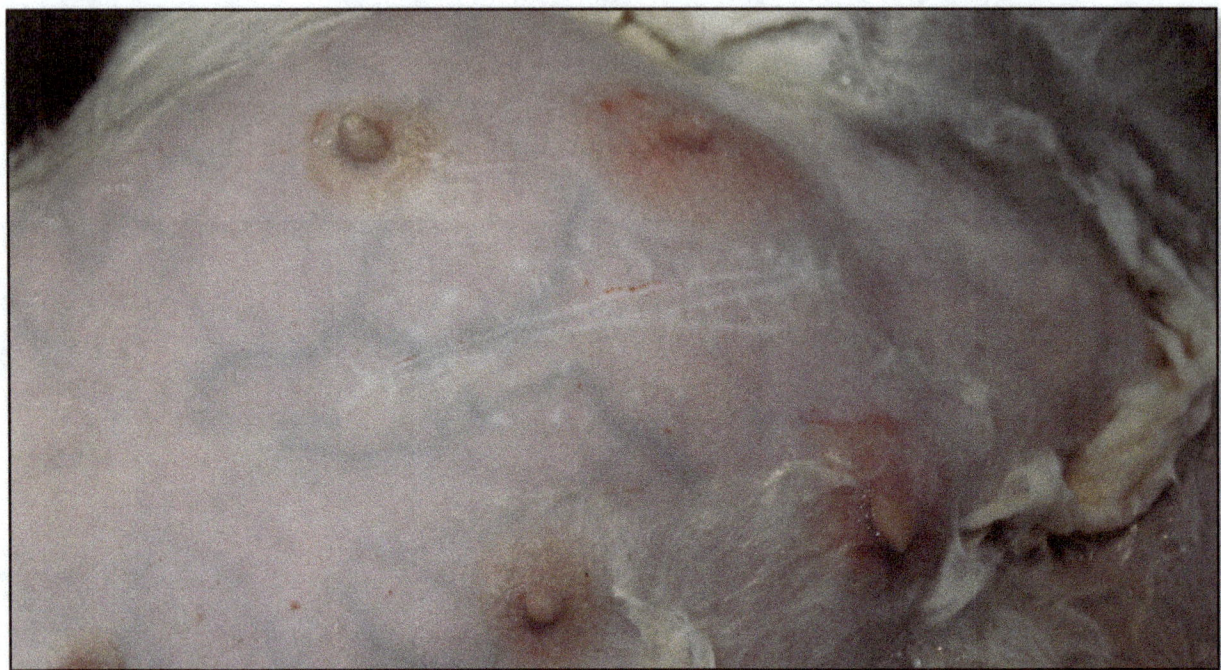

Three scars from previous caesarean sections are clearly visible on this bitch's abdomen whilst being prepped for her fourth caesarean section

9.3. Post-operative care

Although post-operative care is primarily a veterinary matter, this discussion is necessary because breeders will in all probability have to assist their veterinary surgeons if intervention is required after-hours. This assistance is welcome, especially if the intervention takes place at an hour when veterinary support staff members are off-duty.

Post-operative care of the bitch is crucial because fatalities usually occur within 12 hours of surgery. After the completion of surgery, the bitch must be monitored with the endotracheal tube in place. When the coughing reflex returns the tube can be removed. At this stage increased vigilance is important, particularly in brachiocephalic breeds. In these breeds it might be necessary to pull on the tongue or to hold its mouth open until the bitch is fully awake and breathing is unrestricted. Intubation and anaesthesia can cause a swelling in the airways and restrict already narrowed airways even further, which can result in hypoxia and even death.

Direct visual monitoring in the recovery room is vital even if the bitch is fully awake. Respiration rate, mucous membrane colour and capillary refill time should be continuously assessed during this time. Fluid therapy (drip) should continue until the bitch is haemodynamically stable. The bitch must be checked for post-operative haemorrhage and if the bitch is stable and ambulatory (able to walk and move around), she may be discharged into the care of the breeder. This is usually about 2 hours following surgery. The breeder should only place the puppies with the bitch once she has settled into her nursing quarters and is aware of the puppies.

Some anaesthetic protocols involve epidural anaesthesia, sedatives and post-operative pain control, all of which can affect the bitch's motor skills and therefore her ability to avoid injuring her puppies. It is important that the breeder remains present for a period of time, at least for as long as it takes to ensure that the puppies are safe from injury and that the dam calmly performs her nursing duties.

9.4. Resuscitative aids in neonates following caesarean section

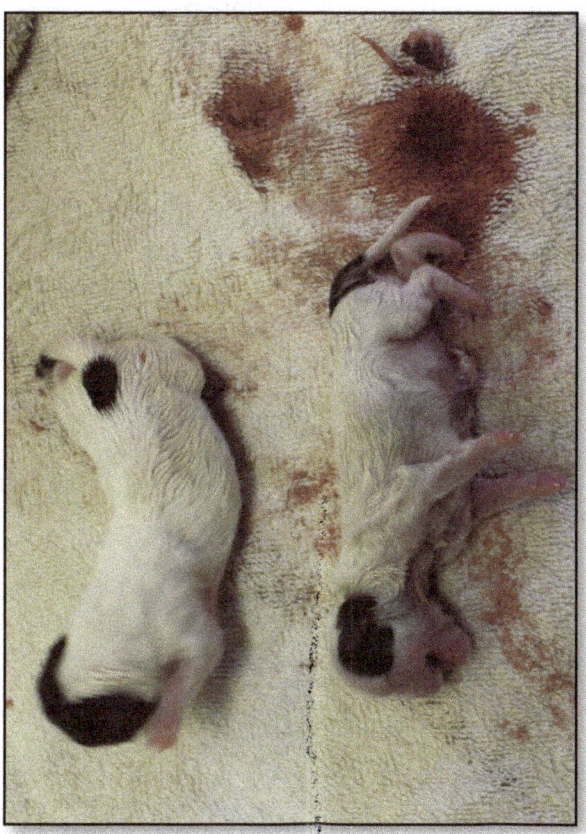
Strong puppies vocalising and moving at birth

It is important to ensure that the puppies breathe immediately after birth. Strong puppies will breathe easily, cry and move around within minutes after natural birth or delivery by CS. The factors that can influence vigour in puppies which were delivered by caesarean section are, either: dystocia and associated poor oxygen delivery to the foetus before the caesarean section was performed, or the use of cardio-respiratory suppressive anaesthetic protocols, or the inadequate execution of resuscitation techniques following the birth, or a combination of all three. The resuscitation techniques involve clearing the airways of fluids and drying the puppies whilst also rubbing the thoracic wall. There are resuscitative drugs which stimulate respiration and increases cardiac output, but their routine use is questioned. Specific drugs which reverse the effects of the anaesthetic agent are indicated and very helpful in initiating and restoring normal cardiorespiratory function in the puppy.

9.5. Concepts which require explanation relevant to size of puppies

9.5.1. Synchrony of ovulation

In poliovular species, (species which normally have several offspring in one litter) such as the dog, the question may arise over what timeframe ovulation occurs. If this time frame was very long it may follow that puppies of different gestational age may be born in the same litter. If this time frame is very short then ovulation may be considered a synchronous affair. Synchrony of ovulation in the dog needs be discussed and should convince the reader that differences in puppy size or apparent maturity and/or gestational stage has little to do with ova presumably having been released at so vastly different times to account for different sizes and apparent puppy maturity or lack thereof. Numerous studies concluded that ovulation in the bitch occurs over a period of 24-48 hours. For all practical purposes, it may be assumed that all puppies within a litter are of identical gestational age. The difference in puppy sizes in the same litter may be explained in most cases by genetic variation or other factors.

9.5.2. Prematurity

Prematurity refers to offspring born before they were full term. Estimation of neonatal maturity is based on the subjective assessment of the amount and extent of hair cover on the face, paws and trunk. The ear appears to be the last part to be covered by hair during foetal development. Puppies that have clear evidence of hair on their ears should be considered full term and the ones without are not. Premature puppies are usually weak and have difficulty breathing. The extremities of premature puppies appear redder, and the toe nails more prominent than for puppies born at full term. Because there is an accelerated growth rate towards the end of gestation in dogs, premature puppies may be significantly smaller than full term puppies even if they only differ by a couple of days. In the absence of accurate parturition dates, it is not possible to categorically confirm that a litter is full term.

9.5.3. Dysmaturity

If it is assumed that ovulation is almost a synchronised affair (meaning all eggs are released almost simultaneously, this within 24-48 hours), all the puppies in a litter should be of similar age. Breeders often make the erroneous assumption that if a bitch was mated twice, let's say 6 days apart, and the resulting litter had 2 puppies which were slightly smaller and 4 bigger, that the big puppies were from

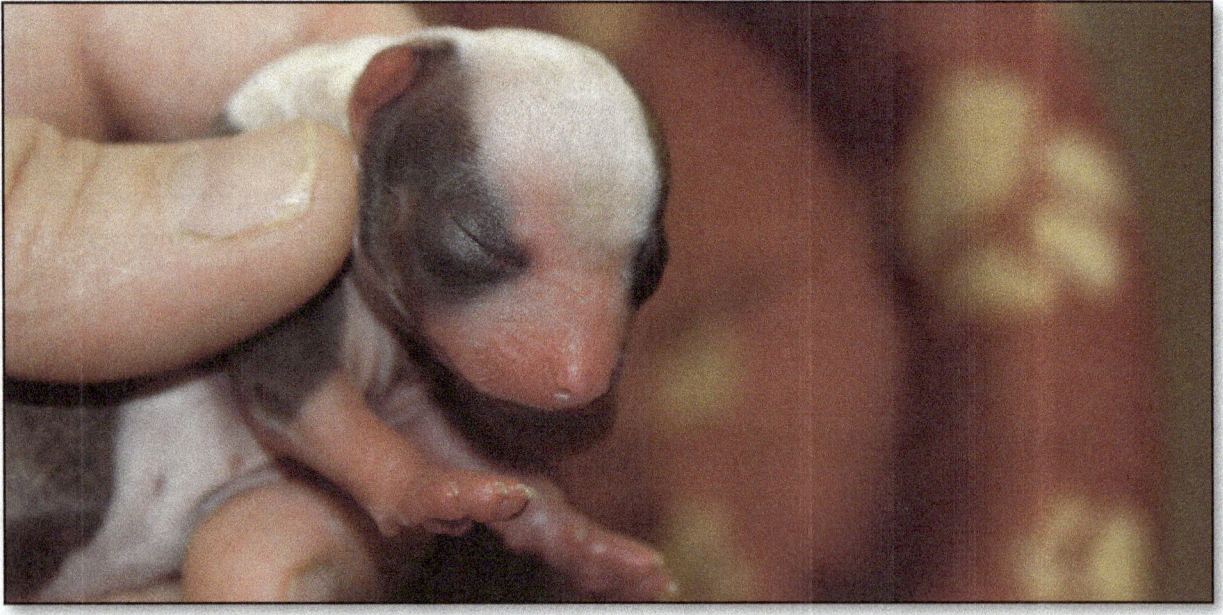
Premature puppy, note lack of hair on face and feet

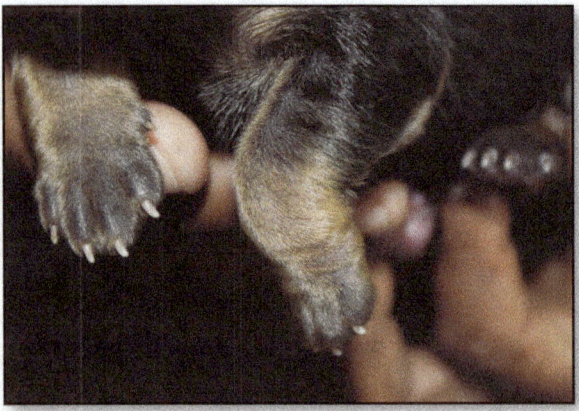 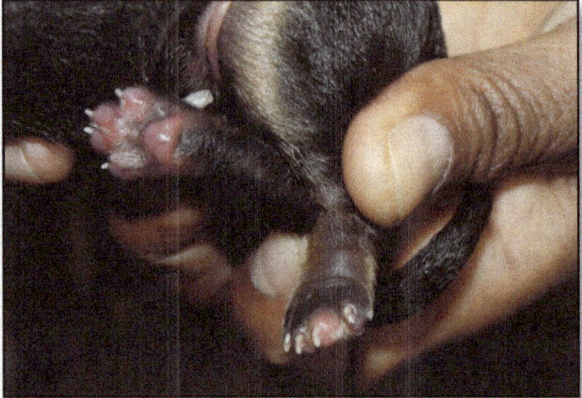
Hair coverage on feet indicating full maturity

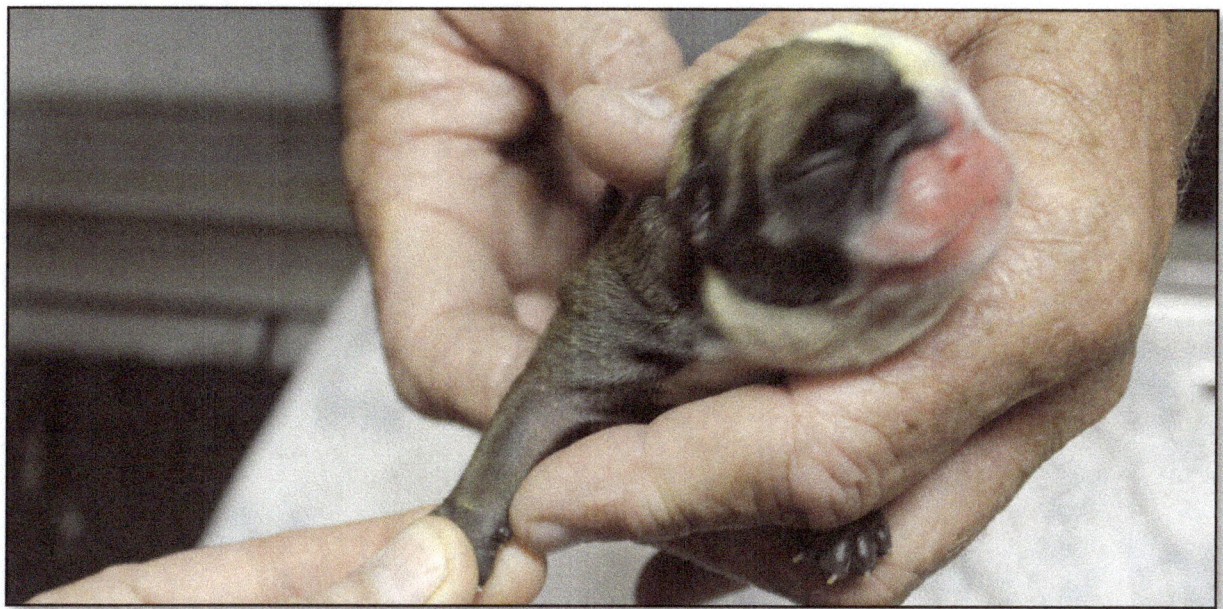
Hair coverage on feet indicating full maturity

the first mating and the smaller ones from the last mating. This misconception is commonly affirmed by the fact that these very same smaller puppies may indeed look less mature than the bigger ones judged by hair coverage. This phenomenon is explained as follows. These puppies are of identical age but did not develop at the same rate as their litter mates because of some factor that impaired the oxygen or nutrient supply of the smaller immature looking puppies. These puppies are also not premature because they were born in the presence of full term puppies so they must have spent the same time in the womb. These small and immature looking puppies are termed dysmature puppies (not fully developed but yet full term).

9.5.4. Superfoetation (pregnancy with foetuses of different age)

Superfoetation occurs when a pregnant female, already carrying one or more live foetuses, is bred again, on another heat cycle and a second conception occurs. Although this is frequently reported in ruminants (which have 3 week intervals between heats) it has never been reported in the bitch and is probably not possible in canines. In species where superfoetation is possible, the female animal which is already confirmed pregnant has another cycle a few weeks later, another ovum is released and fertilised, and the animal is pregnant for a second time with another offspring, albeit at a different stage of development. This is known as superfoetation.

9.5.5. Runts

Runts are smaller than average puppies, are weaker, grow slower, mature slower and usually are in poor condition. Most runts usually present as disadvantaged puppies from the first day they are born. On the other hand, some look quite normal at birth and then gradually deteriorate and become runts. Many litters, particularly large litters, include a runt, the causes of which are not clear. The size disparity frequently becomes exaggerated as time goes by because the stronger litter mates push the weakling aside in their attempts to get to the teats. As a result, the runt consumes fewer nutrients, which stunts growth even further. With extra attention, and provided a runt does not suffer from a congenital defect, the puppy will frequently show compensatory growth and catch up with its litter mates. More commonly, though, these puppies fail to thrive and they die before weaning, despite

Chapter 9 Caesarean Section in the Bitch

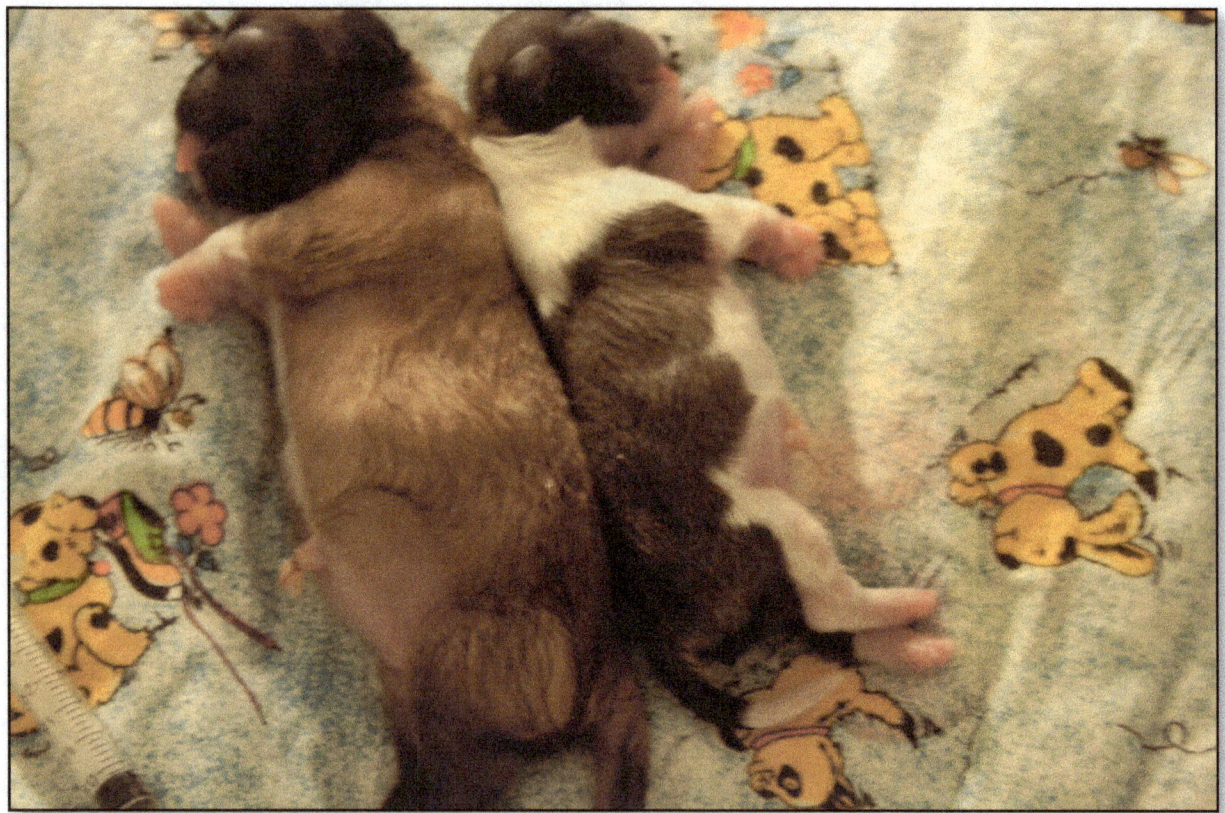
Huge difference in size between these littermates is already visible immediately after birth

nursing and veterinary efforts. Runts should not be confused with dysmature or premature puppies. They are distinguishable in that they are born mature, with all their hair present, and then start showing ill thrift and poor growth later on.

9.5.6. Twinning
Unlike humans, dogs are a polytocous species (species which have more than one offspring in a litter) and so heterozygous offspring within a litter is the rule. Homozygous twins (identical twins) are twin offspring which are formed when an embryo splits in two. Although breeders claim to have found two puppies in one sack, and consequently suspect that twinning has taken place, it has not yet been proven scientifically. Puppies that do indeed share foetal membranes are not necessarily identical twins. If homozygous twinning does indeed occur in dogs, it is likely to be confirmed sometime in the near future through DNA profiling. To date, no scientifically confirmed twins have been reported.

9.5.7. Sharing of placentas
The author has photographic evidence of puppies which shared a placenta and gestational membranes. This has not yet been reported in scientific literature. In this specific case, the puppies were of different gender and therefore the possibility of identical twins is excluded. It is assumed that this finding is extremely rare. Furthermore, such finding is probably only possible when puppies are delivered by CS. During normal birth, once the puppy advances into the birth canal, the umbilical cord is likely to tear away from the sibling and the bitch is likely to detach the puppies from each other, when she bites open the sack and starts to clean them. The sharing of placentas has oddity value more than anything else. It does however show that the number of puppies is not necessarily equal to

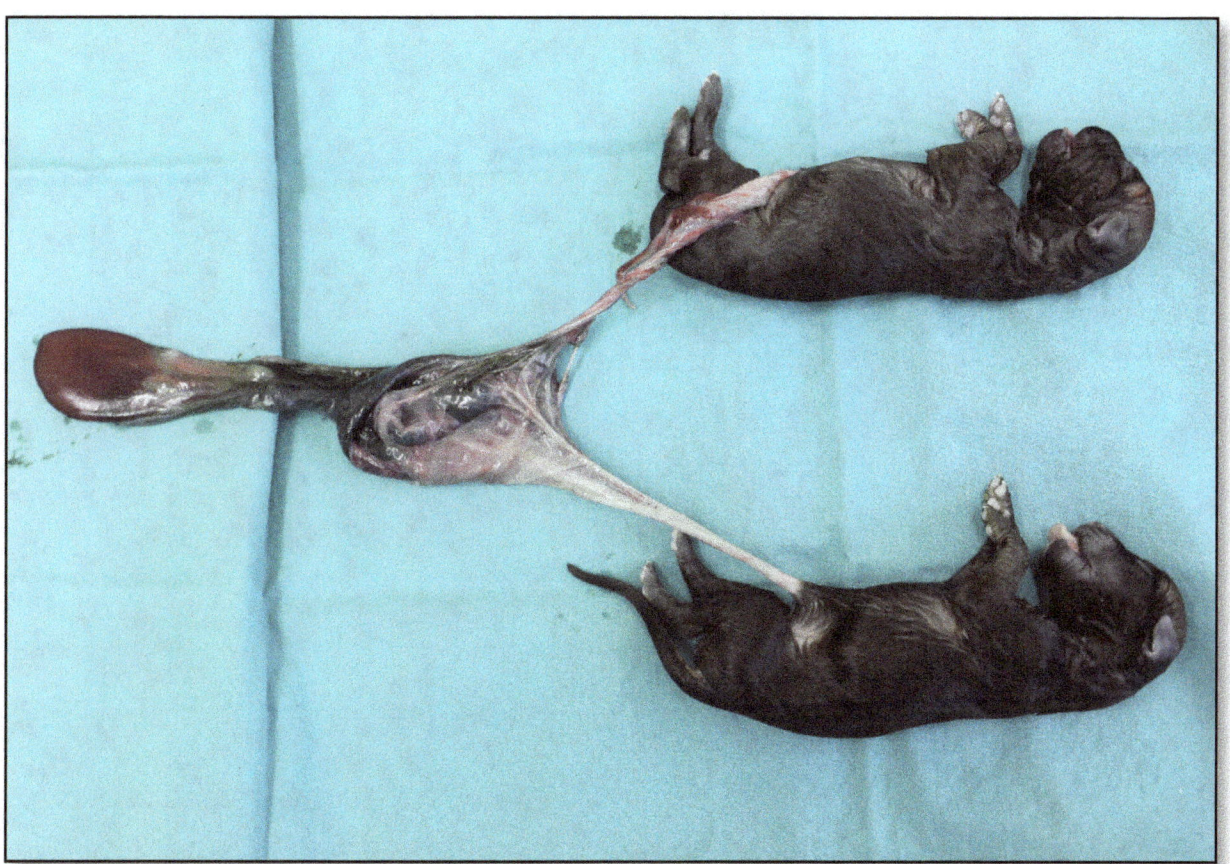

Puppies sharing placentas which indicates that identical twins may be possible in dogs but is still under investigation

the number of placentas or placental attachment sites. There can be more puppies than placentas or placental attachment sites in dogs. The genetics of puppies which share a placenta are currently under investigation and the possibility that they are mosaics is not excluded.

Chapter 9 Caesarean Section in the Bitch

Chapter 10

Reproduction in the Male

10.1. Puberty in males and age of first breeding

Puberty signals the beginning of the stage of the animal's life when reproduction is first possible. Factors affecting puberty include nutrition, environment and breed. Similar to the bitch, on average, males reach puberty at the age of 7-12 months for small to medium breeds (extremes are 6-24 months) and 12-18 months for larger breeds. Clearly poor nutrition and suboptimal condition (bodyweight) will delay puberty. The presence of dominant individuals and hierarchal status of the male can influence both testosterone levels as well as onset of puberty in some species. In nature, in many species, it makes sense that in the presence of a strong dominant male, a younger male's puberty be delayed. This is nature's way of protecting the younger males from attack and allows the young male to fully develop and minimise risk of mortal danger and injury before challenging or threatening the dominant male. In a dog colony it is speculated that the presence of a dominant individual may delay puberty by a short while, suppress testosterone levels in postpubertal males and suppress exhibition of normal libido and mating behaviour of subordinate males in proximity of dominant individuals.

Most males will display sexual interest at an age earlier than onset of puberty. Thus the age at which the young male puppies start exhibiting sexual interest does not always coincide with sexual maturity and presence of optimal number of mature sperm in their ejaculate. This does not mean that an over-zealous six-month-old puppy is "safe" to mate as he may very well surprise the breeder by siring a large litter with his sister. It just means that many breeders erroneously assume that if their young prospective stud puppy starts showing sexual interest, it will necessarily be sexually mature.

It is not harmful if a young prepubertal male ejaculates and this will not compromise future fertility. It is advised that breeders have any prospective stud checked to confirm presence of mature sperm in adequate number before they start using them on their own and other bitches.

10.2. Spermatogenesis

Spermatogenesis is the process of sperm (seed) genesis (production) and this process occurs within the testicles. The process starts off with the stem cells (spermatogonia) which multiply to provide the precursors of sperm. Spermatocytes result from meiosis which is a process of division which results in the production of haploid cells from diploid cells. In the final steps of development they acquire a tail and cap and are released in the seminiferous tubules as sperm. The entire process takes about 6-8 weeks. This has important implications. Spermatogenesis occurs at a few degrees less than body temperature in the dog and most mammals. This lowering of temperature is achieved by the testicles which are situated outside the body in a scrotum which has its unique temperature regulation mechanisms. A fever caused by a disease or condition will affect the entire generation of future sperm and it may take 6-8 weeks after the fever bout, for the stud's sperm count to return to where it was originally.

The sperm is genetically different from the body and the latter may identify it as foreign. This is why the sperm reside in a tubular structure which is isolated from the immune system via the blood-testis barrier. If this barrier becomes compromised through trauma or inflammation, the body may produce antibodies against its own sperm which may lead to infertility.

Spermatogenesis is a continuous process and there are always a given number of sperm in production. Sperm production should be viewed as a production line in a factory. The sperm travel from the testis to the epididymis where part of the development of the sperm takes place and it also acts as a temporary storage vesicle for a limited number of sperm. As the sperm is produced it slowly moves through the tubules of the epididymis. Sperm which is not ejaculated may end up in the bladder and some dead sperm is resorbed in the epididymis. If a dog has not ejaculated within the week or so before semen collection, there might be sufficient dead sperm in the ejaculate to negatively impact on the quality of the sample. Therefore it is advised that the collection be repeated on the same day or following day. This may improve the quality of the sample and is important when collecting semen for purposes of semen evaluation, semen storage and artificial insemination using chilled or fresh semen.

There is not an exact time period that spermatogenesis arrests. Although it is true that both men and dogs can produce offspring into advanced age, it is also true that their semen quality may start deteriorating and in many cases spermatogenesis may even arrest. As a rule it may be said that semen quality may start to decline in older studs (eight and older) but there are certainly examples of older dogs with very good semen quality.

10.3. Vasectomization

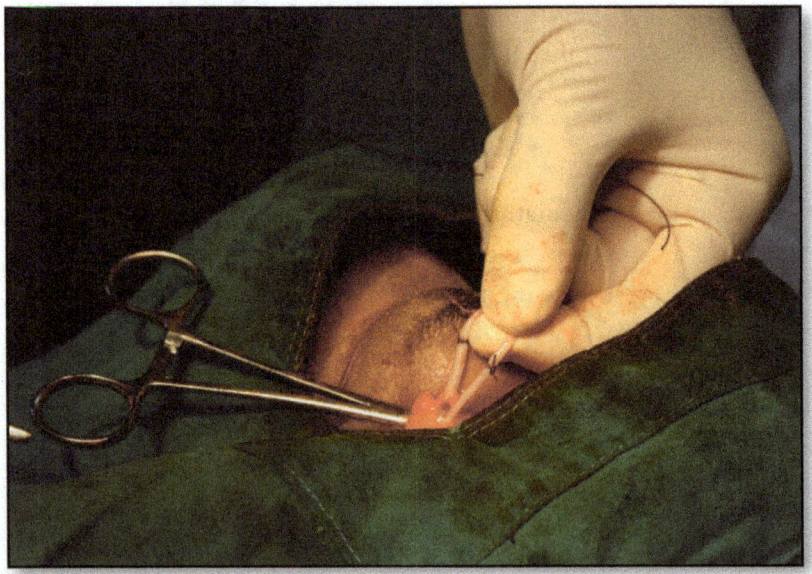

Vas deferens is being tied off during vasectomy

Vasectomy means tying off the sperm ducts of the testicles. Vasectomized dogs are rendered infertile but they will still have good libido and will indeed still mate. Vasectomy is sometimes requested for service dogs, where both breeding and castration is unwanted. Vasectomised dogs still have normal testosterone levels. Some breeders often want a teaser dog which can assist them in identifying heat in bitches. A vasectomized male may be very helpful in identifying bitches which normally show very little external signs of heat. Vasectomized males are ideal because there is no danger of unwanted pregnancies. Some breeders vasectomize young puppies to enforce breeding restrictions. It is extremely difficult, and in most cases impossible, to reverse a vasectomy. Sperm which are produced in vasectomised dogs cannot escape the testicles and can therefore only be removed by resorption inside the testicles.

10.4. Castration (neutering)

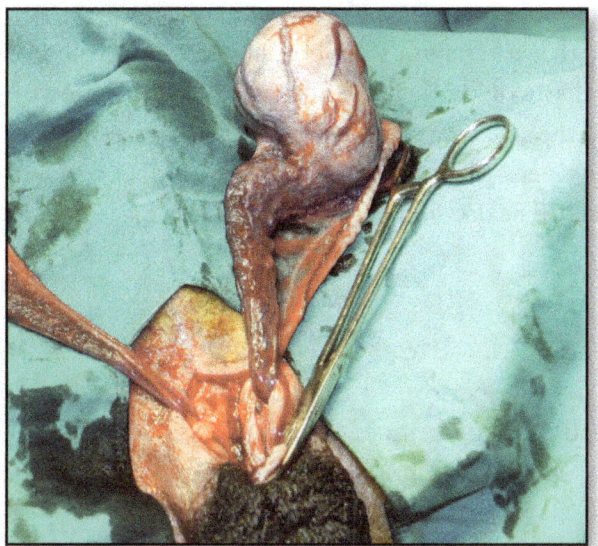
Castration

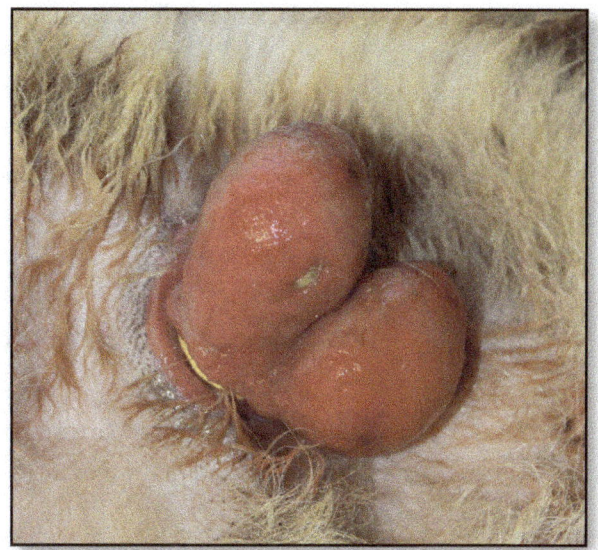
Castration gone awry using unaceptable method

Castration involves the removal of the testicles. It brings about infertility and it removes the main source of testosterone in a male dog. Castration has numerous advantages other than the fact that it renders the dog sterile.

Urine marking is effectively controlled in most males and roaming and interest in bitches which are on heat is also inhibited. Most castrates will have no libido and, therefore, have no interest in mating a bitch, but there are exceptions. Castrated males, particularly those with sexual experience prior to castration, can still have sufficient sex drive to mate a bitch. Although they are able to ejaculate, only prostatic fluid will be emitted and therefore such a mating cannot be fertile. Although it is commonly advocated that castration is highly effective in reducing aggressive behaviour in male dogs, this is not true. At the very most, castration takes a slight edge off a dog's aggression. Castration helps to lower the incidence of prostatic hyperplasia, testicular neoplasia and perianal adenomas.

Castration also has its negative effects. A very small percentage of dogs develop urinary incontinence (spontaneous urine leaking) after castration. There is proof that both males and females have slightly reduced energy levels and drive. This is probably the main reason why dog-people are reluctant to sterilise a male which they are competing with. Nevertheless, the neutering of a male dog does not render it useless for protection work or guarding. Castration does however contribute to obesity in susceptible dogs. It is proven that castration slightly increases the risk of prostatic cancer, but it is questionable whether this fact justifies advising against the routine castration of dogs.

The age at which castration surgery is performed requires discussion. The reasons why early castration is requested are in essence the same than those put forward for bitches, as discussed in 6.1.2. Contrary to common belief, early neutering does not stunt the growth of a dog but actually slightly extends it. Radiographic evidence indicates that early neutered animals are actually slightly taller than their non-castrated counterparts. Fierce opposition is sometimes directed against early castration in large breeds. This is because some breeders purport that castrated dogs do not develop sufficient breadth of chest, which then causes orthopaedic problems. Whether this is true or not, requires further investigation.

Chapter 10 Reproduction in the Male

Some dog owners (mainly men) find the emasculated look of an empty scrotum too much to bear. For those, the option of implantation of neuticles exists. Neuticles are prosthetic testicular implants for neutered dogs. Some hold the view that they serve no purpose other than to entertain human vanity, and therefore question the ethics of their use. Others argue that it removes an important reason why people elect not to neuter male pets, thus allowing castration that would otherwise not have been permitted by their owners. A last word on castration is probably that the advantages for the dog's long term health and behaviour far outweigh the disadvantages in home kept pets. Most breeders however do not routinely castrate their males once they have stopped breeding them. The decision to castrate is usually made if there is a behavioural or medical reason to do so.

10.5. Breeding soundness examination of the stud

Breeding soundness examination (BSE) of the stud may be performed to confirm fertility prior to purchase or sale, as part of an infertility investigation in breeding kennels or to check the suitability of the stud as a candidate for semen donation in assisted reproductive techniques (chilled and frozen semen).

The stud may significantly contribute to poor fertility in a breeding colony. Studs are often excluded as suspects of poor fertility. This is because breeders often erroneously assume that a stud "must" be fertile because he recently produced a large litter. One large litter is not an indicator of optimum fertility. Consistently impregnating 80% of bitches (large number) resulting in normal sized litters, is however an indicator of good fertility.

Purchasing a stud for any substantial amount without insisting on a reproductive soundness examination including semen evaluation is not a sound business principle. Many apparently "fertile" studs may indeed be sub-fertile. Mating bitches to sub-fertile males will result in poor conception rates. The semen evaluation should occur within a short interval from date of purchase of the stud. This is because the stud's fertility may have changed recently due to any number of reasons. The breeding soundness examination may be limited or extensive. The minimum BSE should include examination of the testes, epididymides, spermatic cords, prostate, penis and prepuce, general health check and semen evaluation. More advanced examinations include culture of semen, examination of foreign cells in semen, brucellosis testing and ultrasound examination of the reproductive tract or even endocrine testing.

10.6. Semen collection

One might want to collect semen from a stud for purposes of semen evaluation or artificial insemination. Although it is quite easy to collect semen from most stud dogs, aggressive and nervous dogs often do not cooperate. Some fail to attain an erection, do not ejaculate or produce an azoospermic sample. It is sometimes impossible to collect semen from overly aggressive and nervous dogs. On the other hand, a lacklustre libido also presents a serious impediment to semen collection. The presence of a bitch in heat might elicit more sexual interest in the male and facilitate semen collection. Sometimes a stud dog is more interested in its owner than in the bitch. In these cases it might be helpful if the owner leaves the collection room. The collection room should be a quiet room with no dogs in full view of the donor dog. A bitch familiar to the stud dog is better than an unfamiliar bitch. If it is required, and only in exceptional cases, drugs can be used to assist in semen collection. These drugs may settle down the stud dog, help attain an erection, help with ejaculation or help increase the libido. After the semen is collected it is very important to confirm that the penis has returned to its normal size and that it is fully retracted into the prepuce. Failure to do so may lead to priapism and penile injury.

Chapter 10 Reproduction in the Male

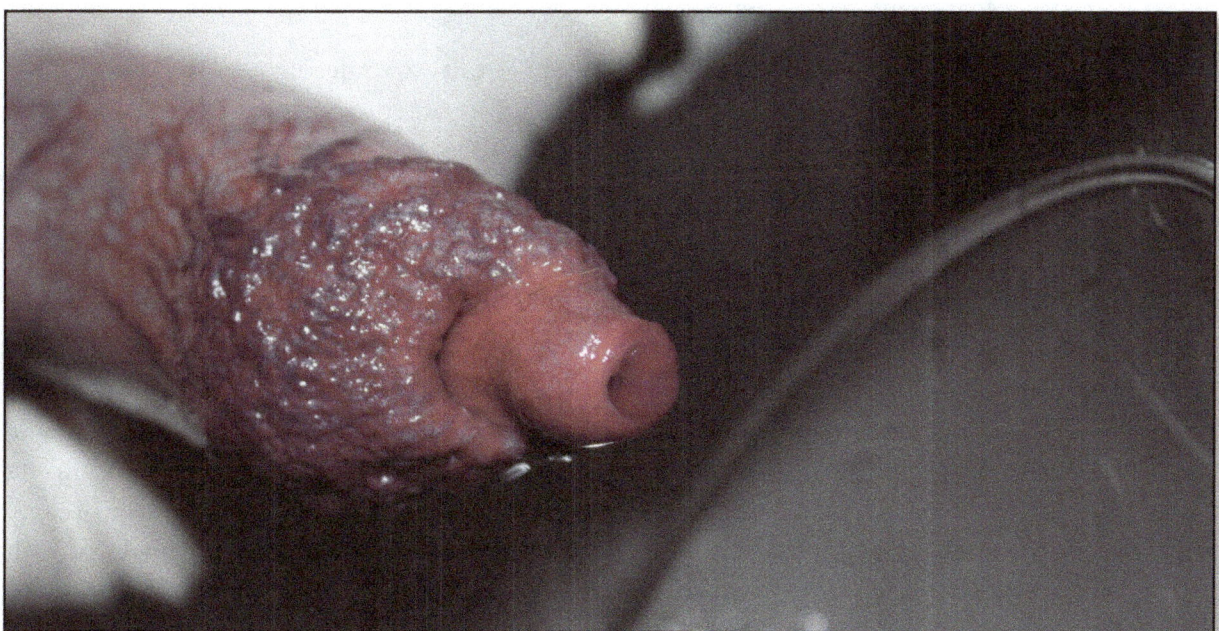
Semen collection

Semen can be collected directly from the testicles immediately after castration or euthanasia, using specialised techniques. This semen, if of adequate quality can be used to impregnate a bitch or be cryopreserved. Collection of semen in this way is highly unusual and the procedure would have to be performed at a centre where all these skills are available and planned ahead of time.

10.7. Semen quality

The semen quality is evaluated by comparing the semen parameters against a set of parameters known to be associated with good fertility. Macroscopic examinations of the volume and colour of the semen, and microscopic examinations of sperm motility, sperm concentration, sperm morphology, sperm number, pH, cytology, and alkaline phosphatase activity are usually performed.

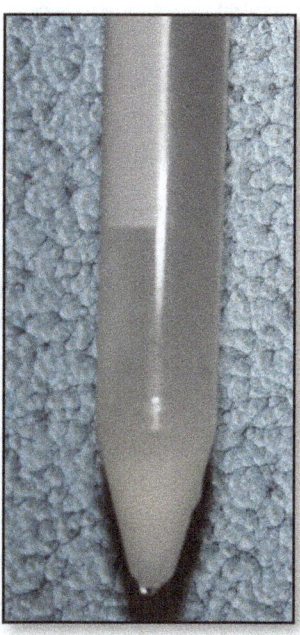

A dog's ejaculate consists of 3 fractions as explained in 5.11. The volume of the ejaculate will depend on the size of the stud dog and can range from 0.5 ml – 4.5 ml; 0.5 ml-4.0 ml; 2.0-40.0 ml respectively for the first, second and third fractions. The total number of sperm in the ejaculate can vary between 300 million to 2 billion. Generally, testicular size and weight is an indication of the dog's sperm producing capacity. Scrotal width, as an indicator of testicle size, has been documented for many breeds and a stud dog's scrotal width is then compared to known values. In a normal ejaculate, 70-80% of the sperm should be motile and 80% should have normal morphology. Sperm motility should be evaluated immediately. Alkaline Phosphatase (ALP) is an enzyme that is produced in the epididymis and normal levels are around > 5,000 IU/L. Low ALP levels (1,000 IU/L), are an indication of either incomplete ejaculation or epididymis duct occlusion.

Semen collected in tube, note dense part at the bottom of tube usually indicating good concentration of sperm with less dense portion above showing prostatic fraction of the ejaculate

Chapter 10   Reproduction in the Male

10.8. Poor semen quality

Poor semen parameters are frequently the cause of subfertility or infertility in stud dogs. True infertility (total inability to produce offspring) can be due to either azoospermia (total absence of sperm in the ejaculate) or severe sperm abnormalities as evidenced in a spermiogram (semen analysis). Absolute infertility is rare in dogs. Suboptimal fertility (subfertility) though, is much more common. Subfertility in the stud dog is normally associated with either: poor sperm motility, low sperm counts, poor sperm morphology or a combination of all these parameters. A reduced number of live progressively motile sperm reduces the availability of sperm for fertilisation, which in turn results in reduced fertility. This occurs because a minimum number of sperm are required to fertilise a bitch. Although the absolute minimum number of sperm required in fresh dog semen (deposited intravaginally) is not known, it is speculated to be around 100 million live progressively motile sperm. It is difficult to understand why such immense sperm numbers are required to fertilize a very small number of eggs. Nevertheless, breeders should not underestimate the importance of these minimum sperm numbers required. This is important because some studs have ejaculates of such poor quality that it is truly not worthwhile to use the dog as a stud. If breeders insist on using such a stud dog, artificial reproductive techniques might provide better results. It is also important to realise that as sperm numbers increase above the minimum number, both pregnancy rates and litter size will improve until it reaches a maximum. Under normal circumstances, given normal bitches and stud dogs, in excess of 80% of bitches will conceive and have normal litter sizes when using healthy studs with good semen parameters. In contrast, when a sub-fertile male is used, some bitches may conceive with normal sized litters but most will either not conceive or have small litters. Therefore, the fact that a particular stud dog has sired a litter, does not imply that the stud dog is optimally fertile. Veterinary surgeons are often asked to investigate why a bitch did not conceive, as she was put to a stud of "proven" fertility. In many instances, examination of the bitch reveals no abnormalities, while on the other hand, evaluation of the stud dog's semen, reveals very poor semen quality.

It is seldom possible to establish the exact cause of poor semen quality. Some drugs are known to deleteriously affect semen parameters and should be avoided. Most drugs, though, will only have a temporary effect. Disease, endocrine (hormonal) conditions, and longstanding fever can also negatively affect semen parameters. In most cases, if the cause is reversible, it will take 6-8 weeks to return to normality, but up to 6 months if the cause is more serious. It is advised that the dog be rechecked before being put to stud again. In certain breeds, particularly giant breeds, poor semen parameters seem to be inherited. It is prudent to take note of this aberration and select against it, in cases where a genetic origin is either confirmed or strongly suspected. If breeders do not select against poor fertility they are likely to exacerbate the problem and become more reliant on veterinary assistance to improve results through the use of artificial reproductive techniques. Intervention by artificial means does not (per se) imply genetic deterioration of semen parameters. This is because many causes of poor semen quality have nothing to do with the genetic makeup of the dog.

Whatever the cause of poor semen quality, a dog should be thoroughly examined for genital (reproductive) soundness. It is not possible to certify a dog sub fertile or infertile based on an examination of a single sample. If the semen quality is good, a single collection is adequate for certification purposes, but if the semen quality is poor, it is recommended to repeat collection and evaluation on 2-3 occasions, a couple of days apart. Even then it is recommended that the dog be retested, and that semen is collected a month or two later to confirm previous poor results.

If it is categorically established that a stud dog has poor semen parameters, it is only fair that the owner of such a stud dog informs everyone who wishes to use the stud of the fact.

10.9. Treatment of poor semen parameters

If a clear underlying cause can be determined of the poor semen parameters, this can be treated and fertility should be re-established. Testicular degeneration as well as testicular atrophy are frequent causes of the poor semen parameters and are often attributed to ageing and unknown causes. The prognosis is usually guarded.

It has been proven that Zinc, vitamin E and C, L-carnitine, L-arginine, glutathione, selenium, co-enzyme Q10, folic acid, carotenoids, N-acetylcysteine, omega-3, omega-6 and omega-9 fatty acids all resulted in a statistically significant increase in both live birth rates and pregnancy rates in various species when used in males with suboptimal semen. Breeders should however not have unrealistic expectations of many popular "sperm aiding" products. Some of these products often make very "promising and exaggerated" claims of increased fertility and improved sperm quality. In cases where poor quality semen has been confirmed and has not improved despite attempts at treatment, it is highly improbable that it will improve. In most cases, the stud's semen deteriorates with time.

Artificial insemination using intra-uterine techniques and proper timing may improve results using poor semen.

10.10. Daily sperm output (DSO)

This discussion is important because it clarifies the impact of frequent matings on the stud dog's sperm reserves and fertility. The daily sperm output refers to the number of potentially fertile sperm which can be produced by the testes each day. DSO is influenced by age, testicular size and individual variation; all probably predetermined by genetic factors. The DSO can only be established by taking the average daily sperm count over several days. The DSO is an accurate measurement of sperm production (spermatogenesis). Although most dogs aged 8 or older may have decreased DSO, there are exceptions to the rule and some studs of 11 years may still have excellent semen parameters. For small, medium and large breeds this number respectively on average is 290, 490 and 800 million sperm per dog per day.

It is important for breeders to understand that sperm is eventually evacuated from the testicles irrespective of whether ejaculation took place or not. Under normal circumstances, the fate of the old sperm is resorption within the testicles and passive transport into the urethra and the bladder. Therefore sperm which is not ejaculated is disposed of through resorption within the epididymis or transported to the bladder. There is a small sperm reserve that resides within the tail of the epididymis of the testis and this reserve is greatly reduced after a single ejaculation. This reserve is replenished within 24 hours.

The duration of sexual rest does not influence DSO but it might influence the sperm numbers and sperm quality in the ejaculate, on the day of collection. By resting (4-5 day) the sperm count may increase by about 25-30% for one day or so and thereafter the stud's sperm count will be approximately equal to his DSO again. What this implies is that the normal stud has little to gain from sexual rest. Many breeders may have heard of "old sperm" which may have accumulated after sexual rest (10 days

Chapter 10 Reproduction in the Male

or more). This refers to old and degenerate sperm which reside in the sperm reserve of the testis. A single ejaculation is usually sufficient to rid the stud of these old and degenerate sperm. It is important that this single ejaculation is not less than 1 day and not more than 7 days before semen is collected for semen evaluation or for freezing purposes.

The practical implication is that the normal healthy stud with a normal DSO can mate daily for several weeks without deleterious effect on its semen parameters. It is however more likely that this frequent mating schedule will result in temporary lack of sexual interest. More than once a day matings is not harmful to the stud or his sperm producing tissues but will result in slightly lower sperm counts in the ejaculates from which the dog can recover in a few days, irrespective of how long the twice daily mating had continued. When using normal males of good fertility, twice a day mating is unlikely to adversely affect conception rates. This is in contrast to the notion by breeders that an "overworked stud" is likely to result in poor conception rates. When a stud is collected twice in short succession (1-2 hours), the second ejaculation will contain 70% of the sperm numbers attained in the first ejaculation. This is often practised to maximise sperm numbers when collecting semen for freezing purposes. Twice a day semen collection or matings should only be used under special circumstances and not as a routine. Besides reproductive repercussions there are also ethical concerns and allegations of exploitation when maintaining such extensive use of a stud.

In summary, healthy studs can comfortably mate daily for some weeks or every alternate day indefinitely without any deleterious effect to his sperm number, quality and fertility. This may however not be true for dogs which are not reproductively sound and have either poor semen quality or inadequate DSO or both.

Many registering authorities however, will not allow the registration of more than a finite number of litters for any one given male over any given 12 month period. Breeders should acquaint themselves with and abide with these regulations.

10.11. Superfecundation (multiple sires of one litter) achieved by multiple sire matings

Superfecundation is a scientific term for a litter where more than one sire is represented in the litter. Superfecundation occurs when two or more eggs which were ovulated during a single cycle are fertilized by spermatozoa from different males. It results in a litter of which some puppies are from male A and others from male B. It does not matter who mated the bitch first or second, all that matters is whether the male's spermatozoa were still motile and fertile at the time of optimal fertility. Theoretically, more than two sires are possible. If this is the case, it is termed heteropaternal superfecundation. This is quite common in stray dogs. Dogs can theoretically produce litters where every puppy in a litter has a different father.

Superfecundation can be accidental or deliberate. Deliberate superfecundation is achieved by multiple sire matings. There are many instances where multiple sire breeding (natural mating or AI or both) is wanted. Before the advent of parentage testing, superfecundation was not allowed because registration procedure requires the identification of the true sire. In most countries, parentage testing is now possible, which makes superfecundation a viable option. Blood sampling from the dam, sire A, sire B (or even more sires), as well as blood samples (buccal or other DNA containing sample) from each individual puppy needs to be submitted so that parentage verification can be done. The question arises as to why any breeder would want to practice superfecundation and why veterinary surgeons would assist breeders to achieve this? The discussion that follows will endeavour to provide the answer.

10.11.1. Using two or more sires with poor semen parameters on one bitch

A sire with compromised semen parameters is defined as a sire which does not produce semen of optimal quality. This may be because of age, disease, infection, trauma or any of a number of unknown reasons. These males will either have sperm abnormalities, low sperm counts or poor sperm motility. Using these studs will result in lower conception rates. In some breeds this may be a real problem, particularly if there are not many sires available in any geographic area. This set of circumstances is not uncommon in some scarce breeds. For instance, the breeder may have two studs e.g. Irish wolfhounds, (there are many other examples particularly in the giant breeds where this problem is more common), of which the semen is of suboptimal quality. These breeders may have already failed in attaining pregnancies using these males individually. Furthermore as previously explained, bitches may reach an age where it becomes crucial that she becomes pregnant because of age or in order to maintain uterine health and prevent pyometra. If it is not possible to use optimally fertile studs on such a bitch, the breeder may elect to use two (or even more) sires on such a bitch in order to increase chances of conception.

10.11.2. Using compromised semen or stud of poor fertility in combination with a semen of optimal quality

In this example the bitch is bred (natural mating or AI) to a stud which is known to be of suboptimal fertility or inseminated with semen of known poor quality or insufficient quantity. The latter is a set of circumstances which present itself very frequently when frozen semen inseminations are planned. These breedings should obviously be timed using the best methods (hormone profiling). Using the latter will enable the breeder to have upfront knowledge of the fertile period of the bitch. The bitch is then bred with mentioned sub fertile stud or inseminated with semen of poor quality or insufficient quantity, till just before the anticipated end of the bitch's fertile period. This offers the compromised semen enough time to potentially fertilise the available eggs. Just before the end of the fertile period the same bitch is then bred to a stud of known optimal fertility. This allows the better semen to fertilise any eggs which may not have been fertilised as yet by the first breeding attempt. Using this method, the most desired stud or semen from artificial insemination (but less fertile one) is given the benefit of the largest part of the fertile period to fertilise the eggs and potentially sire the puppies. However, if his sperm did not achieve this, the eggs have another opportunity to be fertilised before they age and degenerate. This practice of multiple sire breeding enables the breeder to use the most desired male but if he was unable to achieve fertilisation, the breeder may at least have another chance of a pregnancy albeit it with the less desired stud. In this case the bitch has less chance of missing a breeding opportunity and retaining uterine health. Typical examples are using a stud of poor fertility on a bitch first, then a stud of optimal fertility or using frozen semen (which normally is of poorer fertility than fresh semen of good quality) and just before the end of the fertile period using fresh semen or natural mating, both of known good fertility. In the opinion of many reproductive specialists this is just another tool to improve conception rates. Breeding authorities which are currently not registering dual sire litters should be encouraged by their members to strongly reconsider this stance.

10.11.3. Concerns of breeding authorities regarding multiple sire breeding

Some breeding authorities do not allow deliberate dual sire breeding. Their concern is that the random use of deliberate dual sire breeding selects for poor fertility parameters and goes against the principle of keeping the breed reproductively sound. The concern is justified and it holds true for most artificial reproductive techniques in use today. Artificial reproductive techniques, such as A.I., intra-uterine inseminations, multiple sire breedings, supportive hormone therapy to induce ovulation or sustain pregnancies, assisted deliveries and caesarean sections all add to selection for poor reproductive health. Many of these bitches or stud dogs would not have been able to produce offspring without assistance. All assisted reproductive techniques, in essence, oppose natural selection for good fertility parameters.

In defence of these techniques however, it needs mentioning that reproductive traits as a general rule, have low heritability potential (usually less than 20%). It also needs consideration, against the background of their worldwide frequent use, that reproductive specialists have to remain on the cutting edge of technology regarding artificial reproductive techniques otherwise they could be seen to be antiquated.

The diversity and size of a breed's gene pool must be taken into consideration when a ruling whether or not to allow the use of artificial reproductive techniques is made. For instance, in most countries, owing to the German Shepherd Dog breed's popularity, the genetic pool and diversity might be large enough to justify restrictions on, for instance, dual sire matings. The situation for the many other minor breeds (especially giant breeds with known fertility problems) is very different.

Artificial reproductive techniques, in these breeds, help to maintain the little diversity which there still is and it also helps to keep the population size up. It must be mentioned that some breed authorities allow the registration of puppies from accidental dual sire matings; however, penalties are attached if breeders do transgress. Notwithstanding this, the ruling does open the door for breeders who wish to circumvent the prohibition of deliberate dual breeding by staging an accidental mating. The last word on dual sire breedings is that it was never intended to be or is likely to become routine in any breed.

10.12. Prostatic disease

Prostatic disease is discussed in detail. This is because prostatic disease can frequently signal the end of the stud's reproductive career and in some cases be fatal. Knowledge of prostatic disease can help the breeder make informed decisions.

10.12.1. Benign prostatic hypertrophy

Not unlike men, older intact dogs also frequently suffer from prostate problems. The dog is however more likely to suffer from benign prostatic hypertrophy (BPH) which is enlargement of the prostate as opposed to prostatic neoplasia in humans. It is estimated that by the age of 6 years over 60% of intact males have BPH and the incidence keeps increasing from then onwards.

Initially dogs show no symptoms. As the condition progresses, the signs of prostatic hypertrophy will typically be constipation and frequent urination of small amounts at a time. A small stream of urine is voided instead of a strong stream, together with dripping of urine and small specs of blood visible at the prepuce at the end of urination. The semen may also be blood-tinged. It is important to determine what the nature of the dog's prostate problem is. If breeding is no longer desired, castration is the treatment of choice. If a breeder still wants to breed with the affected stud dog, medical treatment can be attempted. Lifelong medical management is required using a drug which blocks the conversion of testosterone to dihydrotestosterone. As is the case with humans, this drug can cause reduced libido in susceptible individuals. It is probably best to treat the stud dog until the dog has reached the end of its reproductive career, and then castrate them.

10.12.2. Prostatitis

Prostatitis refers to an infection of the prostate gland. Most dogs which suffer from prostatitis also suffer from BPH because BPH predisposes the prostatic gland to infection from ascending bacteria in the urogenital tract. Again, the treatment of choice is castration. If the breeder wishes to still breed, specific drugs to treat the bacterial infection (if present) and drugs to reduce prostate size are available. Treatment for prostatitis in most cases should be regarded as an interim measure until the stud dog reaches the end of its reproductive career. At that point it is wise to castrate the dog to decrease the chance of recurrence. The symptoms of prostatitis are similar to BPH with the exception that dogs suffering from prostatitis usually have more blood in the urine and are febrile. Appropriate long term antibiotic treatment for the bacterial infection is indicated together with the treatment of the BPH. Prostatitis is rare in castrated males. Prostatitis can predispose dogs to prostatic abscesses.

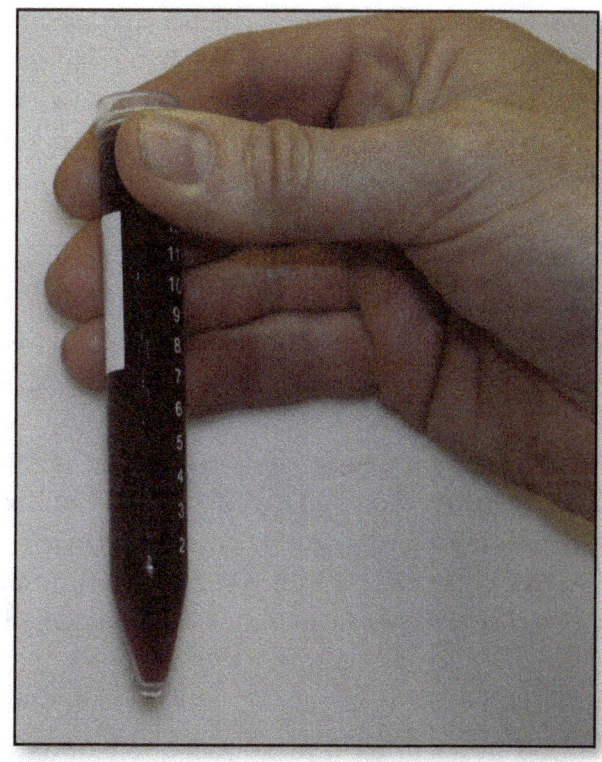

Red discoloured sperm frequently associated with prostatic disease

10.12.3. Prostatic and paraprostatic cysts and prostatic abscesses

In dogs, cysts may be found inside the prostate gland itself (prostatic cyst) or outside but adjacent to the prostate gland (paraprostatic cyst). Most prostatic cystic conditions are incidental findings and are often asymptomatic. The veterinary surgeon should at this point attempt to distinguish between the various types of cysts. Cysts may later become abscessed and pose a very serious threat to the dog's life. Surgery to remove cysts, drain abscesses or even total prostatectomy may be required. This surgery is very high risk but may be crucial to saving the dog's life. Castration is strongly advised, particularly if a dog has prostatic cysts.

10.12.4. Prostatic cancer

Prostatic neoplasia (cancer of the prostate) is a rare condition which can befall both neutered and intact male dogs. However intact male dogs seem to have a slight decreased risk. It is a serious condition that can metastasise (spread) to other organs. Castration does not slow the progression of prostatic neoplasia. Although a total prostatectomy or chemo- and radiotherapy can help, the prognosis remains poor. Tests for early prostatic cancer detection in humans are already available but the development of such tests for dogs is a work in progress. The symptoms are similar to those of BPH. Treatment options are limited and the chances of recovery is poor. In the end, the best option is most probably a total prostatectomy.

Chapter 10 Reproduction in the Male

10.13. Testicular conditions

10.13.1. *Cryptorchidism (undescended testis)*

Cryptorchidism is defined as failure of one or both testes to descend into the scrotum at the time normal for the species of interest. Cryptorchidism (hidden testis) is the preferred term. In contrast, monorchidism (single testis) implies that one testicle did not develop at all, a condition which has not been reported in male dogs. Monorchidism and cryptorchidism are often used erroneously as synonyms. Cryptorchidism may be unilateral or bilateral and the undescended testicle may be inside the abdomen or inguinal canal and are then known as cryptic testicles whereas if they are found outside the inguinal canal, they are referred to as ectopic testicles.

Cryptorchidism is congenital, caused by a genetic defect and inherited as a sex-limited autosomal recessive polygenic trait. Although the condition is obviously seen only in male dogs, both males and females can carry the gene for cryptorchidism and can pass the gene on to their offspring. Homozygous males are cryptorchid. The meaning of this terminology is made clear in the chapter on genetics (Chapter 16).

Dogs with two undescended testicles are infertile whereas unilateral cryptorchids show variable semen quality. Most will have good libido and exhibit male behaviour because undescended testicles produce testosterone. Although cryptorchids are usually sub fertile, they may produce offspring. Because the condition is of genetic origin it is not advised to breed with affected dogs and it is best not to breed their parents either as they are known to both carry the gene.

Although there is speculation of environmental causes or contributing factors to cryptorchidism, they are ill-defined and rare. For instance, it is theoretically possible that any cause of inflammation or adhesions in the inguinal canal or scrotum, such as trauma to the inguinal region may prevent normal testicular descent or indeed cause the testicle to be retracted again up the canal. This is extremely rare and would be very difficult to prove. Therefore, for all practical purposes, any dog which has one or more undescended testicles is to be considered a cryptorchid due to genetics by default.

Contraction of the cremaster muscle can pull the testis from the scrotum into the inguinal canal if the puppy is stressed but this is a temporary phenomenon.

Although some breeds appear to be over represented, any purebred or mixed breed dog may be affected. Reported incidences of canine cryptorchidism usually vary from 1-8% but higher incidences in some breeds have been reported.

The age of examination for cryptorchidism is of importance. In the normal dog, the testes pass through the inguinal canal by 5 days after birth and by 10 days most testicles will be in the scrotum but not later than 6 weeks. It is true that some testicles will still descend after the age of 6 weeks but this should be regarded as delayed testicular descent and considered abnormal. These testes are usually situated in an inguinal location at first examination and later be positioned permanently in the scrotum. The genetics of delayed testicular descent have not been investigated but it is sound advice not to breed from dogs suffering from delayed testicular descent until proven otherwise. This is because it is speculated that breeding from such dogs may increase the incidence of cryptorchidism. Because the inguinal canal closes to the passing of testicles by the age of 6 months, it is not possible for a testicle to still come down after this age.

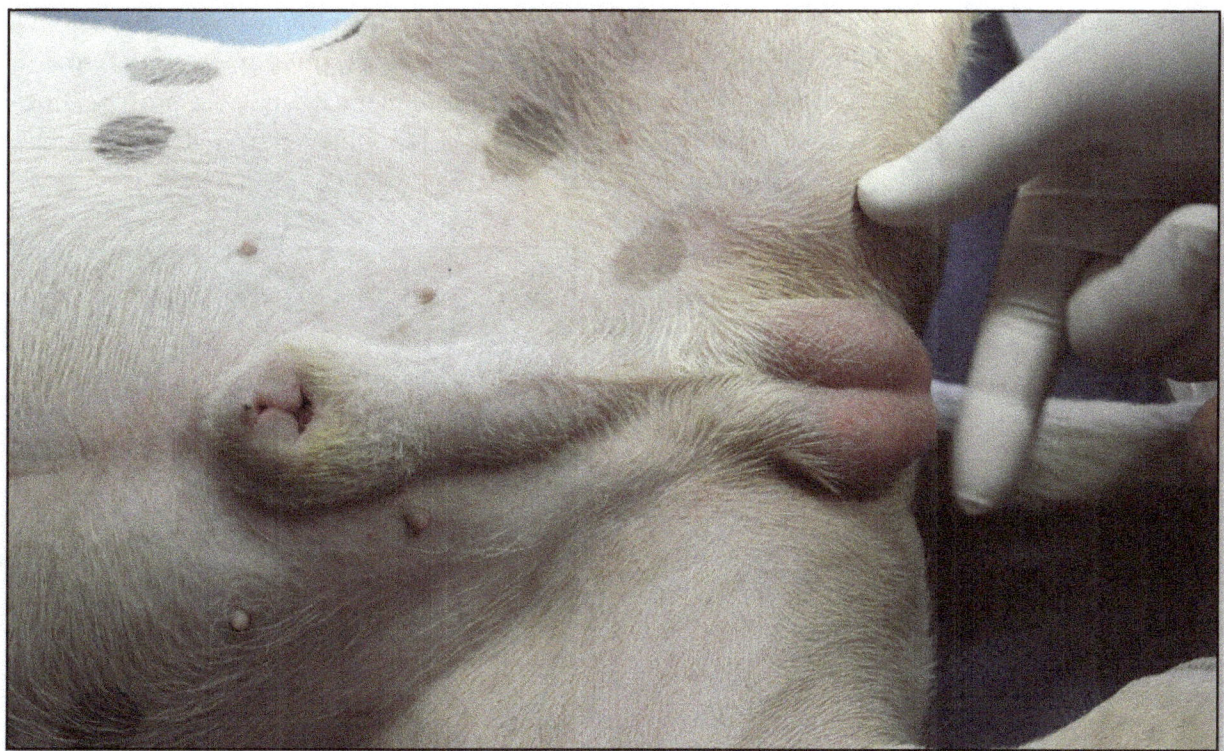
Intact male

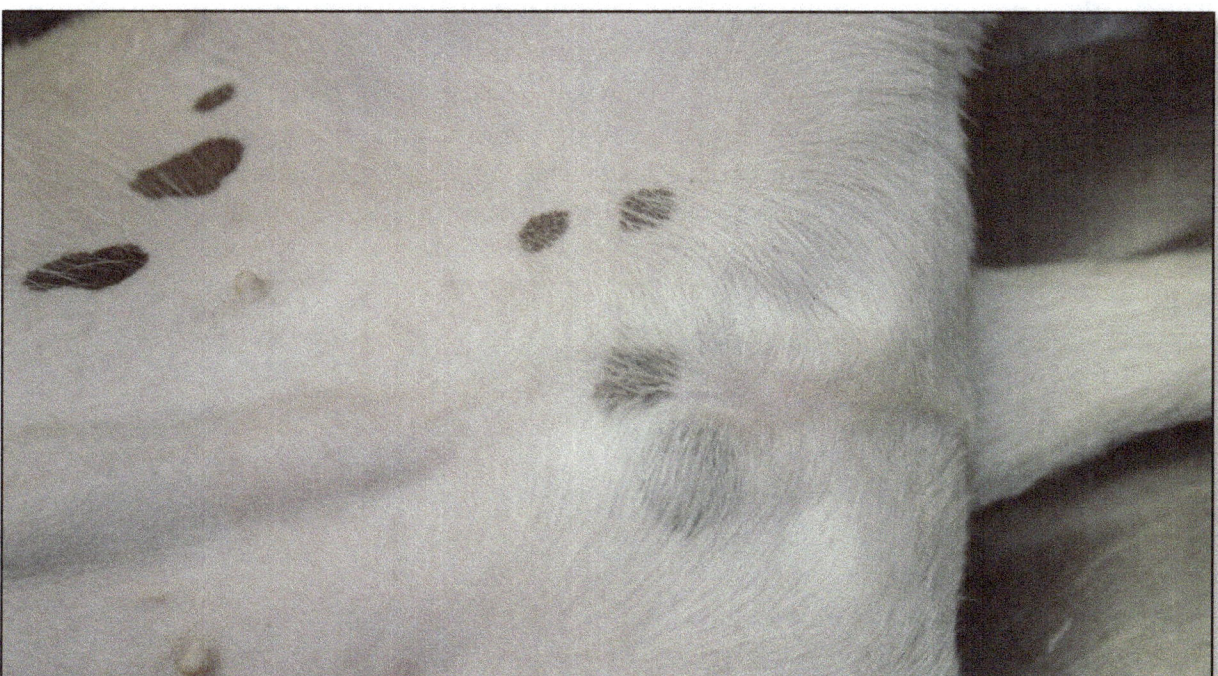
Bilateral undescended testis in puppy

The diagnosis of cryptorchidism is by visual inspection and careful palpation of the scrotum and inguinal region in dogs. Due to the larger testicular size, this examination is easier in large and medium breeds. In small breeds but particularly in toy breeds, it may be very difficult to consistently and accurately count both testicles at 6 weeks of age. In these breeds it may be better to evaluate the dog at 3 months of age. The best way to palpate a testicle is to pick the puppy up under its two forelegs and turning the puppy on his back and lifting the dog from the examination table at about 45° with the table. It may take some experience not to confuse inguinal lymph nodes with testicles. In young dogs the testes can move freely between the scrotum and inguinal canal. Cryptorchid dogs are at increased risk for the development of testicular neoplasia and should be castrated (both testicles removed) preferably at an early age of 6 months onwards.

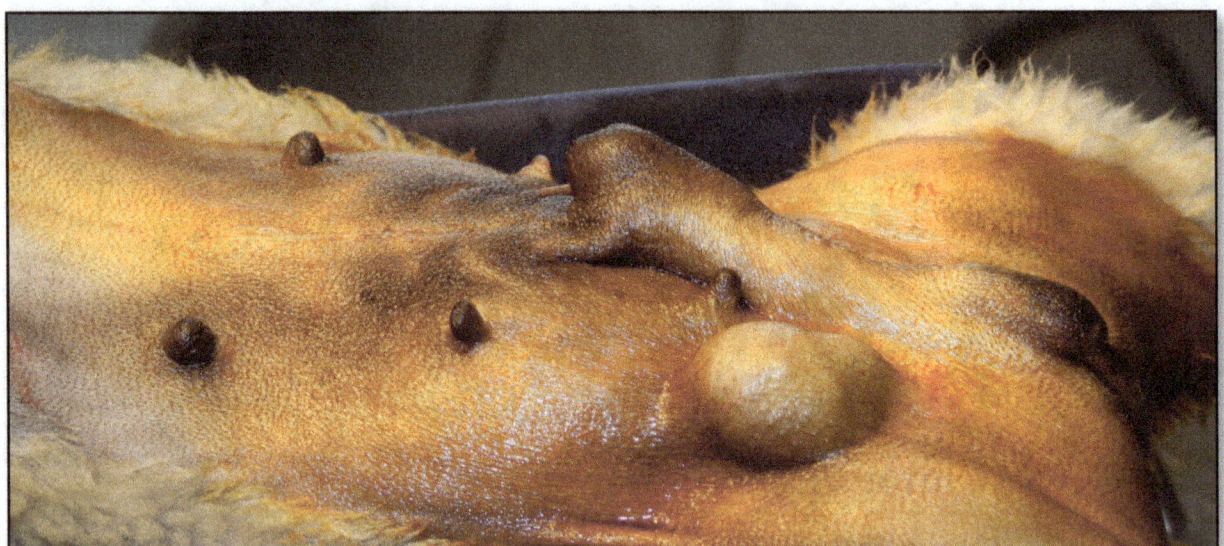

Cryptorchid male, note testicle in groin that is also enlarged

Orchiopexy (surgical correction) of the retained testis in the scrotal sac has been described in the literature, but is not recommended. The ethics of this may be questioned as it corrects (disguises) genetic fault. Removal of the cryptorchid testicle and placement of a prosthetic testicle has also been performed. In countries where such intervention is legal it is advised that the dog is vasectomised. Hormonal therapy has been reported to "force" the testicle down but is usually associated with poor success.

10.13.2. Testicular torsion

Testicular torsion is a condition where the testis twists around by 180 degrees or more causing constriction of blood flow to the affected testis. The testis swells and becomes painful. By the time the condition is detected, the condition is usually irreversible and the testis needs to be surgically removed. Following surgery these dogs can be bred from.

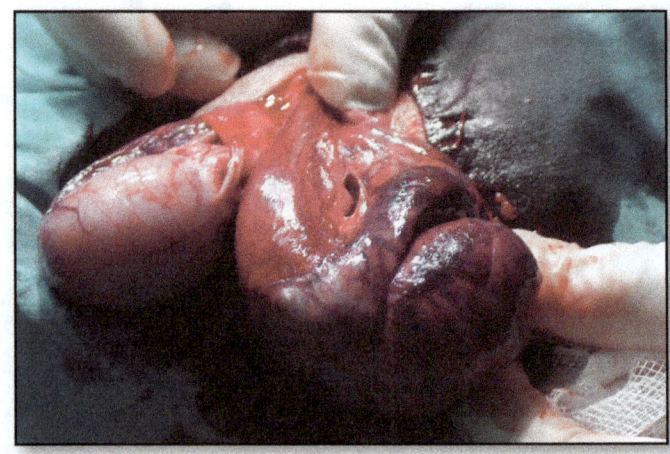

Testicular torsion. The twisted testicle is red and swollen

10.13.3. Testicular infection (orchitis) and epididymitis

Orchitis results from bacterial infection of the testes and its structures. Infection may be spontaneous or result from trauma in the region i.e. penetrating wounds. If breeding is no longer required, castration is recommended. If the reproductive capacity is to be retained, antibiotic therapy may be attempted. Surgical removal of one testis (hemiorchidectomy) is indicated where treatment fails and only one testicle is involved.

The infection might also be located in the epididymis which is the tubular system that transports the sperm from the testes to the tube (vas deferens) which leads them to the ejaculatory apparatus. Inflammation or trauma of this structure may lead to an obstruction which results in an accumulation of sperm near the site of the injury. This in turn may lead to an immunological reaction and give rise to what is known as a sperm granuloma and results in inflammation and swelling of the epididymis. This will lead to infertility of the affected testis. Response to treatment for this condition is usually also very poor and may lead to the need to surgically remove the affected testicle.

10.13.4. Testicular trauma

Testicular trauma may result from dog fights, penetrating wounds, motor vehicle accidents and many more possible causes. The trauma may be restricted to one or both testicles. Invariably the trauma will lead to inflammation, haemorrhage and in many cases infection of the testes, epididymis and scrotum as well. Prompt treatment will be required using anti-inflammatory agents and antibiotics. Again when breeding is still desired, the attending veterinary surgeon may attempt treatment first. Failing that, surgical removal of the affected testicle is indicated and castration if both testicles are affected. In cases where there is an apparent recovery, it is strongly advised that a semen evaluation is performed to confirm potential for fertility.

10.13.5. Testicular neoplasia (cancer or tumours)

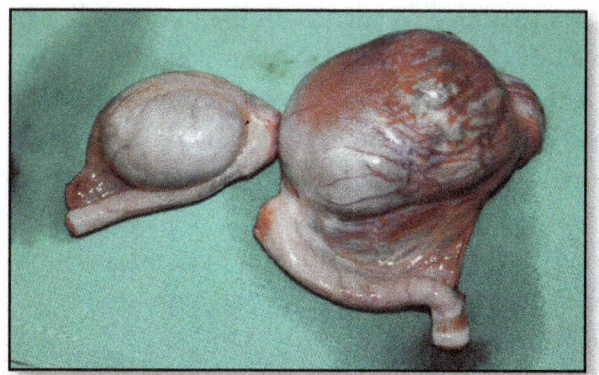

Normal and cancerous testicle

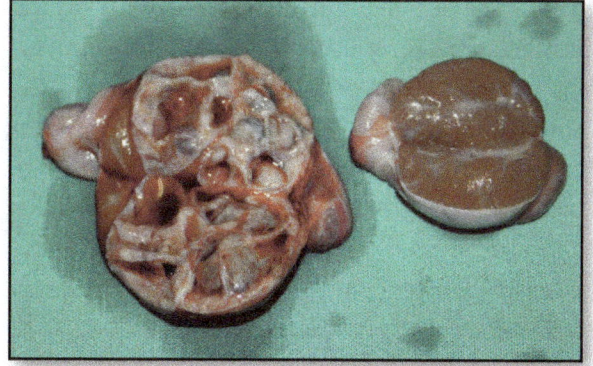

Normal and cancerous testicle in cross section

Although many cancers can affect the testes and its surrounding structures, three main types of testicular cancer occur in dogs. Mostly older dogs are affected. Testicular cancer usually affects one testicle but both may be involved. If breeding is no longer intended, castration is indicated and is usually curative if diagnosed early. This is because testicular cancers other than sertoli cell tumours generally have a low potential to metastasize (spread). Depending on the type of cancer which affects the one testicle, the contralateral (other side's testicle) may become infertile as well and prostatic disorders may also arise from one or both testicles which have a tumour. It is therefore of prime importance that the affected testicle is surgically removed as soon as the condition is diagnosed.

In short the three main types of testis cancer (neoplasia) are sertoli cell tumours, seminomas and interstitial cell tumours.

Chapter 10 Reproduction in the Male

A Sertoli cell tumour is a tumour of the sertoli cells. These are the cells which aid in the development of the spermatozoa. Sertoli cell tumours may occur in a normally descended testis but are far more frequent in cryptorchid testes. These tumour cells have a high tendency for metastasis (spreading to other parts of the body). This tumour produces excess production of oestrogen and this in turn may lead to anaemia, alopecia (hair loss), feminization and the attraction of other male dogs.

Seminomas are tumours of the cells which actually form the spermatozoa (spermatogenic cells). These tumours may produce oestrogen or androgens (testosterone and testosterone like substances) and lead to hormone associated side effects and also tumours of the anus (perianal adenomas). Interstitial cell tumours are tumours of the interstitial cells (Leydig cells of the testicle) which are the cells which are responsible for the production of testosterone.

10.13.6. Testicular hypoplasia

Testicular hypoplasia (the failure of an organ or body part to grow or develop fully) is when one or both testes are unusually small. It is a rare condition and is suspected to originate during the developmental stage of a foetus. These dogs can display normal sexual behaviour and libido, even if both testes are affected. Dogs with one affected testis have lowered fertility, but if both testes are affected the dog is infertile. There is no known treatment for this condition. Because the condition is rare, and uncertainty exists whether testicular hypoplasia is genetically linked; the breeder, in consultation with their veterinary surgeon, should decide whether or not to breed with affected dogs. It is not necessary to remove a hypoplastic testis unless there is other pathology which must be addressed.

10.13.7. Testicular degeneration

Testicular degeneration is the medical term ascribed to an abnormal change in the functionality of testicular tissue. It usually develops after puberty, even in apparently normal dogs which have sired many litters. One or both testicles can be affected. Although trauma, infection or an inflammatory condition can cause testicular degeneration, it frequently develops spontaneously in middle-aged dogs as an aged related condition of unknown origin. Initially the dog will be asymptomatic but as the condition progresses, the testes become smaller and softer. Again, although the dog might display good sex drive it will have poor fertility or be infertile. Treatment is usually only successful in cases where a clearly discernible underlying cause can be identified. In most cases dogs are unresponsive to treatment, but particularly so if the testicular degeneration is age related.

10.13.8. Inguinoscrotal hernia

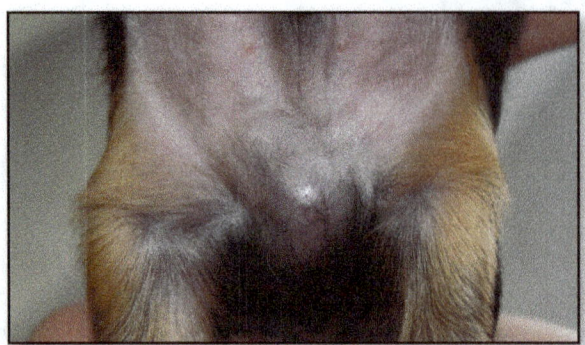

Inguinoscrotal hernia

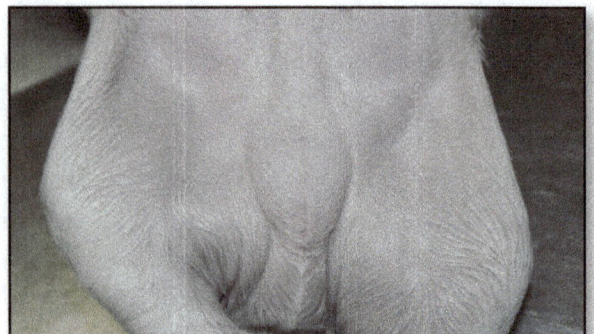

Scrotal hernia in young puppy on first glance it appears that the sack is filled with two testicles but close examination reveals presence of fluid and omentum in the scrotal sack

This hernia occurs when a portion of the intestine loops into the scrotum. It is a rare condition which may occur due to congenital abnormalities or trauma. Affected dogs present with swelling of the scrotum which may or may not be painful. Surgery involves narrowing the inguinal ring to prevent recurrence of hernia. This surgery is not without risk as the blood supply to the testis at the side of the surgery may be affected causing it to become inflamed and become infertile. This surgery may be rather tricky. This condition may be bilateral (on both sides). Due to the strong suspicion of a hereditary basis, castration is advised during surgical correction of the hernia. (Scrotal hernias are also possible).

10.13.9. Hemiorchidectomy (removal of one testis)

Many testicular afflictions end up with the removal of one testis (hemiorchidectomy) and for this reason it requires comprehensive discussion. It is also clear that not removing the testis can affect the other testicle's sperm producing ability. Breeders should ask the attending veterinary surgeon for a certificate which states that the dog, indeed, had two testicles at the time of surgery, and what the medical reason for the hemiorchidectomy was. It is wise to do so, because breeders might be expected to prove that the dog was not a cryptorchid in the first place.

It is obvious that the stud dog's semen count will reduce significantly if one testicle is surgically removed. The extent of which varies. Semen evaluation is, therefore, a logical follow-up procedure. This examination should take place not before 6 weeks following hemiorchidectomy. This allows for full recovery of the stud following surgery. In cases where a cancerous testicle, which might have affected the prostrate was removed, a three month recovery period is required. Depending on the result of the semen evaluation, breeding recommendations can be made. In general, if a dog had good semen parameters prior to the hemiorchidectomy, the prognosis for achieving pregnancies with that stud dog is good. Many hemi-orchids have produced many litters of normal size, even in advanced age.

10.14. Penis and prepuce conditions

10.14.1. Phimosis

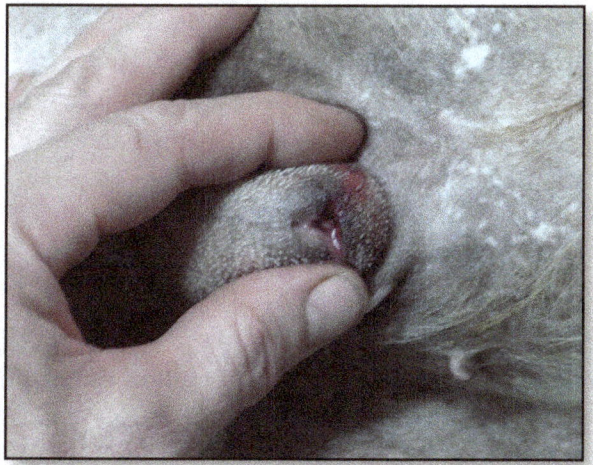

Stenosis (phimosis) of preputial opening

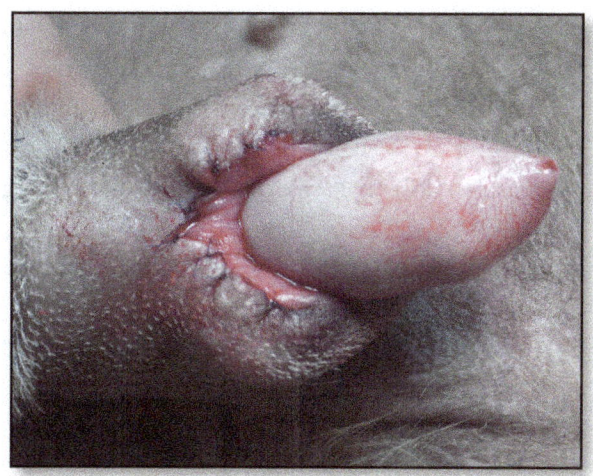

Repair of phimosis

Chapter 10 Reproduction in the Male

Phimosis is the inability to extrude the penis. Stenosis (constriction) of the orifice (opening of the sheath) of the penis is the most likely cause. This stenosis can be congenital or acquired. It is usually impossible to extrude the penis of a prepubertal animal as the penile epithelium is fused to the internal preputial sheath until puberty. Typically in phimosis, the dog may sometimes get an erection and find it difficult to retract its penis. In this case the dog will get another condition which may become an emergency, namely paraphimosis. The reduced sheath opening size can be surgically corrected. Heritability of this trait is not known.

10.14.2. Paraphimosis

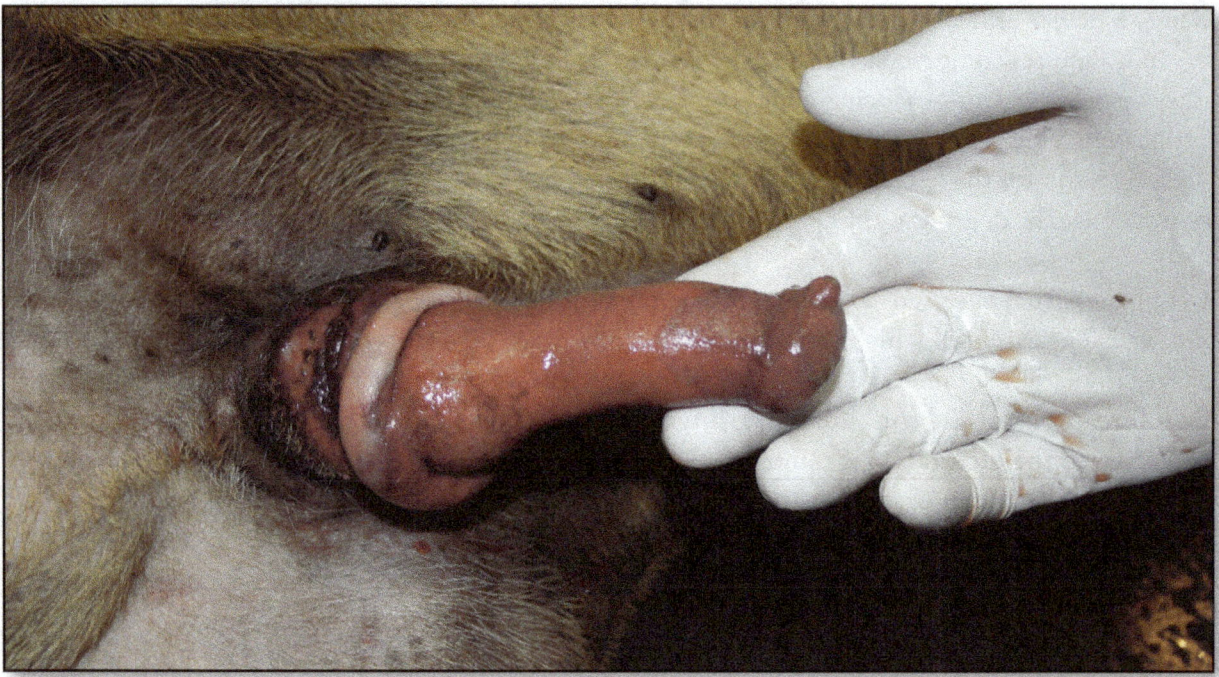

Paraphimosis

Paraphimosis is the protrusion of the full length of the penis outside its sheath (prepuce) and the dog is unable to retract the penis back into its sheath. The cause, in most cases, is unknown but a small preputial orifice can cause trauma to the penis during mating, which in turn, can cause paraphimosis. Long coated dogs with long hair on the preputial orifice are more prone to develop this condition because the hair can get stuck to the erect penis and when the penis disgorges, the hair pulls the skin of the preputial orifice inward, curling the skin in on itself, and thereby reducing the diameter of the orifice. This smaller orifice opening can then lead to paraphimosis. As with phimosis, treatment involves surgical correction.

10.14.3. Balanosposthitis

Balanoposthitis is the term used for an inflammation and or infection of the head of the penis and the surrounding sheath. In severe cases the penis is ulcerated and discoloured. This condition must not be confused with smegma, which is a normal yellow discharge of the penis. Intact dogs have more smegma than neutered ones. Some dogs are more fastidious than others and lick their prepuce clean; however, excessive cleaning and licking should alert the breeder to the fact that something might be wrong. A dog with an excessive discharge or one that cleans and licks more than usual must be investigated by a veterinary surgeon.

10.14.4. Priapism

Priapism is a term used for a persistent erection of the penis. Irrespective of cause, a persistent erection lasting longer than several hours will lead to drying of the mucous membranes, inflammation, infection and compromised blood flow to the tissues and finally possible loss of its penis if not attended to.

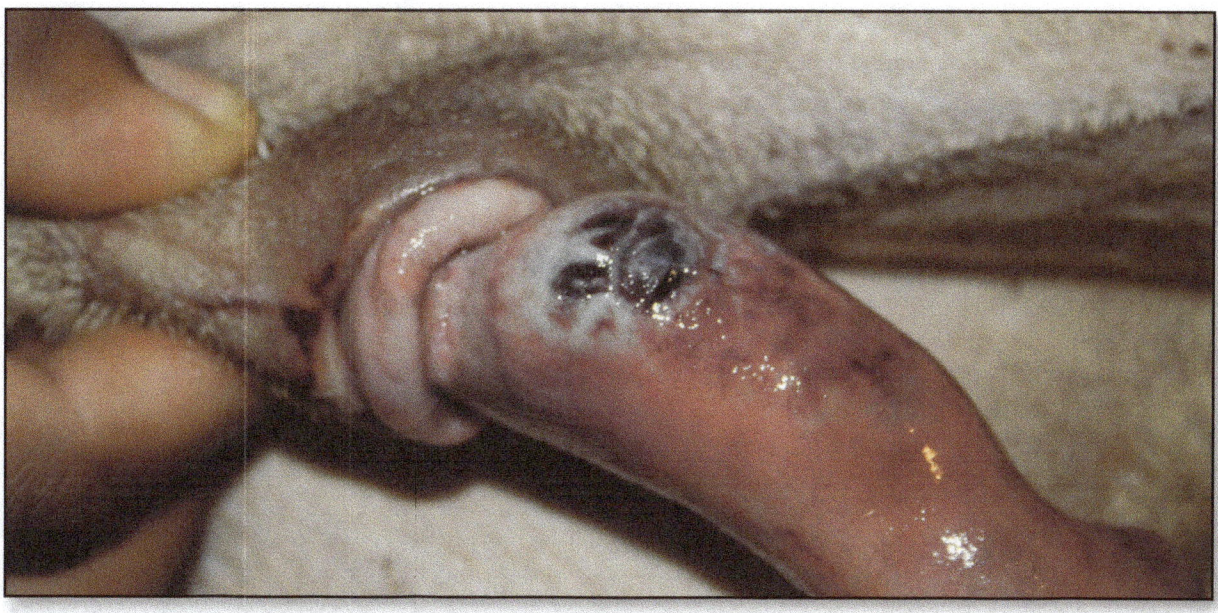

Penile trauma

10.14.5. Persistent frenulum

The internal sheath of the prepuce and the epithelium of the penis are fused in neonates by a membrane called the frenulum. In dogs this band separates around puberty. Failure of a portion of this membrane to separate results in a persistent frenulum. This condition is very easy to correct surgically.

10.14.6. Urethral prolapse

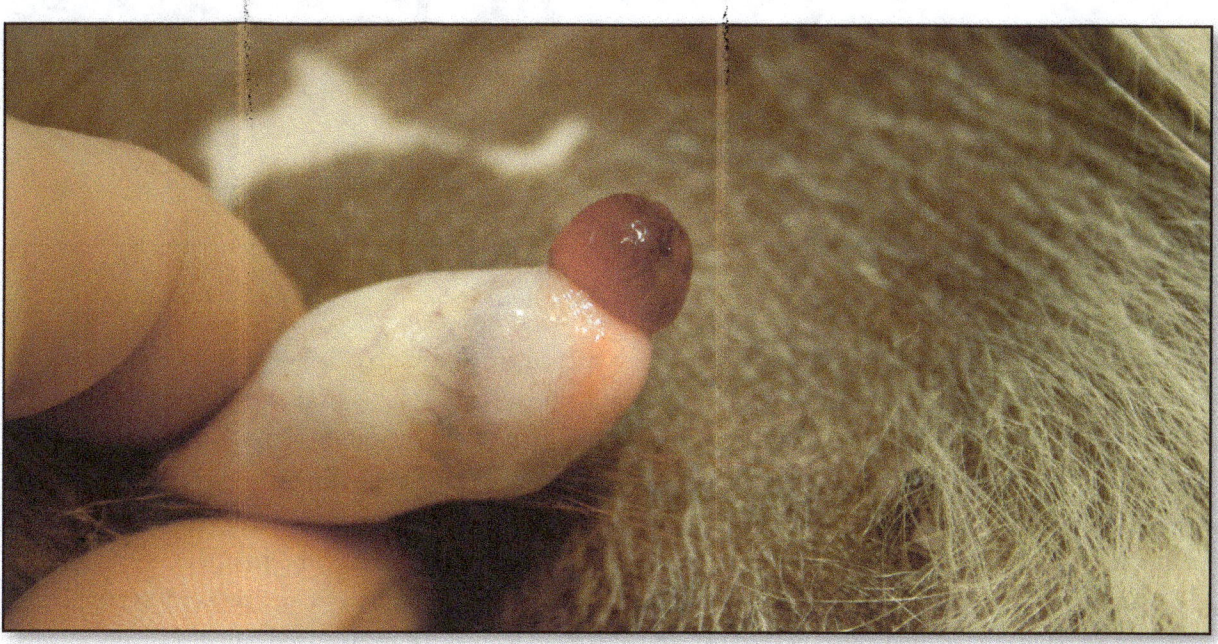

Urethral prolapse

Urethral prolapse is when a small piece of the urethra lining, right at the tip of the dog's penis, bulges out. It presents as a red to purple pea sized mass which protrudes from the opening. The breeder will most likely just see blood dripping from the penis sheath. It is a rare condition which can befall any male dog. It is more commonly diagnosed in younger dogs and brachycephalic breeds seem to be over-represented.

Although medical treatment can cure the condition, surgery is more likely to succeed. Recurrence is common following medical treatment but uncommon following surgery. It is vitally important not to expose the dog to in-season bitches for at least 3 weeks following surgery. This is because serious bleeding is a real risk if the dog should get an erection before the surgical site has fully healed, even worse, the entire surgical procedure can be undone if this happens. Fortunately, there is medication which can be administered to reduce the risk of erections. Once a dog is fully recovered from surgery, it can return to stud without any problems. Although some breeds are over-represented, which suggests some hereditary base to the condition, it is probably unnecessary to discriminate against an affected male if the dog is considered to be a superior specimen.

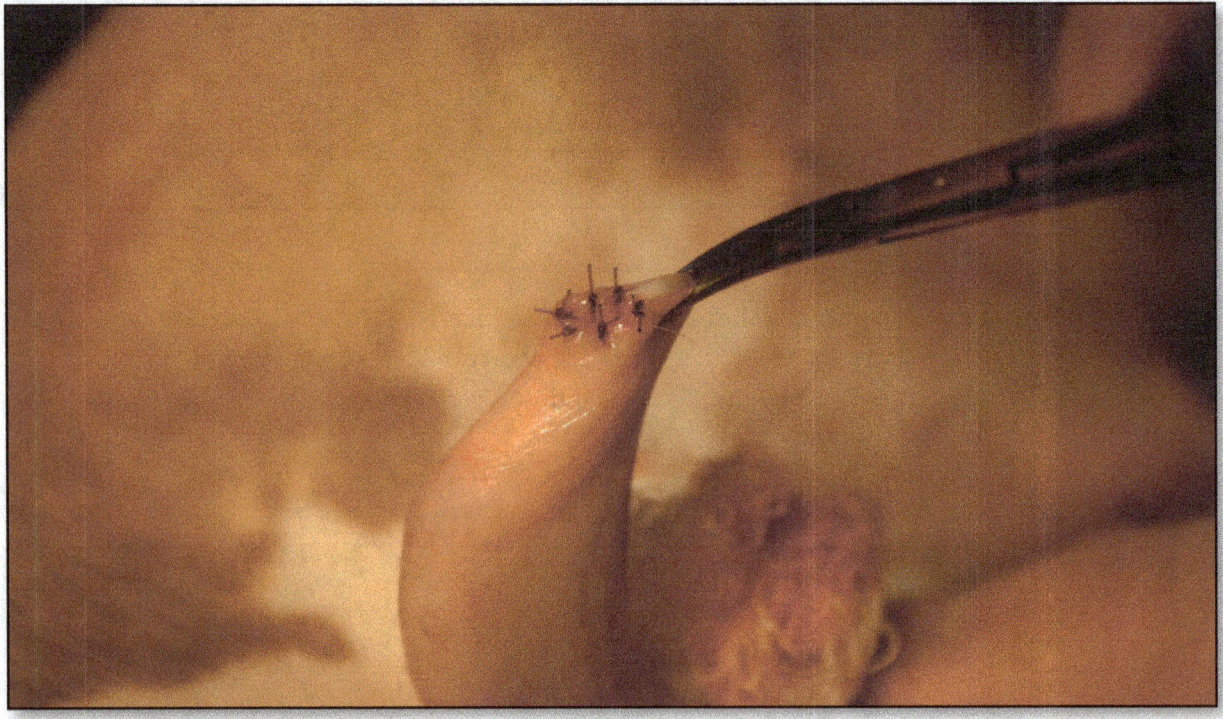

Urethral prolapse repair

10.14.7. Transmissible venereal tumour (TVT)

As the name implies, this is a tumour which may spread from dog to dog by contact during coitus or licking of genitalia. Both males and bitches may be affected. The tumour may be solitary or multiple and is almost always located on the external genitalia, although it may occur in adjacent skin as well as on the mucous membranes of the mouth, nose and eyes. The tumour may arise deep in the prepuce or vagina and be difficult to see. In the bitch it may lead to bleeding of the vagina and misdiagnosis of the bitch being on heat or suspecting another problem. The incidence varies from relatively high in some areas where free roaming dogs are abundant to very rare and even extinct in other areas. TVT is medically curable but needs to be carefully monitored once introduced in a colony to ensure its eradication.

10.15. Libido

Libido refers to sex drive, sexual interest or willingness to mate. Complex behavioural factors play an important role in the expression of normal libido. Confidence and good socialization are vital to good libido. Males which are anxious or fearful, submissive, imprinted on humans only, or find themselves in an unfamiliar environment are likely to display poor libido. Males are more likely to be confident in familiar surroundings; therefore, bitches should be brought to the stud and not the other way around. Even so, aggressive bitches, an individual dislike in a bitch, a previous unpleasant sexual experience and too frequent mating can affect a male's libido. Physical factors which negatively influence libido are disease, poor nutritional condition, over-exercise, arthritic conditions or any other cause of pain. Endocrine disorders may also affect libido but these are rare. It is not good practice to randomly administer testosterone or testosterone releasing hormones as it will aggravate the condition. Not only may it affect libido adversely in the long term but also have adverse effects on fertility.

In some cases sexual over-use brings about lacklustre libido, but sexual rest usually resolves the problem.

A stud dog's lack of interest or refusal to mate might have nothing to do with poor libido, but rather be due to an individual idiosyncratic (inexplicable) dislike of a particular bitch. This condition is confirmed when the same stud on the same day is quite willing to mate another bitch that he likes. Stud dog owners should not dismiss poor libido out of hand. Breeders often defend a stud dog's reputation by insisting that their dog's lack of interest and unwillingness to mate is due to the fact that the bitch is not ready to mate. These breeders will insist that their stud only mates if a bitch is truly ready. Such "picky" males might exist, but if they frequently refuse to mate bitches, the owners should face the reality that they probably own a stud with poor libido.

If males still display poor libido at the age of 30 months the prognosis for improvement is poor. In many cases the cause of poor libido remains unexplained (idiopathic poor libido). Lacklustre libido can be very frustrating and in most cases difficult, if not impossible, to solve. "Love potions" which promise increased libido are unproven. Good libido can be sustained in old age but it generally declines as stud dogs age.

Chapter 10 Reproduction in the Male

Chapter 11

Artificial Reproductive Techniques

The word artificial by definition implies intervention in a process. Artificial reproductive techniques refer to intervention using advanced technologies to manipulate reproduction and genes. To some, this intervention is viewed as wrongful interference with nature. Humans have made a lot of progress since they moved away from their existence as hunter-gatherers to modern farmers. We have developed technologies to manipulate each and every aspect of our existence.

There is the opinion that it might be wrong (unnatural) to assist dogs with artificial insemination because by doing so we are artificially propagating the very same genes which prompted the assistance in the first place.

Reproductive data in dogs seem to suggest that the heritability of reproductive traits e.g., fertility, litter size, semen quality and early postnatal survival is low, with values ranging between 0.1-0.2. What this means is that even if a breeder was to select for or against reproductive performance, the genetic progress or decline is likely to be very slow or negligible. By virtue of cost, time and personal preference, artificial reproductive intervention, however, is not for every breeder.

11.1. Artificial insemination using fresh semen

Artificial insemination (AI) refers to the deposition of semen into the female reproductive tract by means other than natural mating.

11.1.1. Intravaginal use of fresh semen

The main reason why breeders resort to fresh semen artificial insemination is inability for coitus (mating) to take place. Many breeds have a conformation which may impair coitus, lack athletic ability (mating dexterity) or inability to penetrate. Some dogs may suffer from arthritis or physical disabilities. Vestibulo-vaginal obstructions, behavioural factors, inexperience, premature ejaculation, size and weight incompatibilities, heat cycle abnormalities, spread of venereal disease and splitting the ejaculate between two or more bitches are all reasons for AI. Lacklustre libido on the day is a very common reason for A.I.

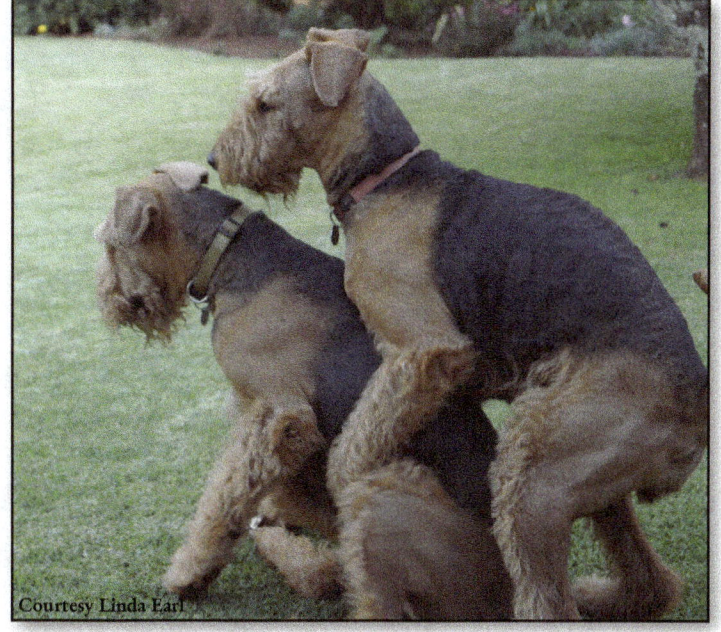

Bitch continues to squat at mating attempts and remains uncooperative until end of her season

Chapter 11 Artificial Reproductive Techniques

Freshly ejaculated semen has limited ability to survive and therefore should be used within less than half an hour of collection. Fresh semen has to be handled with the respect it deserves. Insemination utensils must be clean, sterile and nontoxic to sperm and kept at temperatures to avoid cold shock. Success of AI will depend on semen quality used, semen dose used, fertility of the bitch and proficiency in determining the optimal insemination times. Two inseminations have proven to be more effective than one irrespective of method of timing used. More than two inseminations are only required when less accurate timing methods are used. If no timing methods are used, the bitch should be inseminated once every 48 hours throughout the fertilization period (see 5.15). The insemination dose should preferably be the entire ejaculate and contain 100-200 million (preferably not less than 100 million but certainly not less than 50 million) or more progressively motile sperm. Ejaculates can be split to inseminate two or more bitches simultaneously as long as the semen quality is good and the minimum insemination dose is respected. Breeders often get frustrated if the veterinary surgeon insists on repeat visits in order to optimise the time of insemination. This is because the optimum time is frequently later than what the breeder expected. In dogs where all the parameters are normal (good semen, normal cycle, good insemination technique, good timing), the results achieved are generally good and can be expected to at least equal those of natural matings where the same conditions applied. Under these circumstances, both should result in conception rates around 80% or a little more. Veterinary surgeons involved in canine fertility will however report results poorer than this. This is mainly because breeders will often present bitches which have repeatedly failed to conceive and clearly have underlying fertility problems. Breeders also insist on using semen of questionable quality and then some breeders fail to comply with appointments to inseminate on given days. Typically the veterinary surgeon may require access to the bitch every alternate day for 12 days or longer in some cases.

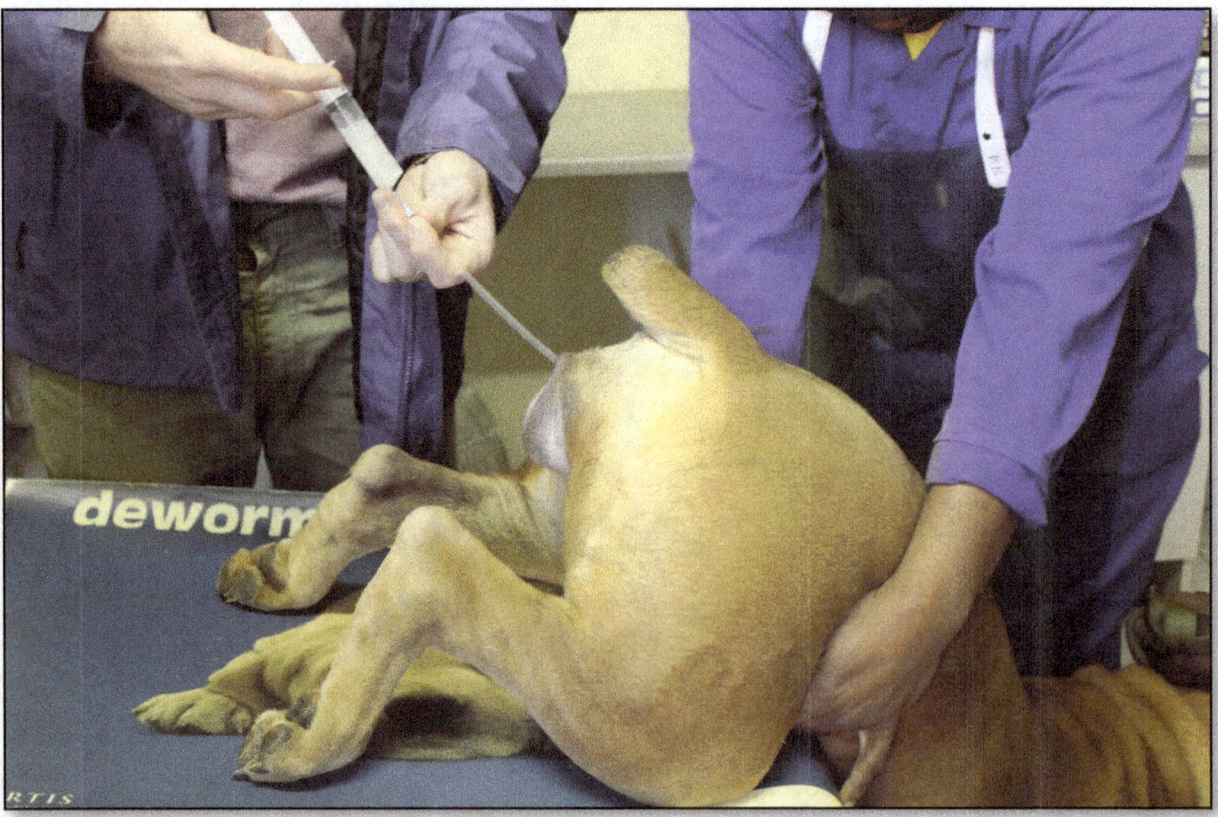

Artificial insemination using fresh semen intra-vaginally

11.1.2. Intra uterine use of fresh semen

This method involves the collection of fresh semen and depositing it directly into the uterus via either surgical, trans cervical or laparoscopic techniques. This method is only recommended when the breeder insists on using a stud with semen quality which is particularly poor. It is also sometimes used by fertility specialists in bitches which fail to conceive as it enables the veterinary surgeon to directly inspect the uterus, ovaries and its structures and this may be of diagnostic value.

11.2. Artificial insemination using chilled semen

Chilled semen, also called fresh extended semen, is fresh semen which has been processed; extended with a special media, gradually cooled to, and kept at 4-5°C during transit in a special container. When kept in this way, the sperm cells are nourished and protected and remain fertile for about 2 days. The main indication for using chilled semen is to inseminate a bitch which is geographically distant from the stud. Chilled, extended semen is a cheaper alternative than frozen semen. This method requires a veterinary surgeon to monitor the oestrous cycle of the bitch in order to determine, one to two days in advance, when the fertilization period is likely to start. This veterinary surgeon must determine when the semen should be collected. There should also be a veterinary surgeon available on the stud's side, to collect the semen and treat it correctly.

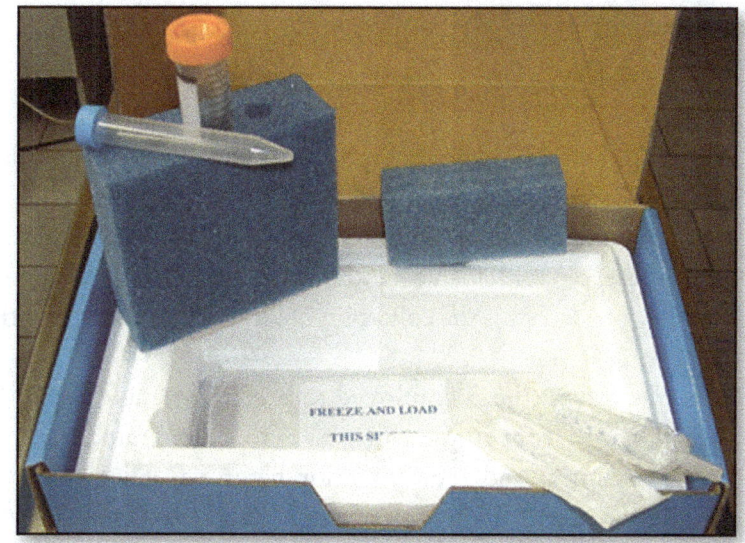
Equipment used for chilled semen

The use of chilled, extended semen is popular in those parts of the world where a reliable transport network exists. Results using this method vary, but are generally poorer than with fresh semen and are estimated at around 70% conception rate under ideal conditions. In deciding whether to use chilled semen the owner should weigh the cost of this procedure and possible reduced conception rate against the time and money spent to transport the bitch to the stud.

Chilled semen is normally deposited intravaginally but intra uterine insemination could also be performed if the quality so dictates.

11.3. Artificial insemination using frozen semen

Frozen semen involves the collection of fresh semen, extending it with cryoprotectants (diluent that protects sperm from damage during freezing) and cooling it down to -196°C in liquid nitrogen and keeping it there indefinitely.

The semen may be packed in vials as pellets or straws. Due to the cost involved, some breeders wish to form a small syndicate and jointly purchase frozen semen to have a bitch inseminated. Not

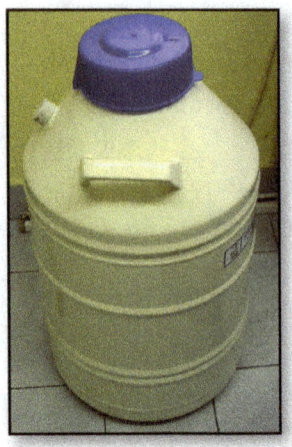
Liquid nitrogen canister

all clubs permit the registration of puppies conceived by frozen semen insemination and breeders should familiarise themselves with such rules.

Results using frozen semen vary but given that good quality frozen thawed semen is used, the bitch is fertile and that good timing methods have been used, a 65% conception rate is plausible albeit with slightly smaller litter sizes. In deciding whether to use frozen semen the breeder should weigh the cost of this procedure, and possible reduced conception rate, against the cost of the purchase and importation of a puppy with the same genetic superiority as the semen. Frozen semen AI does not damage the bitch's reproductive tract and the procedure cannot alter her future reproductive performance.

Semen destined for freezing purposes is best collected using collection by digital manipulation and better samples (higher sperm yield) are achieved in the presence of a teaser bitch (preferably one the stud is familiar with). Semen may also be collected using electroejaculation under anaesthesia but this method is usually reserved for semen collection of wild animals. An interesting method of semen collection in extra ordinary conditions is the collection of semen following castration by flushing the cauda epididymis.

This method has been employed to preserve semen of studs with high breeding value that require euthanasia or from studs which need to be castrated for medical reasons. The entire procedure is highly technical and requires prior planning. The conception rate obtained with frozen-thawed epididymal sperm is lower than that of ejaculated frozen-thawed sperm.

11.3.1. Reasons for semen freezing

The breeder should convince themselves that they have good reasons to either preserve semen from an individual stud or to want to use frozen semen in one of their bitches. The most common reasons to freeze a dog's semen is to preserve genetic material from a perceived genetically superior stud for future use and to transport semen over long distances for use at a convenient time. Cost factors and genetic value should be the main considerations. Some breeders wish to preserve semen to "insure" themselves against possible loss of the stud's fertility or death of the stud. Considering that the freezing process kills a considerable percentage of sperm, it would make sense that the sperm must be very good to start off with if one is to expect reasonable sperm at the end. Therefore the semen donor must have good semen quality. Semen of poor quality should preferably not be frozen unless the breeder is willing to live with the considerable risk of very poor results.

11.3.2. Age of stud at freezing

Ideally, younger dogs' semen, at peak fertility, 3-5 years old, should be frozen preferably before the age of 8 years. Many dogs older than 8 years may have semen which is not of sufficient quality to freeze, but there are exceptions on both ends of the scale. Some breeders elect to freeze semen of young dogs prior to them having proven genetic superiority. In these cases, semen is frozen from the stud whilst still in his prime and the breeder may retrospectively decide to use or discard the frozen semen.

11.3.3. Freezability of dog semen

Despite good quality, in some rare cases, semen from otherwise healthy studs with good fertility may freeze poorly. The exact reason for this is not known. Older studs may be more prone to poor freezability than younger dogs. Freezability can neither be predicted nor assumed and should thus be confirmed.

11.3.4. Number of ejaculates which need to be frozen
As discussed previously, large numbers of sperm are required to successfully inseminate a bitch. Given good quality semen, one ejaculate is usually sufficient to inseminate 1-3 bitches (medium to large breeds). In small breeds 2 ejaculates may be required to render enough sperm to inseminate one bitch. As the dog can easily manage 2 ejaculations within a short time span with minimal sperm number loss, the breeder should consider having two ejaculates frozen simultaneously as this will reduce cost.

11.3.5. Number of inseminations
Depending on the number of sperm available, two inseminations should preferably be performed 24 hours apart per heat cycle. Although ideal, this is not always possible and some experienced reproductive specialists do report good results using a single well timed insemination. Breeders should liaise with their veterinary surgeon to discuss the breeding units (straws or pellets) required to inseminate their bitch.

11.3.6. The insemination method and site
Frozen semen is severely compromised following thawing and has a life span in the order of hours rather than days. This makes both the timing of the insemination and its deposition site critical. The sperm's journey through the female reproductive tract towards the fallopian tube where fertilization takes place is associated with massive loss of sperm numbers and requires "athletic ability", energy and longevity. Frozen-thawed sperm have reduced ability in this regard of these and therefore their journey towards their goal should be made as short and unobstructed as possible. It would therefore

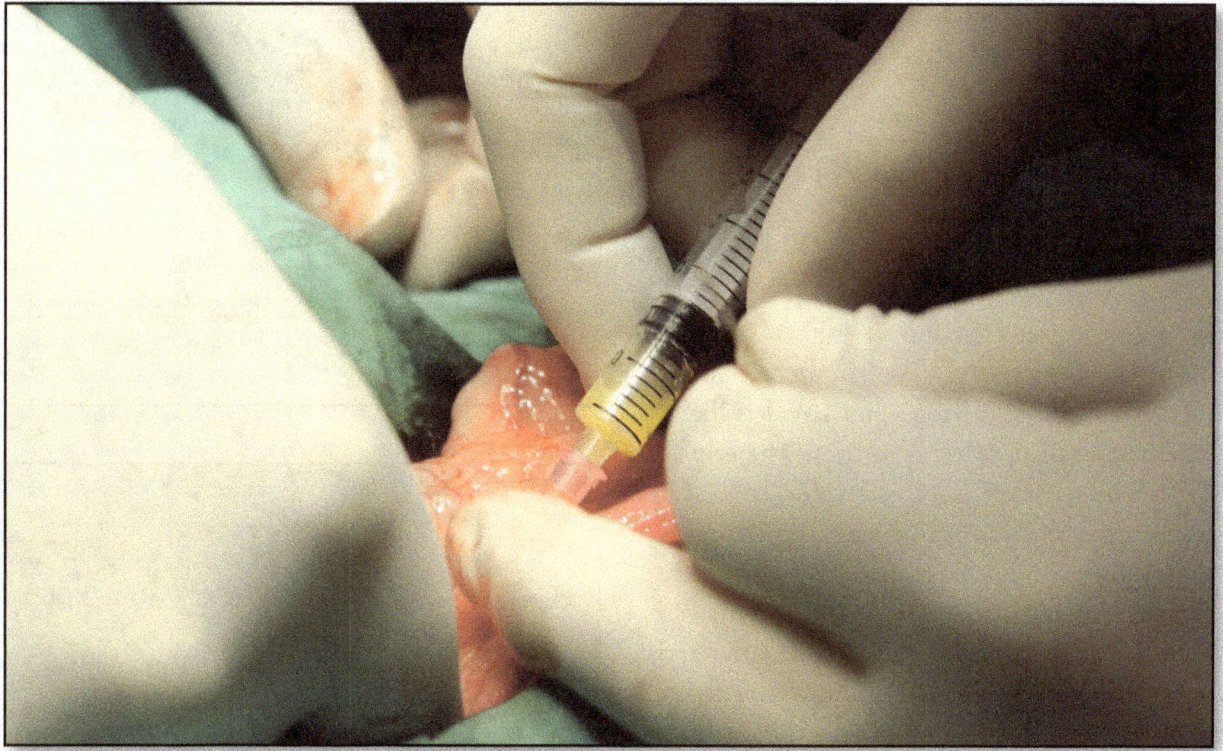

Surgical intra-uterine insemination

make sense that better results are obtained by depositing the semen directly into the uterus. The bitch may be inseminated into the uterus by various means. The surgical methods involve anaesthesia and a small incision into the abdomen. The sperm is then injected directly into the uterus. Although considered invasive, this is a very reliable method to ensure that the semen is deposited where it was intended. Another distinct advantage of this method above all others is that it offers the veterinary surgeon to evaluate the uterus and ovaries for pathology which could otherwise have been very difficult or impossible to diagnose. Intra uterine insemination using laparoscopic equipment also requires anaesthesia and involves inserting needles into the uterus under direct visual control. The latter two methods are considered invasive methods which involve both anaesthesia and entering the abdominal cavity. This inherently carries with it associated anaesthetic and surgical risks.

Less invasive methods of semen deposition entail the use of the "Norwegian catheter" or endoscopic equipment in order to traverse the cervix and deposit the semen into the uterus through the vagina. This is the so called trans cervical insemination (TCI) using endoscopic equipment.

The endoscope has the advantage over the Norwegian catheter in that the semen is deposited under indirect visual control. In skilled hands these methods are successful in achieving the deposition of sperm into the uterus but it does fail in some cases. Transcervical deposition or insemination of semen requires cooperation of the bitch. Bitches resisting the procedure may require some extent of sedation. In cases where it fails, surgical methods may have to be employed and the breeder should be made aware of this possibility.

The intravaginal deposition of frozen thawed semen never gained popularity due to variable results albeit that some very good results have been reported using this method.

In some countries, animal rights activists have been successful in banning invasive methods of insemination. This trend is likely to repeat itself in other countries. The ethical debate of whether it is acceptable to resort to invasive methods to achieve pregnancies, is not over. It is therefore likely that intra vaginal insemination using frozen thawed semen will be revisited. Until such time and unless dictated by legislation, most veterinary surgeons will advocate and use the method which works best in their hands.

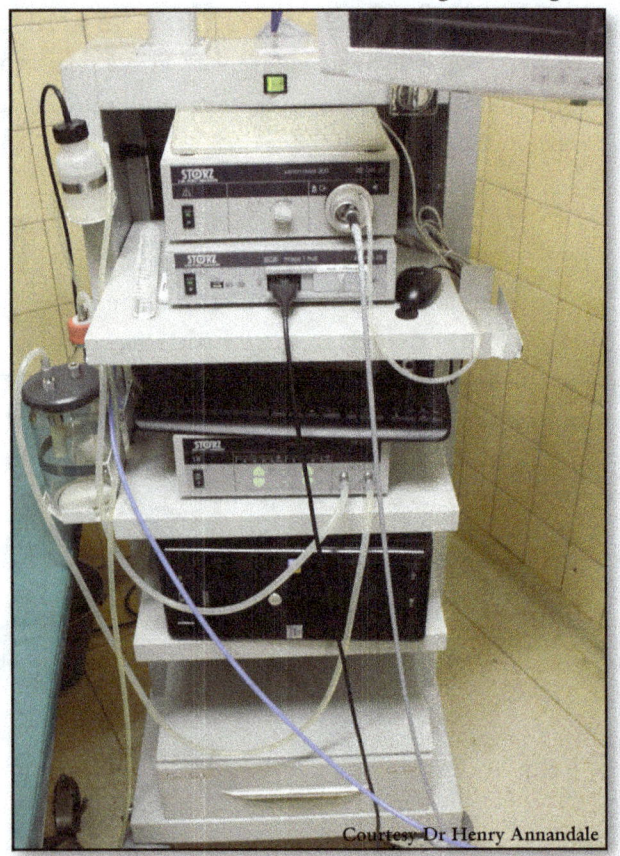

Aparatus required for transcervical intra-uterine insemination

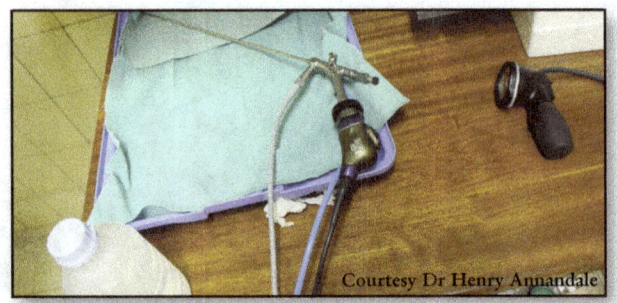

Trans-cervical insemination scope

11.3.7. The number of straws or pellets required (insemination dose or "breeding unit")

The real matter at stake is not the volume or number of straws inseminated. What really matters is the number of progressively motile sperm inseminated. For frozen semen this should be 50-100 million. Some veterinary surgeons wish to refer to this volume as the "breeding unit". For example, if the straws each contained 50 million sperm of which 50% are progressively motile post thaw, then the required 100 million would be contained in 4 of these straws. These 4 straws would then constitute one single breeding unit. Considering that 2 inseminations are required, two breeding units are required to inseminate a bitch twice. In this case, a total of 8 straws would be required. Breeders wishing to inseminate their bitch should consult their veterinary surgeon with regards to the number of straws or pellets to purchase. Semen originating from reputable sources usually comes with data which accurately reflects post thaw motility and recommended number of straws per insemination (breeding unit). In cases where multiple owners jointly own semen, it is advised that they do not split up a breeding unit but rather agree to split up potential puppies from a litter. In order to achieve the intended goal, namely to get a pregnancy from the purchased frozen semen, it is best to buy enough frozen semen to inseminate at two different heats in order to "beat the odds".

11.3.8. Import and export of semen

Depending on the countries involved, trans border import and export of semen may be strictly regulated with a lot of administrative steps to be taken by various individuals and authorities. It is best for the breeder to contact individuals familiar with this process and contract someone to perform all these duties on their behalf. Likewise the transport of the semen and cooled containers should be handled by those familiar with semen transport. The individual freezing the semen should also be informed about whether this semen is intended for local use or export as additional steps then might have to be made that cannot be done after the fact.

11.3.9. Thawing (defrosting) of the semen

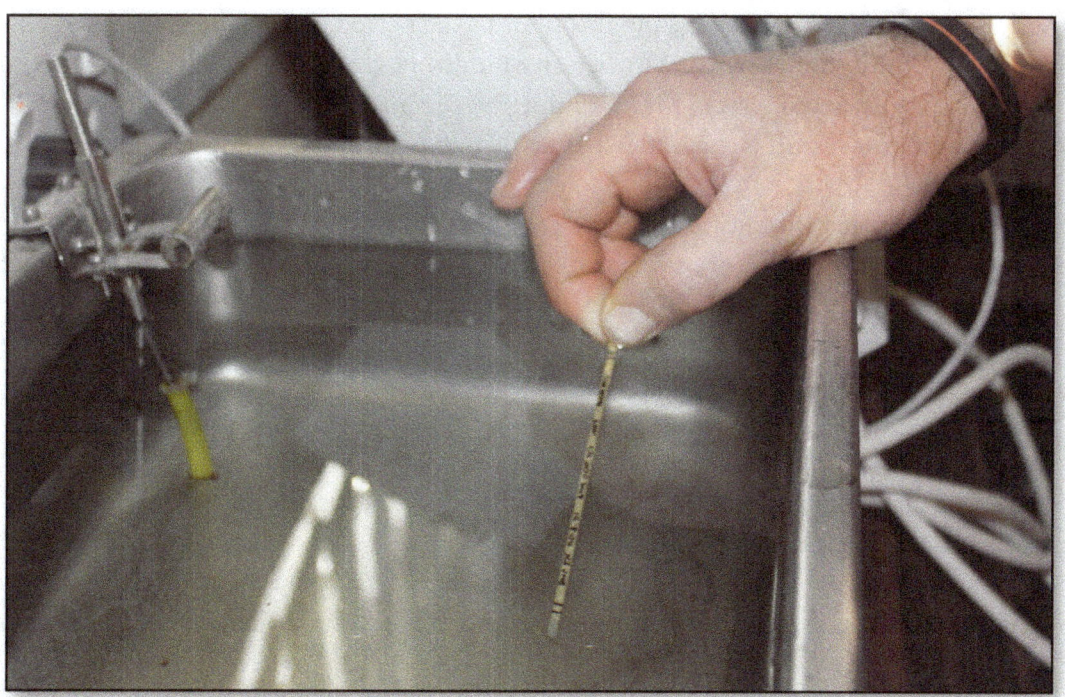

Thawing frozen semen in heated waterbath

Chapter 11 Artificial Reproductive Techniques

The frozen semen needs to be thawed minutes before insemination. There are slow and rapid thawing methods (30 seconds at 37°C or 8 seconds at 70°C). The final choice will be dictated by the recommendations from the person who froze the semen. Some frozen semen also comes with a thawing medium which may have to be used as per instruction. The veterinary surgeon who is tasked with the insemination procedure should be provided with the thawing instructions well ahead of such planned inseminations.

11.3.10. Semen banking

Semen can be stored in liquid nitrogen flasks for a short time varying from several days to several weeks depending on the capacity of the semen flask. It is strongly recommended that long term storage be taken care of by a company which specialises in this.

11.3.11. The ideal recipient of the frozen semen

In order to justify the cost and effort of frozen semen AI, it makes perfect sense that the bitch should be of such genetic quality that it complements the semen's superior quality. Ideally, the bitch selected should be of proven fertility and in her reproductive prime. Young maiden bitches may also be used as second choice. If during the heat monitoring of the bitch, it becomes evident that, the heat cycle is aberrant, the hormone profile is atypical, bitch becomes ill or develops a urogenital infection, it may be necessary to abort the frozen semen AI and resort to the use of fresh semen.

11.3.12. Deliberate superfecundation following artificial insemination

Bitches in which artificial reproductive techniques have been employed, are often reaching the end of their reproductive life span with limited future breeding opportunities. Also, the expected results when using compromised semen (either poorer quality or chilled or frozen semen), are expected to be less than those obtained with non-compromised semen. In these bitches it may be considered to inseminate or mate the bitch using fresh semen after the optimum fertile period, when she has already been inseminated using compromised semen. The rationale is that this bitch then had every opportunity to conceive using the compromised semen because it had been inseminated in the peak fertile period. Some 12-24 hours following this peak fertile period when the bitch was inseminated, there is still opportunity for sperm to fertilize any unfertilized eggs which may still be around. By doing this, the breeder may increase the possibility of pregnancy in that bitch albeit with the less desired sire and uterine health is maintained as explained before.

Clearly, parentage testing is indicated in these cases to confirm paternity. In these cases the DNA profile or DNA samples of the frozen semen donor, dam and second stud as well as offspring must all be submitted for testing and comparison. It is also imperative that the breeder consult with their breeder authorities whether registration of puppies conceived under these circumstances is permitted.

11.3.13. The insemination centre

The selection of the insemination centre will rest upon its expertise in the field, whether it is fully equipped to perform the procedure and whether the centre can render round the clock service. In many cases these centres will be headed by a qualified reproductive specialist or veterinary surgeon with special interest and skills in canine reproduction. Bitches should be presented timeously for early monitoring of their cycle.

11.4. Advanced artificial reproductive techniques

These techniques are included for interest and completeness sake only. They are mostly experimental in nature and are not established well enough for general commercial use.

11.4.1. Embryo transfer

The canine reproductive system appears to be very resistant to manipulation and hence embryo transfer has made little progress. Embryo transfer is a delicate and complex procedure. In other species including man, embryo transfer is commonplace. The techniques of superovulation, recovery of eggs and embryos, synchronisation of oestrus, freezing and storing of embryos or eggs and in vitro fertilization, all need to be well established in a species before embryo transfer can become a viable procedure. This is not the case in the dog. Embryos have been successfully transferred in the dog but the entire procedure remains experimental due to the high failure rate. The commercialisation of embryo transfer in the dog requires more study to optimise this currently inefficient procedure.

Embryo transfer forms part of the dream of animal conservationists to have a "frozen zoo". This involves cryopreservation of male gametes (sperm), female gametes (eggs) and a combination thereof (embryo) for future use in case of the species becoming endangered or extinct. The transfer of embryos to from one species to another (interspecies embryo transfer) is the next step in the quest to save a species from extinction or recover a lost species of which embryos had been preserved.

11.4.2. Freezing canine ovaries

Semen freezing involves preservation of the male gamete. Studies are in progress to successfully freeze the ovaries and eggs from bitches. Further research is required to develop the techniques to successfully fertilise these eggs in vitro (in the laboratory), grow them to the embryo stage and transfer them to a recipient bitch. This is also in its infancy in the quest to create an ovarian tissue bank for severely threatened species.

11.4.3. Cloning

The cloning of an animal involves reproducing an exact replica of an individual. The animal clone therefore has the same genes as its genetic donor. Cloning is achieved by extracting DNA from the donor animal and fusing it with the enucleated egg of the same species. The genetic donor cell may be a cell from an embryo, stem cell from a foetus or a somatic cell from an adult. This egg is then implanted in a surrogate female of the same species. Cloning, using transfer of somatic cell nuclear material is inherently associated with a failure rate frequently exceeding 97% but improvements on success rate is expected in the near future. The high failure is attributed to incompatibilities of transferred material and eggs, failure of eggs to develop, failure of embryos to implant in surrogates and pregnancy failures. Other concerns of cloning are developmental defects and the longevity of cloned individuals but clear answers are not yet available. Some animal activists argue that the extreme cost of cloning is not justified as the resources may be better spent on care of homeless animals. The argument however that pet cloning can or will ever contribute to pet overpopulation and related problems is just not relevant. This is so because irrespective of how efficient highly specialized reproductive techniques as cloning may become, it will only be accessible to a very small proportion of the population and can therefore never significantly contribute to the genetic pool of any animal species. Even if it did, it does not differ from any other form of breeding that involves assisted reproductive techniques which already significantly contributes to farm animal populations. Those defending cloning argue that those very few that can afford cloning help scientists make progress and develop techniques which may in future help preserve endangered species or even reclaim already extinct species. As far-fetched as this may sound, it may actually be possible to reclaim the woolly mammoth, Tasmanian tiger and other species, if viable non degenerate DNA of these species can be found or rejuvenated. Amidst the controversy of cloning, some countries allow commercial production of clones and this service is available to pet owners who wish to clone their pet cat or dog at currently a very high price tag. Another field of interest that holds great promise involves the production of transgenic clones. A non-transgenic animal clone is an animal which is produced (called the clone), from another (called the parent donor) by using its DNA. A transgenic animal clone is one which carries a foreign gene which has been artificially introduced into its genome. Transgenic sheep and goats have been produced that produce foreign proteins in their milk. Also transgenic chickens have been created which are able to synthesize human proteins in their egg white. Lastly, the fascinating field of genetic manipulation holds another possible advantage. This involves therapeutic cloning. The aim of this new field is to create an embryo clone to harvest stem cells from it to treat disease. Again this type of research will provoke attention of human right activists and is an ethical minefield.

11.4.4. Chimeras

In case of mammals, a chimera is an animal which is composed of two or more different populations of genetically distinct cells. Chimeras therefore have four parent cells (or more) which originate from either two fertilized eggs or early embryos which have fused together. This fusion may in exceptional cases occur naturally in some species in very rare cases but this is mostly achieved by genetic manipulation of embryos in laboratories. A Chimera is a mixture of cells within the animal but not a mixture of genes. Goat and sheep cannot hybridize but a goat/sheep chimera has been created artificially that had parts of its body covered with goat hair and others with wool. A chimera may be able to breed successfully but its offspring will be pure (goat or sheep in the mentioned example) depending on what species the reproductive organs of the chimera originated from. To date no chimera of canids has been reported.

Chapter 12

Fecundity (Reproductive Efficiency) in Dog Breeding

Fecundity is the potential reproductive capacity of an individual dog (dog or bitch) or dog population whereas fertility is the natural capacity to reproduce. Fecundity can therefore be seen as a measurement of fertility or reproductive success. In simple terms reproductive efficiency for the breeder is the number of puppies which reach weaning age ready for sale. For the purpose of this text, survival of the puppy till weaning age will be included in the fecundity discussion. A bitch's expected annual puppy production from a breed which on average has litter sizes of 4.4 puppies per litter and cycles twice per annum is 4.4 puppies x 2 cycles per year = 8.8 puppies per year. Because bitches are seldom bred at each heat cycle, it is perhaps more appropriate if fecundity in dogs refers to the result attained for each heat cycle which the bitch is bred.

It is of importance that breeders have some knowledge of the concept of fecundity. It will help breeders identify whether they may have fertility problems and reduced puppy survival or not. If this becomes a widely accepted and used concept, as it has with farmers, benchmarks (norms) for various dog breeds could be set against which breeders could measure their performance.

To achieve this, good record keeping is required. Good records are ones which reflect; ages, bitch name, sire name, dates of breeding, method of breeding, notes on length of heat cycle, date of pregnancy diagnosis and outcome, method used to diagnose pregnancy, date of whelping, number of puppies born live and dead, age and date of neonate death, cause of death if known, number of puppies weaned and results of any post mortems in case of dead puppies. Neat computer programs with many more functions now exist to assist breeders in this. This self-assessment against accepted standards (known litter sizes for the breeds), is required to identify whether there is a fecundity problem or not. Because fertility varies between breeds, one breed should be compared against itself and not against other breeds. Many breeders with serious fecundity problems do not know it. Lack of reproductive success can be very frustrating and financially devastating, particularly if a large number of dogs are in the affected colony. In some cases, a single cause e.g. sub-fertile stud or herpesvirus, can be identified and easily resolved. In most cases however the lack of reproductive success may be associated with a multitude of factors and requires a thorough investigation to identify the causes and finally solve the problem. Both genetic and environmental factors may influence fecundity.

Factors which influence fecundity in the dog are; number of oestrous cycles per year, normality of the oestrous cycles, ovulation rate, timing of fertile period, fertility of stud, embryonal survival, implantation rates, resorption, abortion, stillbirths, weak and underweight puppies, fading puppies and neonatal disease. This book cannot discuss all these factors in detail. Awareness of the major causes and when they occur may help narrow down the number of potential causes. Only the causes in this list which are not discussed elsewhere will be discussed in this section. The breeding soundness examination for studs (10.5) and bitches (5.19) are discussed elsewhere and form an integral part of the investigation into lack of reproductive performance of a breeding kennel.

It is important that breeders have some idea of the "normal" expected mortality rate of puppies in well managed kennels. Stillbirth rates may average 12.9%. Overall mortality rates may be around 19% with the majority of these deaths occurring within the first 10 days of the neonate's life.

12.1. Canine herpesvirus

Canine herpesvirus is found throughout the world in domestic and wild dogs. It is very common in dog breeding colonies and infection rates of 30–100% of dog populations and breeding colonies have been reported. It is speculated that the true infection rates in most countries are higher than generally reported. Despite this, its presence may not be that evident to the breeder because the reproductive effects may go either unseen or be subtle. In kennels which do not breed actively, the virus may have little significance. Most owners of infected breeding colonies do not know it. This is because the virus seldom causes symptoms in the adult dogs. In some cases of susceptible adult dogs or dogs stressed in densely populated kennels and other stressful environments, the virus may cause a mild eye infection and respiratory infection in adult dogs. In rare cases the stud and bitch may have small ulcers on the genitals. For the most part, only the foetuses in the pregnant bitch and puppies 4 weeks or younger will suffer ill effect from herpesvirus. Direct contact with fluids containing the virus is usually required to transmit herpesvirus but aerosol transmission is also possible. Indirect transmission is unlikely because the herpesvirus does not survive long in the environment. The most likely source of infection of the new-born is by oronasal (mouth and nose) contact with secretions of the dam, infected litter mates or other dogs in a kennel. The fate of the dog following exposure to herpesvirus depends on circumstances.

12.1.1. Fate of foetuses from bitches exposed whilst pregnant (prenatal exposure)

A bitch and her offspring may either be susceptible or non-susceptible to herpesvirus depending on her immune status. Bitches vaccinated against herpesvirus or bitches still harbouring natural immunity from previous herpesvirus exposures or recrudescence are non-susceptible and their foetuses will be safe. Bitches without antibodies at the time of pregnancy which get exposed to virus

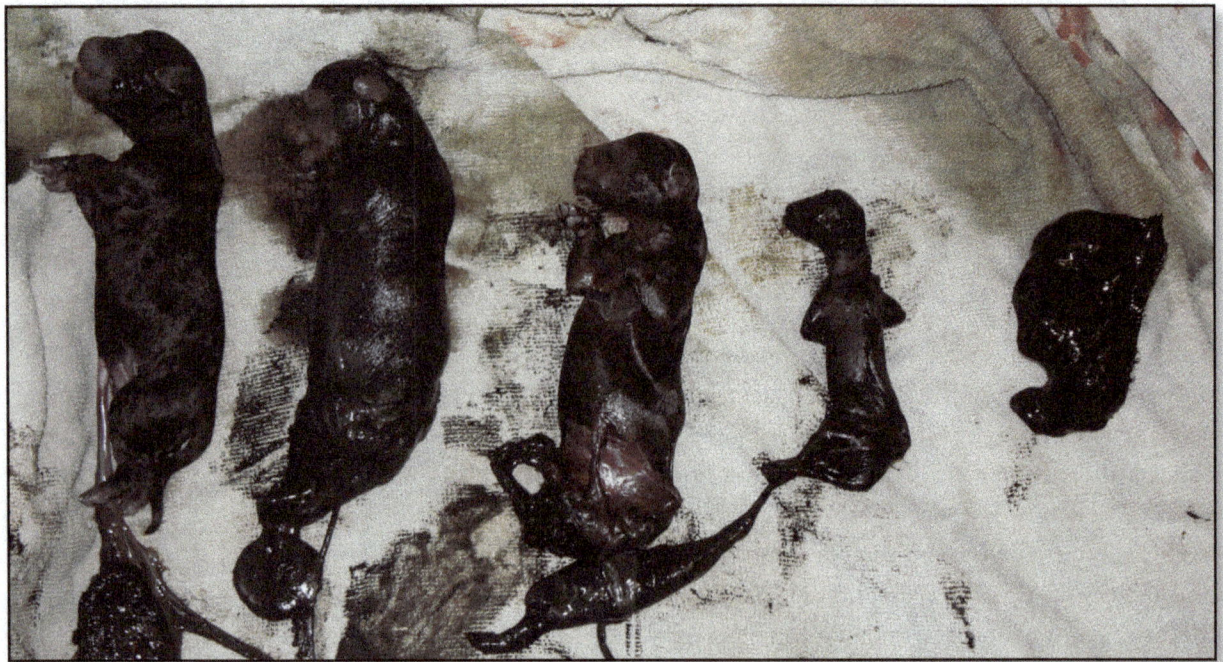

Intra-uterine death of puppies at various stages of pregnancy which is sometimes associated with herpes virus infection

Chapter 12 Fecundity (Reproductive Efficiency) in Dog Breeding

may resorb if the infection occurs during the first 28 days of pregnancy. If the bitch resorbs all its foetuses, the breeder will not know it and possibly think that the bitch did not conceive. If only part of the litter was resorbed the breeder will then only see smaller litter sizes in this bitch. If infection occurs somewhat later in pregnancy, the bitch may either abort, have still born puppies or have weak and underweight puppies which die soon after birth. Not all the puppies infected in utero need necessarily be weak or die. Herpesvirus may single out individuals. Because younger bitches are less likely to have been exposed they are more likely to suffer from reproductive problems following herpes exposure. Bitches having suffered from reproductive failure (fertility problems) associated with herpesvirus are less likely to have future problems but this is not excluded.

12.1.2. Fate of puppies exposed from birth to 4 weeks (post natal exposure)

Puppies born which did not receive colostral immunity from their dams are very likely to fall ill when exposed. These puppies may become infected as they pass through the birth canal. Another source of infection to these puppies is from infected oral and nasal secretions of the dam or any other dog in the kennel which is shedding virus. Transmission in these cases may be by direct oronasal contact with fluids or from aerosol (droplet) infection. Delivery by caesarean section cannot guarantee herpes free puppies but may minimise the risk. These puppies would require hand rearing, colostral intake by tube and total isolation of all other dogs. Therefore, this way of trying to prevent herpes is not always practical or successful. The incubation period is about 6-10 days therefore, puppies infected at birth or very soon thereafter will show illness within the first 7-21 days. Litters in which the onset of symptoms is 7-14 days have a very high mortality rate approaching 100% whilst litters between 14–21 days may have a somewhat lower mortality rate. In the former group the deadly systemic form of the disease is more likely whereas in the latter group the likelihood of the respiratory form is greater. Puppies that die from herpes virus infection are frequently in very good condition because they were doing exceptionally well before they fell ill. The first clinical signs normally seen in the puppies are inability to nurse followed by continuous crying. Their abdomens may appear bloated, are painful to touch and have dark blue discolouration. These symptoms may persist for 1-3 days after which the puppies normally die. Treatment is usually ineffective. Tube feeding, raising the environmental temperature, antiviral therapy and immune serums are all advised but normally do not work. Puppies which survive may suffer from nervous symptoms or myocarditis and succumb to that later. Preventative treatment of in-contact litter mates not yet affected may help. Besides immune-incompetence, inability to thermo-regulate and inability to mount a fever response explains the young puppy's high susceptibility to herpesvirus as opposed to older puppies. As with any cause of reproductive failure and puppy losses, breeders should have this investigated by their veterinary surgeon in attempts to accurately diagnose a cause.

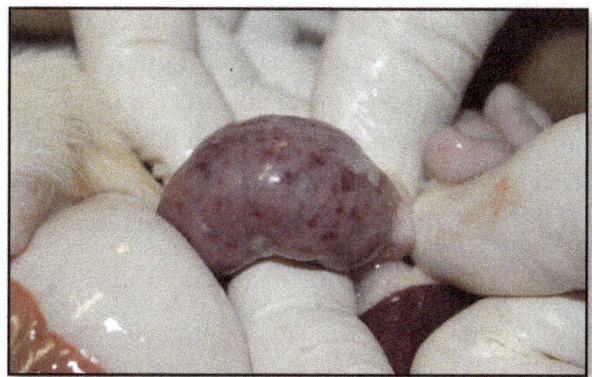

Herpes associated lesions on kidneys

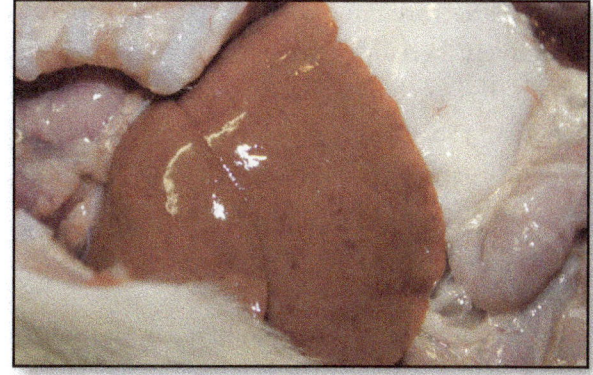

Herpes associated lesions on liver

Chapter 12 Fecundity (Reproductive Efficiency) in Dog Breeding

12.1.3. Fate of dogs older than 4 weeks

Puppies older than 4 weeks of age and any other age thereafter, will either not have any symptoms from the herpesvirus following exposure whatsoever, or only show mild respiratory symptoms. They will develop immunity by producing antibodies against the virus in the blood. This immunity may last for only 2-4 months. A unique feature of herpesvirus infection in dogs is that despite the dog developing antibodies in the blood, the virus does not totally disappear from the dog's body, but rather goes into "hiding" in the ganglia (nerve structure) and remains dormant. Until proven otherwise, it should be assumed that once the dog is infected, most will remain latently affected for life and will be asymptomatic. These latent carriers may falsely test negative against herpes antibody tests. The latent virus may be "awakened" (recrudescence) in the dog's system by numerous stressors after which they show episodes of virus shedding for up to a week at a time in genital or nasal secretions. These stressors may be transport, illness, hierarchical disputes, new introductions or translocation. This intermittent virus shedding may occur at unpredictable intervals over months or even years. Such intermittent shedding assures the survival of herpesvirus in the dog population and in breeding kennels.

12.1.4. Control of canine herpesvirus

Testing at the time of breeding in attempts to eliminate the risk of herpesvirus exposure is useless. This is because most dogs are likely to be positive in any case and negative tests mean nothing because the test does not reveal latent virus in carriers. Vaccination is the only effective control available to breeders. An effective vaccine is available in many countries. Because the immunity induced by the vaccine only lasts 2-3 months following vaccination, it should be administered to the dams whilst in heat and again when the bitch is confirmed pregnant but not later than 10 days prior to the expected whelping date. Ideally, the first herpes vaccination should be administered when the bitch has just entered her season and again about 30 days later. The vaccine has been shown to significantly improve litter size, weaning rates, increase puppy birth weights and reduce early puppy death. At her next pregnancy irrespective of interval, revaccination is required. Vaccination of the stud serves no purpose.

There may be value in collecting colostrum from vaccinated bitches and freezing it in a colostrum bank. This colostrum will then contain antibodies against herpesvirus and could be administered to new-born puppies from bitches which have puppies at risk because they were not vaccinated. This may help reduce losses in case of an outbreak.

12.1.5. Practical significance of herpesvirus to breeders

Venereal transmission is possible but is speculated to be very rare. It may be assumed that the stud plays no bigger a role in transmission of the virus than does any other individual in an infected colony. Canine herpesvirus in dog breeding colonies is so common that breeders should assume that their kennels are infected unless proven otherwise. Breeders who show regularly, have large numbers of actively breeding bitches, groom, run boarding kennels and train dogs on the same premises which they breed, are more likely to suffer from herpes related fertility problems because of higher exposure rates and a more stressful environment. Introduction of herpesvirus into a dog colony which is naïve (has never been exposed before) may lead to serious outbreaks of canine herpesvirus associated fertility problems if this introduction occurs during a time that many bitches are about to be bred or already pregnant.

There is no reason why the breeder should not breed a bitch which produced a litter of puppies which had herpes. Once exposed to herpesvirus her chances to suffer from fertility problems are less at subsequent breedings. Reproductive problems associated with herpesvirus in infected kennels may sometimes come and go mysteriously with intervals of several years. This phenomenon can be explained by immunity that has built up in the dog colony and bitches which were pregnant at any time were either not susceptible because of previous infection whilst not pregnant, or had not been exposed. Some breeders may erroneously think that they are free from herpesvirus reproductive problems because they may have become accustomed to low fertility. These breeders only become aware of the problem once they note improvement following the use of the vaccine.

Absence of evidence of reproductive problems is not proof of absence of herpesvirus infection in that kennel. Given this background, the breeder may now ask what is the relevance of all this to them as breeders and under what circumstances should they vaccinate against herpesvirus. The breeder should consider the following risk benefit assessment. Breeders whom appear to be plagued by reproductive problems such as bitches which fail to conceive, appear to resorb, abort, have weak and underweight puppies or suffer from neonatal deaths should have this problem investigated. If either herpes is confirmed or no obvious cause of the reproductive problems can be found, the index of suspicion is high enough to warrant vaccination against herpesvirus. Some breeders elect to vaccinate their bitches despite not having had previous problems out of fear of devastating losses. It makes sense for breeders whom have already spent a large sum of money on artificial insemination or acquisition of new breeding stock at great expense to eliminate as much risk as they can and to prevent puppy losses by vaccination. Other breeders argue that they will consider control of herpesvirus vaccine if they have experienced losses before they justify cost of vaccination.

In summary, eradication of canine herpesvirus in kennels is not possible but minimizing the risk of losses to herpesvirus is. Minimising stress, isolating pregnant bitches during peak susceptibility (3 weeks before to 3 weeks after parturition) from the general dog population and vaccinating may all aid in this.

12.2. Minute virus of canines

It is appropriate that this virus (CPV-1) be discussed alongside herpesvirus because it may also cause reproductive problems in dogs and may be confused with herpesvirus. The virus is also widespread and 50-70% of dog populations may show antibodies in their blood indicating that they had been infected at some stage. Foetuses may be infected trans-placentally usually when dams get infected in the first half of pregnancy and then the bitch may fail to conceive due to resorption or abort depending on how far advanced pregnancy was. Puppies exposed normally die between 1 and 3 weeks of age with prior clinical signs of respiratory distress and or diarrhoea. Unlike herpesvirus, many affected puppies remain ill for a day or two and make a full recovery. Minute virus of canines may in part be responsible for some "fading puppies". Few laboratories can test for the virus but this situation may improve in time. Currently, the status of minute virus in breeding colonies is unknown and its impact on breeding is uncertain. More research is required to solve the minute virus enigma.

12.3. Canine brucellosis

Canine brucellosis is a zoonosis, meaning a disease of primary interest in animals which may potentially spread to humans. The causative organism is Brucella canis. Transmission of the disease may occur through oral routes or venereal transmission. Transplacental transmission in pregnant bitches is also possible. It is important for breeders to realise that an infected dog may infect others in the colony without sexual contact. The infection causes urogenital infections in the bitch and infection of the testis (orchitis and epididymitis) in male dogs. Infected bitches may fail to conceive, resorb, abort or produce weak puppies which do not reach weaning age. Infected studs may show subfertility or infertility.

A newly infected dog may harbour the infection for a period of months without showing any symptoms.

Failing to test for brucellosis in many countries is considered negligent. Breeders may request a recent (6 months or less) negative Brucella test result prior to contact with their breeding stock. It is important that when testing dogs, they should not have received antibiotic treatment for at least a month prior to testing as this may render false negative results. When testing a suspect colony or individual dog, it may be necessary to test 2-3 times to conclusively prove that the dog or colony is Brucella free. This is because chronically infected dogs may falsely test negative because of fluctuating titres. If the dog however emanates from a known free colony, then a single test may be considered conclusive. Some tests are referred to as screening tests whereas others are considered confirmative. It is important that the breeder consult veterinary surgeons with extensive experience with canine brucellosis. Accuracy of results and how to interpret them is of great importance. This is because the outlook for a positive dog is grave. There is no treatment for the condition and infected dogs remain infected for life. Brucella infected dogs should not be kept in a breeding kennel. These animals should be euthanized or castrated and isolated. As Brucellosis may be transmitted through semen, studs should be tested as well if they are destined for fresh semen artificial insemination. As Brucella may even survive the freezing process, testing of studs used for semen freezing is mandatory in some areas.

12.4. Bacterial infections

Bacterial infections of the urogenital tract may influence canine fertility. The causative bacteria may be foreign or normal flora which become opportunistic pathogens. Breeding establishments where there is a large population of breeding animals all living in close proximity are at increased risk for bacteria which cause infertility. The problem that the breeder may see is mainly poor conception rates or very high mortality rates in the neonates. In some instances there may be clear evidence of bacterial infections such as vaginitis or uterine infection characterised by a vaginal discharge. In others there will be no external signs of infection. As explained in the section on breeding soundness in the bitch (5.19), the breeder's veterinary surgeon should be approached to assist in these infertility examinations. *Mycoplasma spp, Escherichia coli, Enterrococcus spp, Klebsiella spp, Pasturella spp, Bacteroides spp, Streptococcus spp* and *Staphylococci spp* may all be isolated and implicated in infertility in bitches. Isolation and culture of deep vaginal swabs and semen are important examinations towards solving this problem. The transmission of bacterial infections is usually not venereal (transmitted by sexual contact). Although less common, studs may also harbour the mentioned potentially pathogenic bacteria in their reproductive tracts leading to poor conception. They are however seldom involved in the transmission of the bacteria to the bitches they mate. Direct contact between bitches in crowded kennels is the main method of transmission.

These hidden bacterial infections may ascend from the vagina into the uterus and cause low grade infections making the uterine environment unfavourable for implantation or maintenance of pregnancy. In cases where the pregnancy was not affected, the puppies may become infected during birth and die several days later.

When the causative organism is identified and an antibiogram (culture to determine sensitivity to antimicrobials) has revealed the antibiotic effective against it, the affected bitch or stud should be treated. Treatment of in-contact dogs could also be considered.

Unfortunately, many breeders whom suspect that they may be affected by a bacterial infection reducing fecundity in their population resort to self-treating their dogs with antibiotics. The choice of antibiotic is often made on hearsay or internet sourced information. This approach may fail in a large percentage of cases even if bacteria were indeed the cause. This is because the sensitivity of the various implicated bacteria varies so much that this approach has a small chance to succeed. Judicious selection of antibiotics based on laboratory tests is ultimately cheaper and more likely to render good results.

12.5. Obesity of bitches

The chapter on nutrition adequately dealt with the adverse effect on fertility and lowered conception rates and increased risk of dystocia. It is repeated here merely to remind breeders of its importance.

12.6. Selection for fecundity

Although fertility traits are known to be of low heritability, it is nevertheless an important trait which should not be neglected altogether. The value of selecting for fertility is well known in production animals. In dog breeding, fertility as selection criteria is often omitted or in some cases there may in actual fact be selection for reduced fertility. This is because artificial reproductive techniques are applied in dogs of low fertility to improve conception rates. It may be argued that these dogs would not have been able to reproduce without assistance and in this way genes contributing to poorer fertility are "kept in circulation". Selection for miniaturisation is also believed to reduce fertility in some breeds where this practice is popular.

In the broader context both breeders and veterinary surgeons should be more aware of value of selection for fertility traits and perhaps less obsessed with obtaining offspring of the "not so fertile" brood bitches and studs.

Chapter 12 Fecundity (Reproductive Efficiency) in Dog Breeding

Chapter 13

The Normal Neonate

13.1. Birth to weaning

Immediately after birth, puppies will cry, have pink mucous membranes, have strong heart beats and move vigorously. At this stage all the umbilical cords should have been tied off and disinfected using chlorhexidene, iodine or other appropriate disinfectant. Normal puppies will nurse about every 2 hours. Puppies which are healthy will drink and then sleep quietly with the occasional jerky movement. Puppies which cry and move about continuously have some form of discomfort. This may be: hunger, coldness, isolation from the bitch or litter mates, the need to defecate or urinate or burping, bloating, pain or illness. The crying stops as soon as the cause of discomfort has been rectified. If the cause is not rectified, the puppy will in time stop crying, appear limp, have poor muscle tone, become weak, quiet, and finally fall into a coma and die soon afterwards. It is easy to distinguish the latter puppy from a healthy puppy. Healthy puppies which lie still because they are sleeping are very responsive to physical stimulation and will cry and move vigorously whereas unhealthy puppies will not respond to touch. Another easy way to evaluate the wellbeing of a healthy puppy is to evaluate the suckling reflex. This is done by inserting your finger into the puppy's mouth and a healthy strong puppy will immediately suck on it whereas the weak one will either not suck at all or suck weakly. Weight gain is the most reliable and objective parameter to measure progress in neonates.

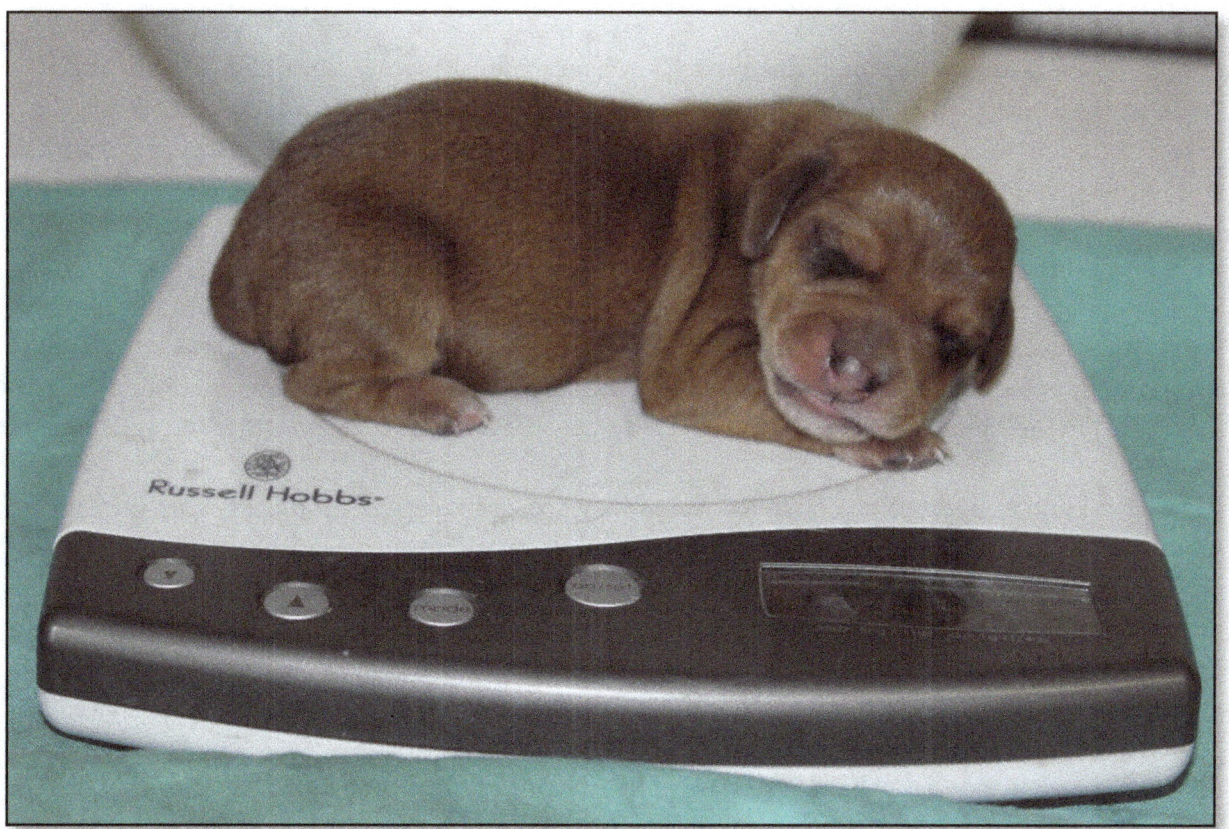

Accurate weighing of puppies, preferably on a digital scale, helps in monitoring their progress

Chapter 13 The Normal Neonate

Every breeder should have an accurate digital scale to record birth weights and monitor weight gain. In the first 24 hours however, puppies may either not gain weight or lose some weight (less than 10% of birth weight). Following that, the weight should increase steadily. Their weight should double in the first 8-12 days. The exact amount of weight gain varies a lot depending on breed and milk production of the dam and many other factors. A rough estimate of normal daily weight gain is 1-1.5 grams per day for every Kg of anticipated adult weight. Thus if the anticipated adult weight is 35 kilograms, the daily weight gain should be around 35–50 grams per day. The growth curve changes with age. Breeders will in time get their own weight gain curves for their breed. As long as there is gain from day to day, things are probably going well. In contrast, puppies which fail to gain weight are either sick or not getting enough milk for whatever reason and will die. The umbilical cord dries and falls off within 2-3 days following birth. For the first 5 days the puppies have extensor dominance meaning that they keep all their limbs forward. The eyes and ears open around day 10-14 and they can usually start standing a few days later. New-born puppies do not have controlled excretion and cannot defecate and urinate spontaneously without stimulation from the dam. The bitch will lick the puppy's perineum (anus area) to stimulate excretion until controlled urination and defecation occurs at around 15-21 days. The puppies' milk (deciduous) teeth erupt between 3-6 weeks but in some toy breeds this may be delayed by a week or two.

Under normal circumstances, if the puppies are growing well, the puppies can be left with the dam to suckle until weaning age. If the dam is not able to provide adequate milk, supplementary feeding of milk formula and creep feeding should be considered. It is important to notice that if creep feeding is practiced, the puppies should be fed water as well in a shallow bowl.

13.2. Dewclaw removal

The dewclaw is the fifth inside facing claw. Dewclaw removal involves cutting off the dewclaw as close to the leg as possible, disinfecting it and applying some pressure on it to prevent bleeding. Cauterising tincture of ferrous chloride may also be used to stop haemorrhage. When performed by a veterinary surgeon, they may normally cauterise the small vessels severed using electronic devices and even insert small stitches. Dewclaw removal may be performed without anaesthesia by some veterinary surgeons whilst other elect to infiltrate some local anaesthetic. Some veterinary surgeons maintain that the needle to infiltrate the local anaesthesia is as painful as the removal of the dewclaw. Most breeds will have a dewclaw on the front feet whilst only some will have dewclaws on their back feet as well. Some members of the giant breeds may have dewclaws which are duplicated or even triplicated in their hind feet. These traits appear to be strongly familial.

Dewclaws in dogs appear to be non-functional as they do not bear weight and neither are they able to hold onto prey as is the case in felines. Their removal therefore is non-consequential. There are breed differences with regards to their presence and desirability to remove them or not. In many breeds either or both of the front or back dewclaws are considered a nuisance and their removal is recommended. The nuisance factor is that in some dogs they do not show natural abrasion and wear down and grow almost 360° into themselves and cause infection. In other dogs they may hook onto objects, tear and bleed.

In cases where removal of the dewclaws is desired, some recommendations are made. Newborn puppies do not have adequate clotting mechanisms until they are about 72 hours old and before then they are at risk of serious haemorrhaging. Therefore it is best to delay the removal of dewclaws till after the third day but not later than the fifth day. This is because some breeds grow very quickly and by 5 days of age, the dewclaw has grown so large that removal is more difficult, bleeds more and removal is also likely to be more painful for the puppy.

There is another very important reason for the delay in time before removal of the dewclaws in puppies. As puppies are born with no immunity as explained in 7.1, the puppy is more likely to develop an infection if the skin is broken and the puppy has not yet received or absorbed all its antibodies.

13.3. Tail docking

Tail docking is a practice which has been performed for many years. In more recent years however, tail docking has become condemned as an unnecessary procedure which mutilates the dog. Others insist that if performed correctly, it is a perfectly humane procedure which may prevent far more distress than it causes.

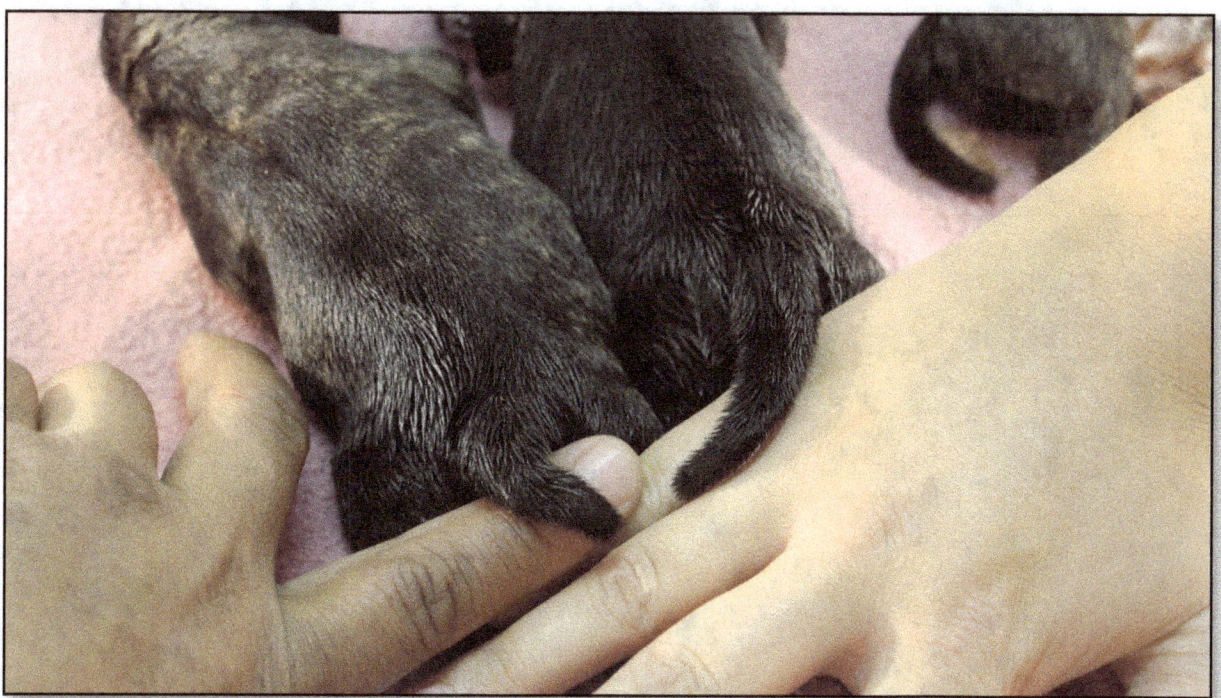

Kinked tails in puppies are seen more frequently in countries where docking is banned because of years of not having selected against these traits

The reasons for tail docking include prevention of tail injuries in gundog breeds working in thick vegetation, increased manoeuvrability in underground holes in terrier breeds, prevention of soiling of perineum in long haired and thick coated breeds and maintaining breed standards. Despite possible advantages, tail docking has been banned in various countries or become frowned upon in others. This is a trend that is likely to spread. The ethical debate surrounding tail docking will not be discussed in this book. It is considered a minor procedure by some, which causes minimal discomfort and it does not appear to adversely affect puppies health in any way. Others maintain that it is an unnecessary painful procedure. It is important for the breeder to familiarise themselves with their local rules and regulations regarding legality of tail docking. In countries where tail docking remains legal, it is advised that breeders consult their veterinary surgeons to perform the procedure or at the very least show them how to perform it. The age of the puppies at the time of tail docking is important for similar reasons as explained as for dewclaw removal in 13.2.

Chapter 13 The Normal Neonate

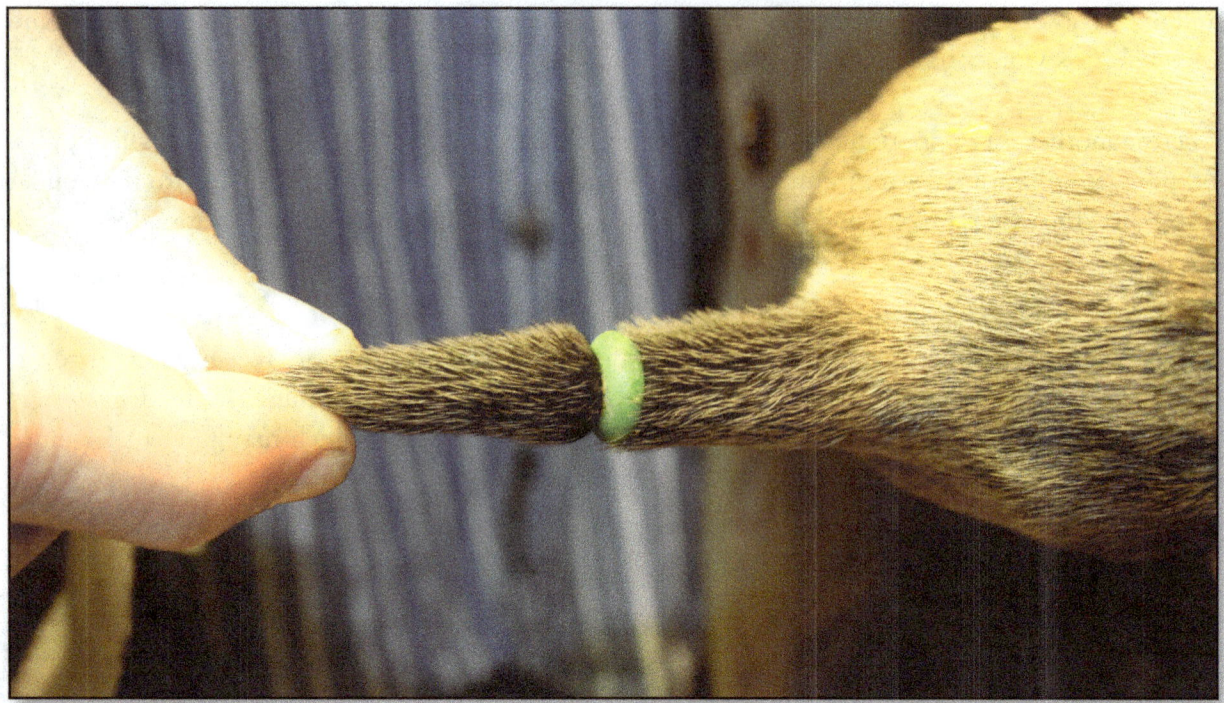
Elastrator ring on tail

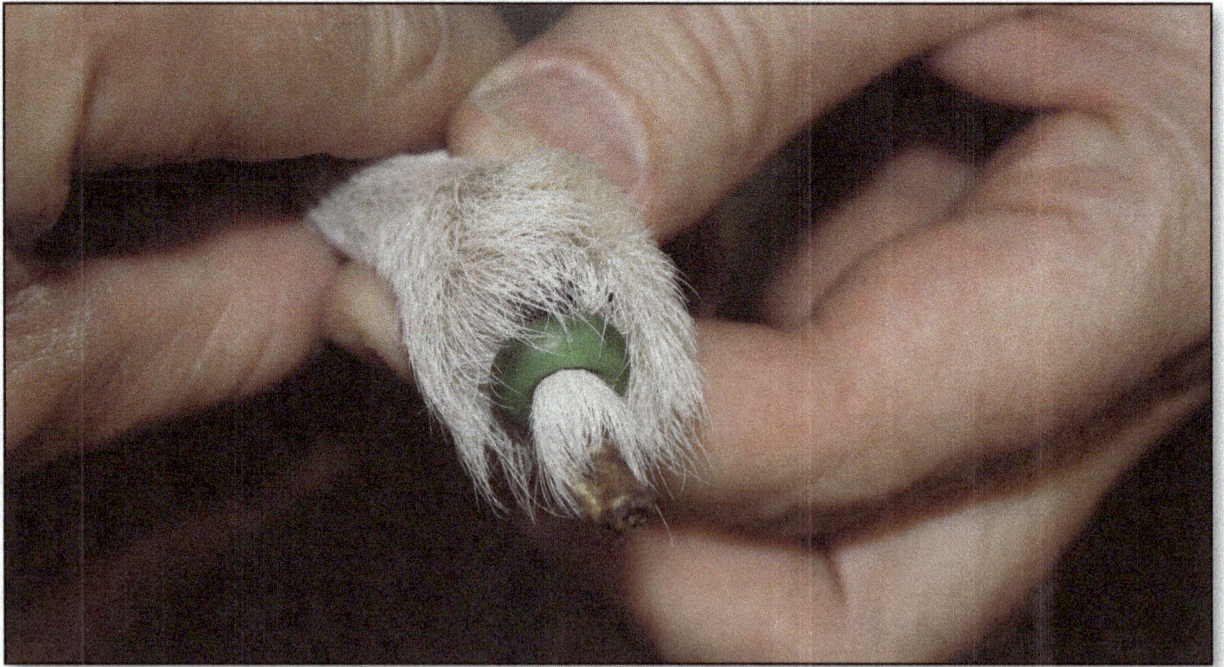
Tail that became necrotic as result of elastrator ring

Some owners whom perform the procedure themselves often have infection, severe haemorrhage and death as a result of docking. Elastic rings as used in small stock are not acceptable in dogs.

13.4. Rearing orphan puppies

The best and easiest way to raise puppies is to have a good dam which does it, as nature intended. They will feed them; care for them, clean them, stimulate excretion and keep them warm. If it appears that the mother has poor milk production but is otherwise a good mother, it should still be considered to have the bitch care for them and only supplement feed the puppies. Poor milk production should be suspected when there is insufficient weight gain and hungry cries from the puppies. There may be a problem with supplement feeding puppies when the dam also still nurses the puppies. When the bitch is the primary feeder of the puppies but the breeder needs to supplement feed them, the trick is to know how much to feed them extra. This is because the breeder has no idea how much milk they are already getting from the dam. The main danger of supplement feeding under these circumstances is over-feeding which may cause severe diarrhoea. Over feeding is particularly likely if the method of milk formula supplementation is tube feeding. The best way to manage this dilemma is to avoid tube feeding and supplement by bottle feed. This way the puppy can regulate its own intake.

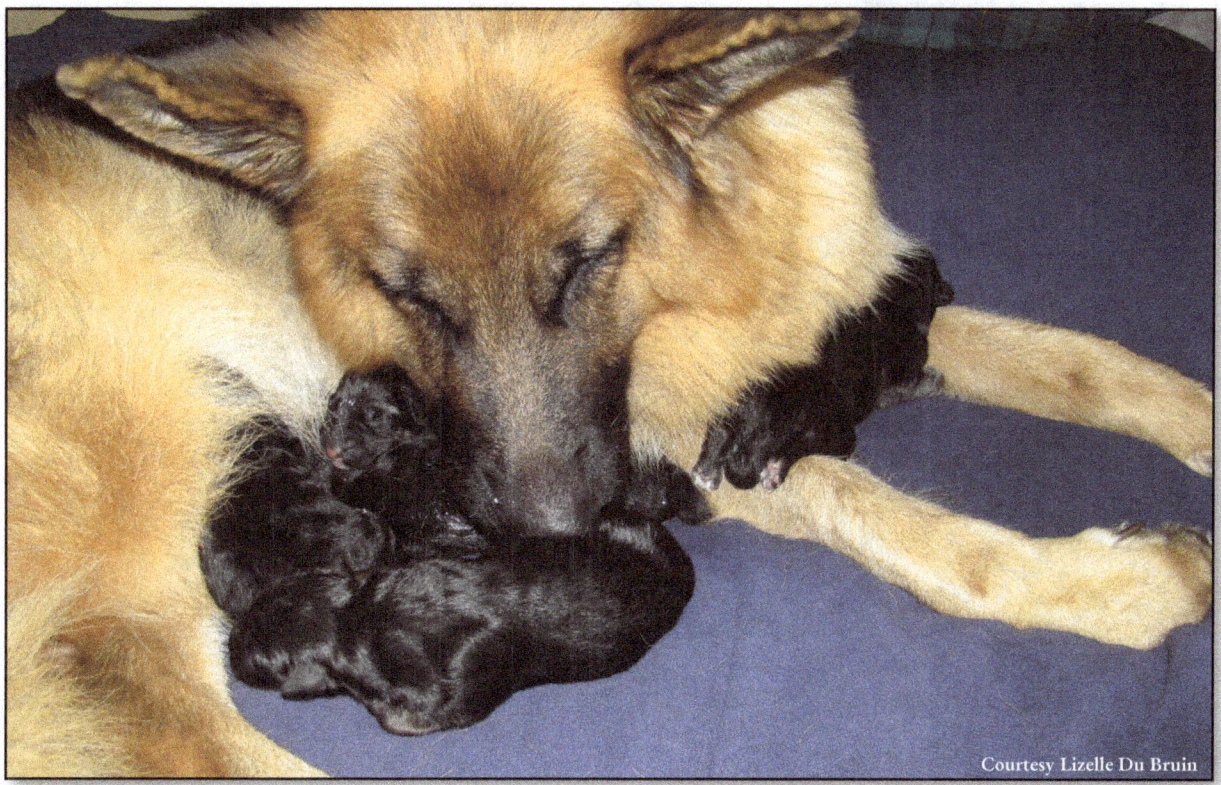

Dog that is exhibiting good mothering instincts

Foster mothers, when available, are the second best choice. Only when neither of this is possible, should hand rearing be practiced. Thus, only hand rear when there is no other option!

Puppies may become orphaned because the dam may be dead, sick, unable or unsuitable to adequately care for her puppies. Poor milk production and poor mothers are the most common reasons for fostering or hand rearing puppies. Irrespective of method of raising the puppies, the breeder should ensure that the puppies have adequate colostrum uptake as discussed in 7.1.

Puppies cannot control their body temperature (thermo-regulate) during the first 3 weeks of life and the environmental temperature must therefore be controlled for them. Normal puppies will crawl towards their mother and litter mates when cold and disperse when hot. For orphaned puppies, the ideal temperatures during the first, second, third and following weeks are 35°C, 31°C, 28°C and 26°C respectively. This can be achieved by using incubators, heaters or lamps. It is important to

Chapter 13 The Normal Neonate

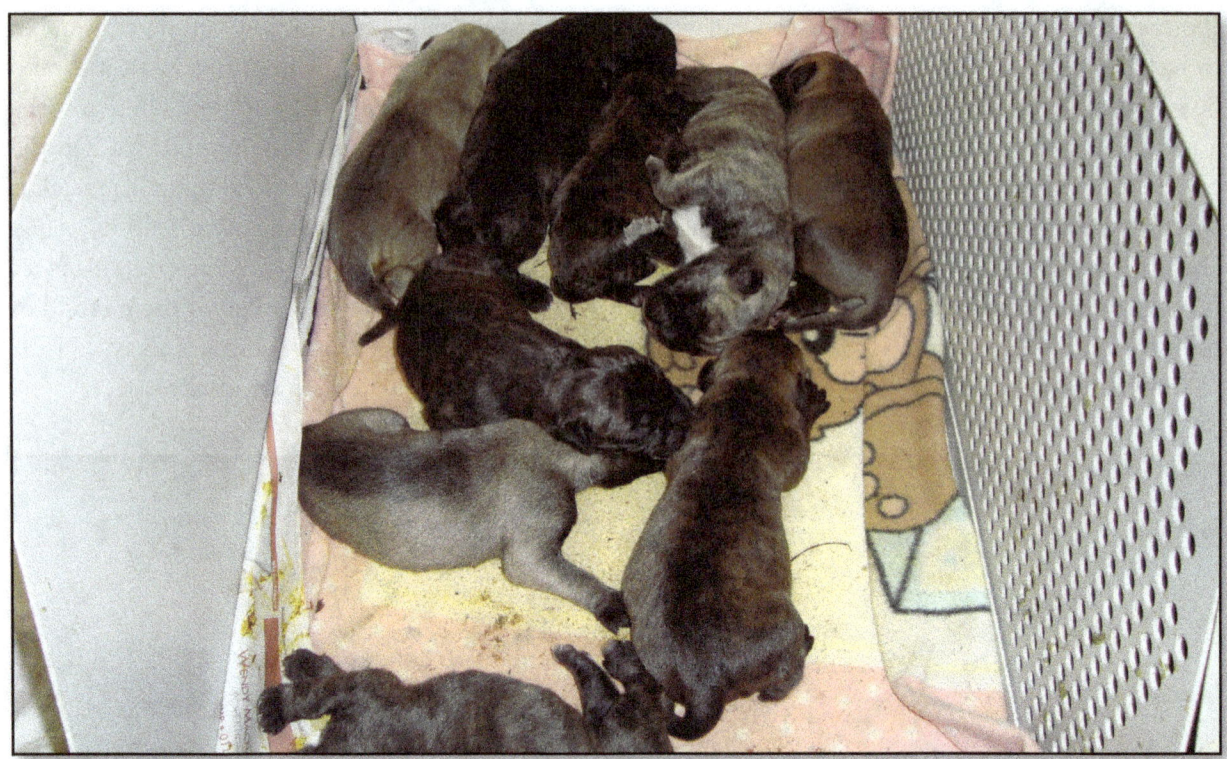
Puppies are spread out and sleeping peacefully in the incubator indicating that the temperature setting is within their comfort zone for their age

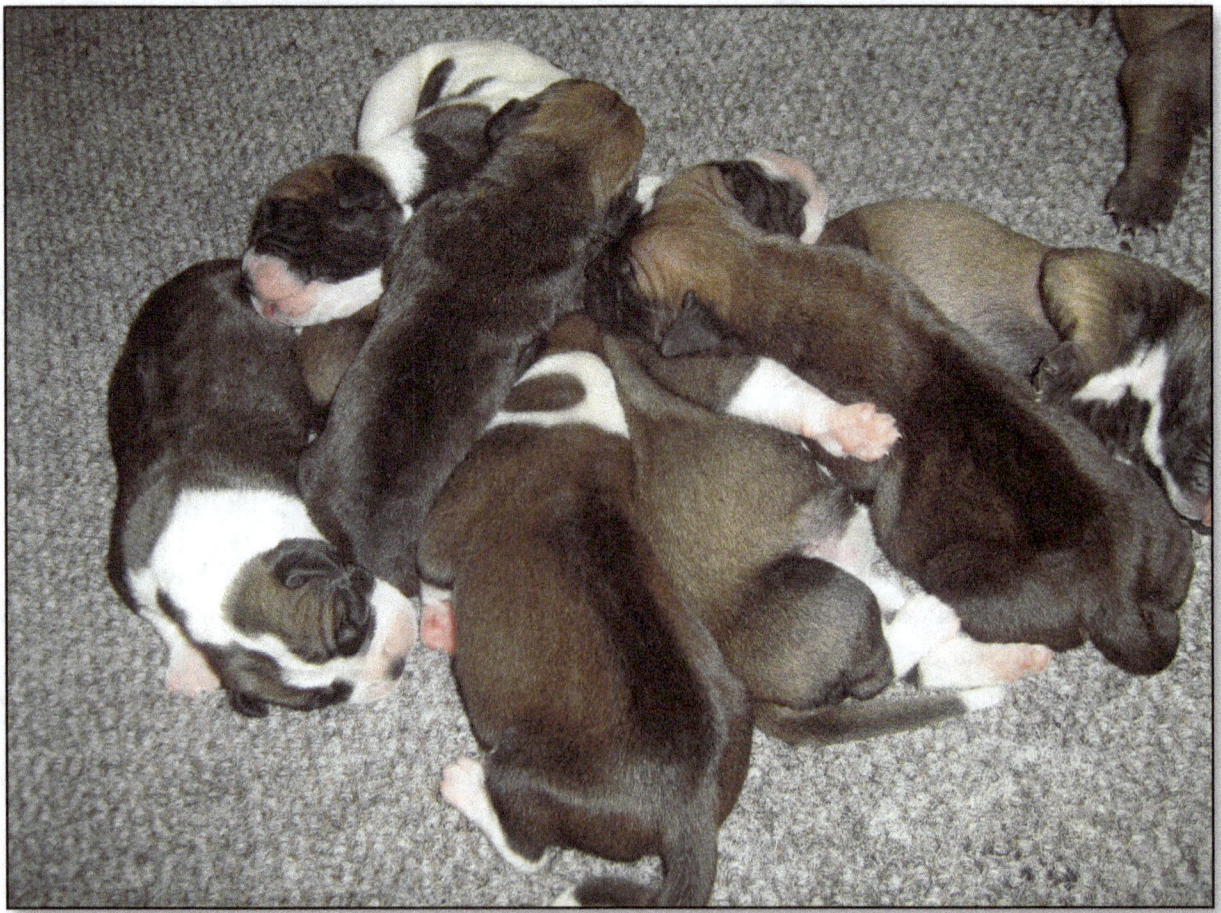
Puppies that are huddled together and keep whining are likely to be cold

make sure that the puppies must have the ability to escape heat if the temperature becomes too hot. During the first 3 weeks the breeder should, after feeding the puppies, stimulate excretion by wiping the perineum and prepuce with a moist piece of cotton wool and drying the skin again afterwards.

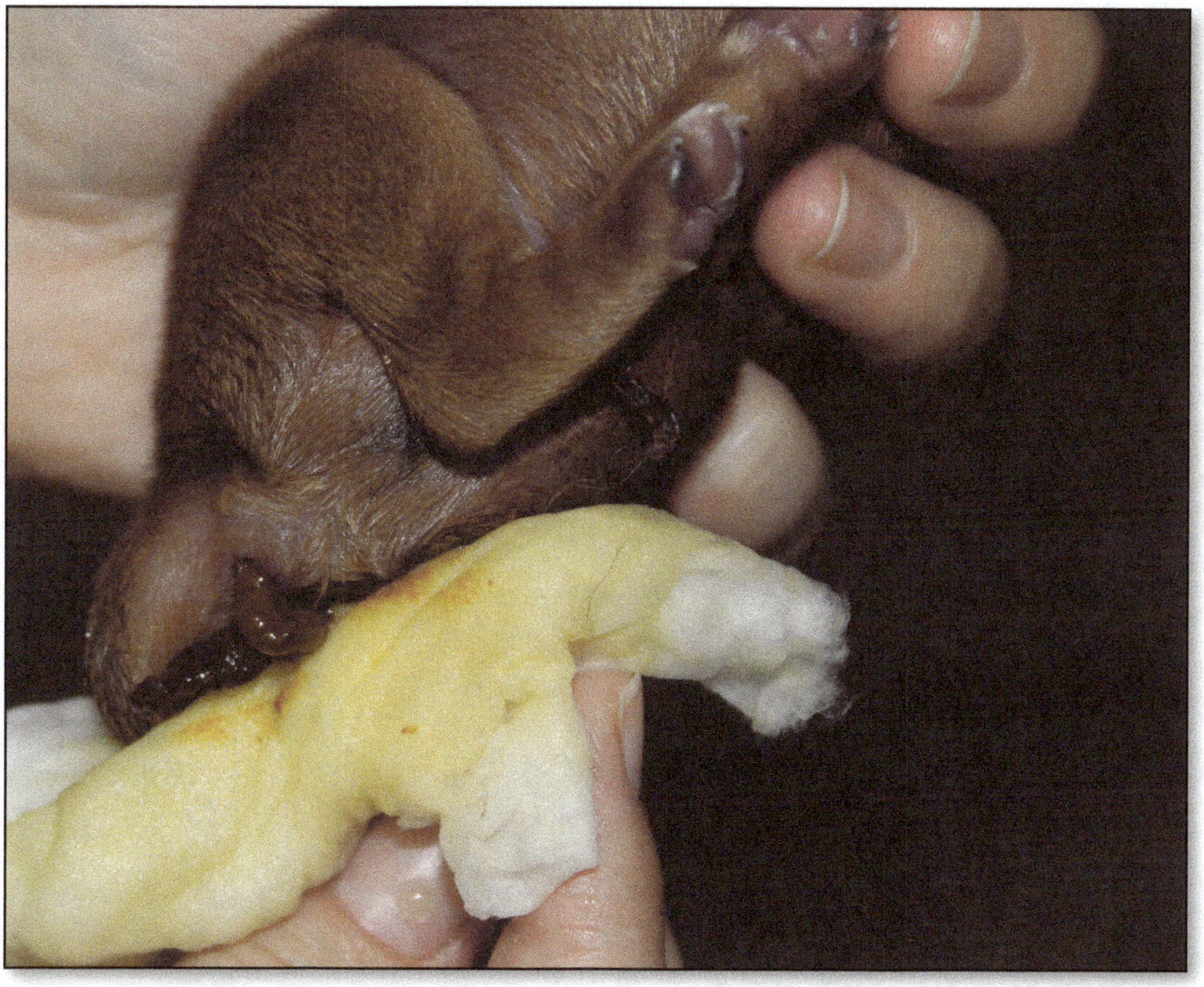

Stimulating defaecation in hand reared puppies

13.4.1. Foster mothers for orphan puppies

Fostering puppies is much easier and more successful than hand rearing if one has a good foster mother. Bitches which are kept together often have synchronized cycles and hence are likely to whelp at more or less the same time. This offers the opportunity to swap some puppies around if there is a particularly large litter. The breeder may even have one bitch rear the entire litter of another when required. The stage of lactation of the foster mother is important. The ideal is that the foster mother is at the identical stage of lactation as the mother of the puppies. This is however seldom possible. Irrespective of stage, the foster mother should have enough milk to ensure adequate weight gain. If insufficient milk production is suspected, supplement feeding may be required

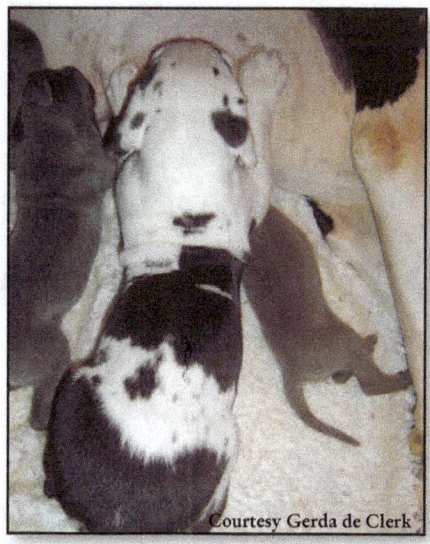

Size matters when fostering puppies

Chapter 13 The Normal Neonate

as explained in 13.4. Foster mothers need not necessarily be of the same breed but should preferably be of similar size. Not all bitches are suited as foster mothers. Puppies must therefore be introduced to the foster mother under careful supervision. If the foster mother has puppies of similar age and size, it is best to take them all away and rub them against each other so that they acquire the same odour before reintroducing them. If the size differences of the puppies are substantial, it may be necessary to remove the bigger puppies to give the smaller puppies uncontested access to the teats and let the puppies of different sizes and or ages drink at separate times.

Breeders should make sure that when fostering puppies that they accurately identify the puppies to avoid incorrect registering. Though rare, pseudopregnant bitches and even spayed bitches with strong maternal instincts may start lactating when exposed to sufficient stimulation of hungry puppies. In some cases, foster mothers may even be of another species.

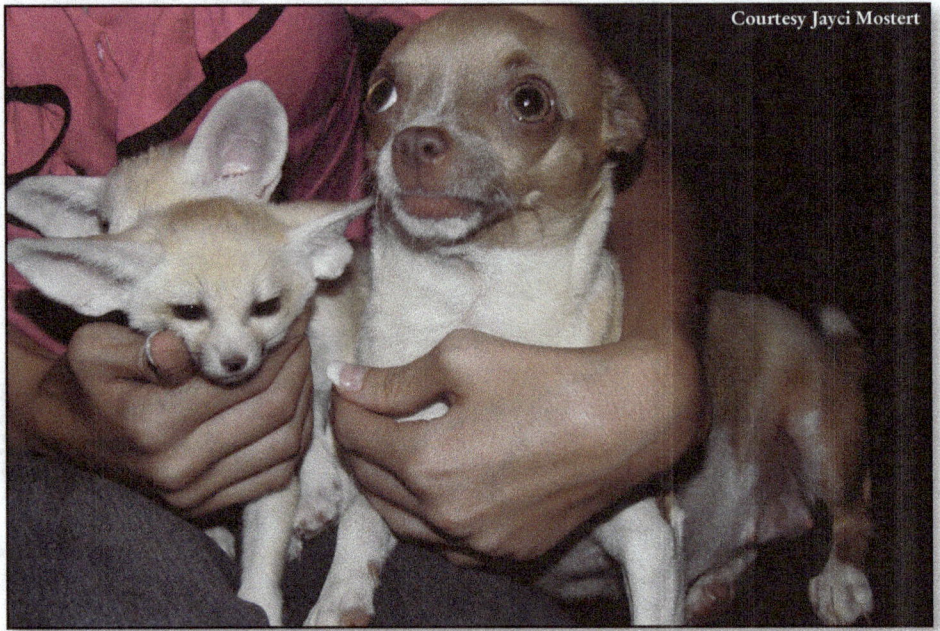
Chihuahua foster mother raised these fennec foxes

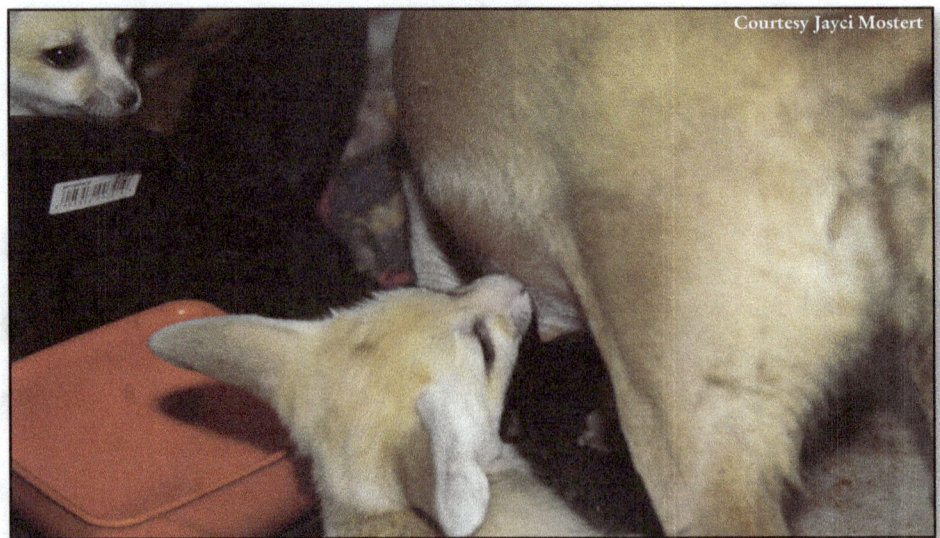
Fennec fox suckling from Chihuahua foster mother

One such example is a breeder of artic and fennec foxes who keeps some Chihuahuas which spontaneously start lactating and readily accept, nurse and successfully raise the fox puppies. Irrespective of source of foster mother, it is crucial that the breeder make sure that the foster mother has accepted the puppies and feeds them well and that the puppies have had colostrum as explained in 7.1.

13.4.2. Milk replacers during the first 3 weeks

Commercial puppy milk formulas are available and are nutritionally balanced to meet the needs of orphan puppies. Homemade milk formula recipes are also available but are not advised unless the breeder is able to fully balance them. Ordinary cow's milk should not be used. The constituents of milk vary widely from species to species. The major constituents which may differ between species are the percentages of respectively, fat, protein, lactose and water. The latter in dog's milk, given in the same order are: 8.3, 9.5, 3.9 and 79%. Only enough milk replacer formula should ideally be made for one feed but if there is any surplus, it should be cooled and rewarmed for the next feed. It should not be stored for longer than 4 hours (till next feed) and not be rewarmed more than once.

The quality of milk replacers differ. It is the author's experience that milk replacers which do not clump easily, are superior to those that do. Poor quality milk formula is one of many causes of diarrhoea and bloating in puppies. Bloating may still be a problem with the best milk formula or homemade formulas. Adding additional fat in the form of cream (5 ml per every 100 ml formula) or tinned puppy starter mouse or high calorie supplement (also at 5 ml per 100 ml formula) may all decrease the incidence of bloating and increase weight gain.

The formula should be made exactly adhering to the instructions. If the amount of water added to the milk powder is too much, the puppy will not receive the correct amount of nutrients for its weight and fail to thrive and grow well. It will remain hungry and cry despite getting correct volumes of milk and feed intervals. If the amount of water is too little, it will dehydrate and die. This is because the concentration of the solids in the milk formula is then too high and an osmotic imbalance occurs. This then leads to so-called osmotic diarrhoea. Simple over feeding of milk formula may also cause diarrhoea. Milk formula must be warmed to body temperature (38°C) prior to feeding.

Feeding the correct amount and at correct intervals is crucial. Instructions in some milk replacer formulas are sometimes vague with regards to amounts which have to be fed. The total requirement of already made up milk formula which the puppy requires is 20 % of its bodyweight over a 24 hour period. The calculated amount can then be divided into 6 meals. So assuming the puppy weighs 300 grams, the puppy needs to consume 60 ml over 24 hours divided into 6 meals of 10 ml each. These guidelines may be used when bottle feeding. Puppies which demand more may be given more. However, if the puppy drinks substantially less than the calculated amount (20% less) the breeder should be alarmed and consider tube feeding.

This feeding protocol is a tested one which serves many breeders well. Many variations thereof exist. During the first week, some breeders wish to feed smaller meals more often (2-3 hour intervals round the clock). This they do because it closer resembles the feeding frequency of puppies at that age. Following the first week they follow the conventional feeding protocol as above. The need to accurately weigh the puppies cannot be overemphasized.

All the principles which apply to human baby feeding bottles should be respected. This involves keeping bottles, teats, feeding tubes and syringes clean and dry as well as using disinfectants and cleaning agents safe for this purpose.

Puppies may be bottle fed or tube fed. In order to maintain a proper suckling reflex it is best to bottle feed as far as possible. Bottle feeding offers the opportunity for the puppy to regulate their own intake and decreases the possibility of tube feeding into the lungs or feeding incorrect amounts. Tube feeding is convenient because it is not so time consuming and it ensures that the puppy receives the required amount. In cases where the puppy is too weak to suckle, tube feeding is the only option. Breeders having or wishing to tube feed should acquaint themselves with the procedure first having their veterinary surgeon demonstrate it on a puppy. If the correct tube and technique is used, it may be a helpful adjunct to rearing puppies.

If breeders notice that the puppy regurgitates the meal they should stop immediately and bring this to their veterinary surgeon's attention. They may have fed the puppy too much or

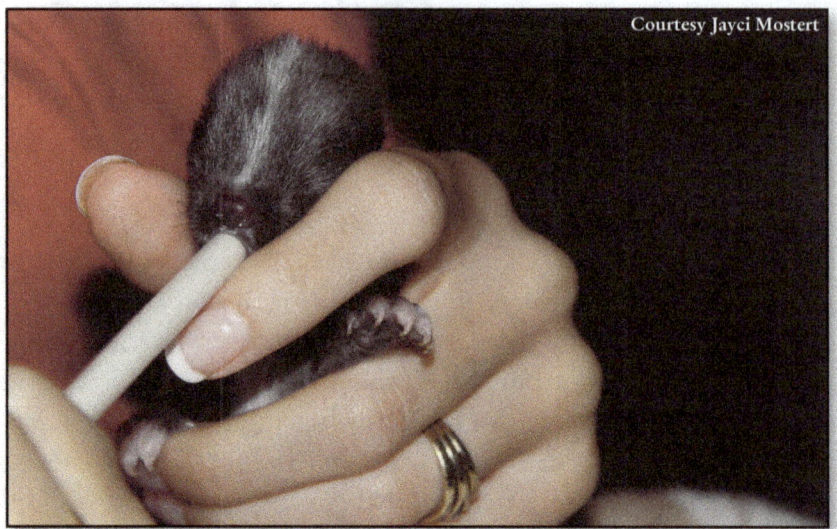
Arctic fox being syringe fed

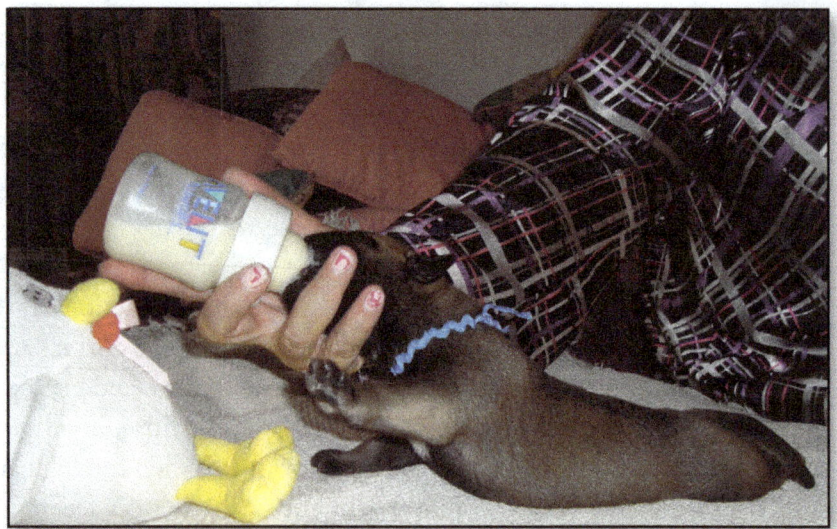
Bottle feeding puppy

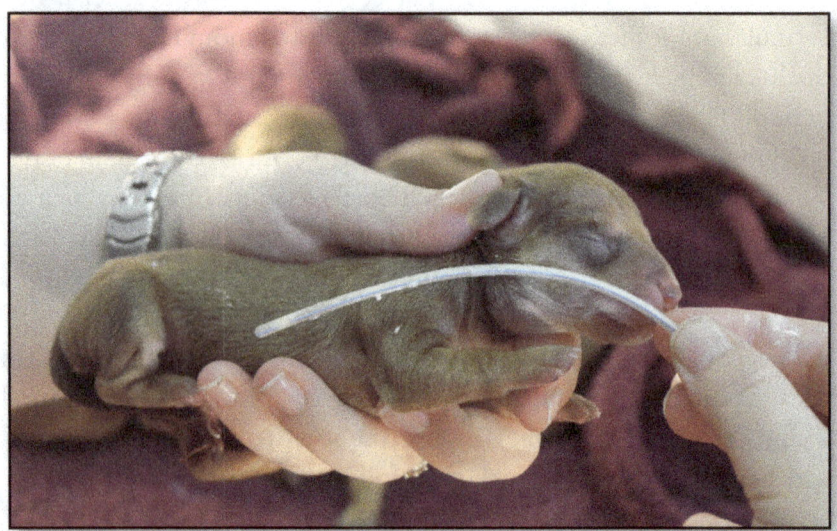
Tube feeding illustrating depth to which tube should be inserted

its stomach contents have not been emptied from the previous meal. Also, tube feeding in excess of the stomach capacity will lead to regurgitation and possible death by aspiration or pneumonia.

Normally, puppies would suckle for 5-6 weeks but it is possible to wean hand reared puppies earlier at 3-4 weeks of age by introducing specially formulated puppy rations (creep feed) designed for this purpose.

13.4.3. Creep feeding

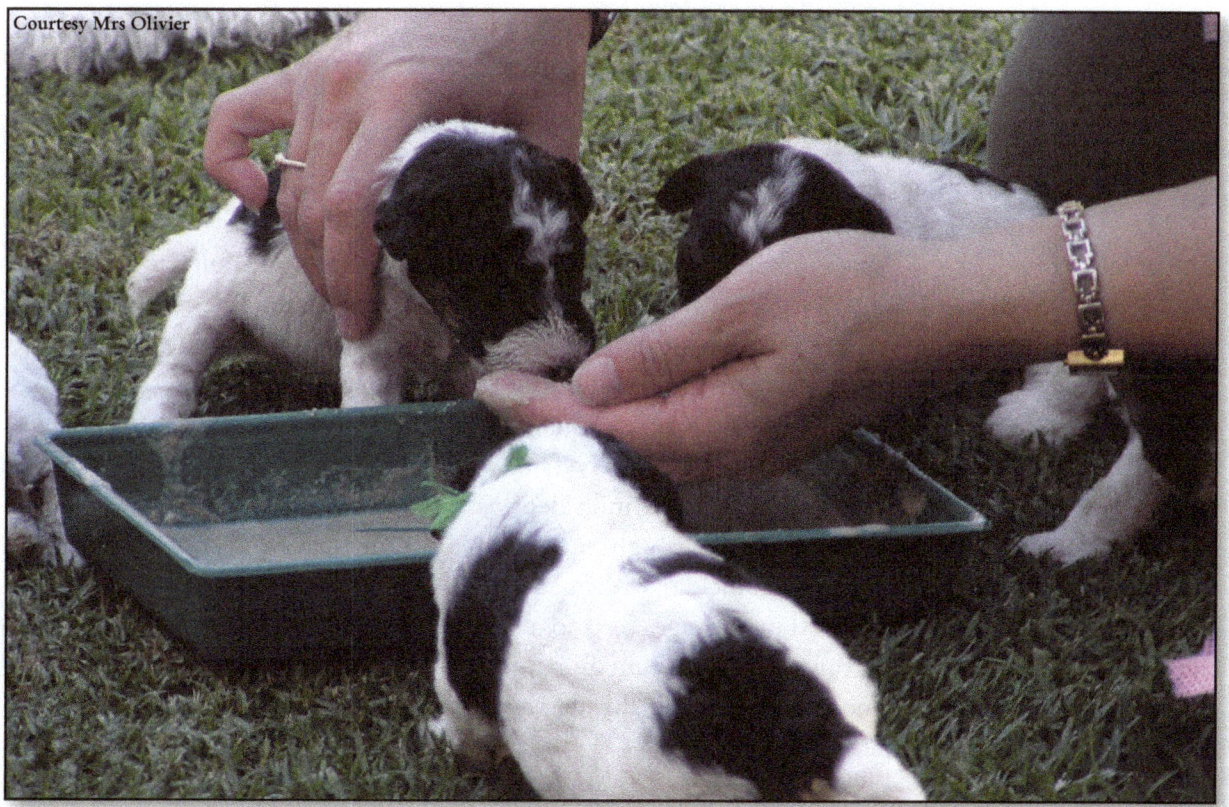

Puppies introduced to creep feeding

Creep feeding is the concept of feeding puppies semisolids at the earliest age which they can consume them. This age varies somewhat but is usually started in puppies from day seventeen. Although still messy, at 21 days most puppies can consume semisolids and by day 24, most will eat well. At about this time, puppies will start walking as well. Top quality creep feeds in the form of porridge, small kibbles or tinned wet food are commercially available. Human baby food is not an acceptable alternative.

Creep feeding has many advantages. It ensures good weight gain in cases where milk production is starting to wane and accustoms puppies to solids in preparation for weaning and rehoming. It is invaluable in cases where early weaning is necessary. Creep feeding is much cheaper and less time consuming and labour intensive than feeding milk replacers. Creep feed may be introduced from 17-21 days onwards and offered 3-5 times per day. Creep feeding is also practiced in nature by wild dogs. African wild dogs will regurgitate their partially digested meat meal in response to the begging of their puppies. In exceptional cases, domesticated dogs have been seen to regurgitate food in response to the whining hungry puppies.

Chapter 13 The Normal Neonate

13.5. Weaning puppies

Weaning refers to the process by which the puppies become independent of their mothers and start meeting their caloric requirements by eating only. The best weaning age for dam reared puppies is 6 weeks and for hand reared puppies it is around 3 weeks. The latter is referred to as early weaning. There are instances where early weaning is advised. This is because some bitches may become agitated, neglect their puppies or even show aggressive behaviour and injure them. Normally, the dam's milk will start decreasing from the fifth week or so, but this may vary widely depending on stimulation from puppies, nutrition of dam and individual differences between dams. Most breeders will introduce creep feeding (13.4.3) from 3 weeks onwards and take the puppies away at around 6 weeks. The best way to wean puppies at this age is to abruptly remove them from the dam.

It is generally recommended that when switching food, it is done gradually by slowly increasing the percentage of new food in the original food.

This is more important in young puppies post weaning, at point of sale, than in adult dogs. Weaning is a particularly stressful time in a puppy's life and at that age they are vulnerable to many causes of diarrhoea. Intestinal upsets are more common in sudden changes. Puppies sold are subjected to numerous stressors, the magnitude of which should not be underestimated. These stressors include, separation from the dam, separation from their litter mates, separation from familiar human contact, adaptation to a new environment, introduction to new family, introduction to new pets, introduction to the bottom of a new pecking order, sudden milk deprivation and introduction to new diets. It is well documented that stress mediated through endocrine and other pathways compromise the immune system. Weaning time also coincides with the time that the maternally derived antibodies start waning. In combination, all these changes lead to a significant reduction in resistance and this opens the way for both opportunistic and specific diseases in this critical period to invade and cause disease. Diarrhoea is a common manifestation during this time but more severe ailments are also possible, these are discussed in chapter 14.

Because puppies are vulnerable to so many problems at the time of weaning, some breeders elect to wean the puppy themselves and only sell the puppy at a slightly older age (9-10 weeks). During the 2-3 weeks that they keep the puppy longer, they accustom the puppy to its new diet and start with the socialization process. Puppies will then also have had more than one vaccination making them less disease prone. Some breeders send the puppy to its new home with a week's or so supply of the food it was on. It is interesting to note the large number of "well trusted" recipes which breeders have as a weaning formula. This formula may contain a wide variety of ingredients including cottage cheese, rice, porridges of all sorts, vegetables, probiotics and many more. Frequently, breeders will have an instruction list which is sold with the puppy. This usually has recommended vaccination programs, deworming schedules and feeding instructions. All too often these feeding instructions contain any number of ingredients followed by a complex homemade recipe. Although the breeder might have the very best intentions and is convinced that it works very well for them, the new puppy owner is unlikely to comply with the instructions. Also, the new owner's veterinary surgeon is unlikely to agree with the feeding instructions given by the breeder, all leaving the new puppy owner very confused. Therefore, it is advised that these feeding instructions be simple and preferably refer to easily obtainable commercial products.

13.6. Selling puppies

The sale of the puppy is met by excitement of both the breeder and new owner. The breeder is content because they have successfully reared another puppy to weaning age and they receive some monetary return. The new owner is excited about the prospect of taking home their cute new puppy. Unfortunately, the excitement of the new owner can be short lived and abruptly changed to disappointment or frank aggression if things inadvertently go wrong. Under these circumstances disputes will arise. This is because the new owners of puppies which develop problems post sale are often very distraught and may not hesitate to implicate the breeder who sold the "sick" puppy to them. These new owners will then often contact the breeder with the news about the sick puppy. Most breeders will at this point try to give advice but it is important that the breeder insist that the puppy be presented for veterinary examination. Giving telephonic advice in retrospect might prove disastrous.

This first news of the puppy's problems is not only a nuisance factor for the breeder but also offers potential for far more disastrous events. All too frequent the breeder may become immersed in a roller coaster of emotions. Depending on the individual personality of the breeder, they may become defensive which usually just adds fuel to an already unpleasant situation. Others will have feelings of inadequacy, feeling they have failed their new owner, feeling guilt, feeling that they may have done something wrong. Post-sale complaints may sour the experience of breeding for some breeders to such an extent that some want to give up breeding altogether.

This situation calls for immediate remedial action on behalf of the breeder. The first question the breeder should ask themselves is where should and can they improve. This book helps to guide the breeders in conjunction with advice from their veterinary surgeons, to address and try and prevent as many post weaning problems and complaints as possible. Breeders should ask themselves what risk can they remove, which can they reduce and which risk they cannot. Once they have convinced themselves that they are doing everything possible to control and prevent as many problems as possible post sale, they should assess the element of risk. For instance, if the puppy was dewormed numerous times and the primary vaccination administered, breeders cannot be made to feel guilty or be implicated if the puppy contracts parvoviral enteritis after sale. This is because there is an inherent risk associated with the breeding and buying of puppies. This risk should be communicated with the new owners and the terms and conditions regarding this sale should be properly spelt out.

13.6.1. Disputes regarding puppy sales

Breeders often end up in unpleasant disputes regarding puppy sales. These disputes may indeed end up in legal proceedings costing everyone unnecessary time, money and heartache. Breeders need to be aware of the notion that many new owners feel that they have paid a high price for the puppy. They may also have the presumption that together with the high price tag comes some form of guarantee. Some of the more common causes of disputes are discussed.

13.6.2. Dispute regarding puppy falling ill post sale

At the time of sale, the puppy was in good condition, appeared healthy, had a good appetite and was lively. However, following sale, any of a variety of events unfold.

Any number of days following the sale of the puppy, it comes down with some ailment. For the purposes of this discussion the example of gastro enteritis is used because it is perhaps the most common

Chapter 13 The Normal Neonate

post sale complaint but any other disease or condition is possible. The puppy is then presented to the new owner's veterinary surgeon who diagnoses a gastro-enteritis. After some 3-9 days or more, the puppy is either dead or healthy again but either way, usually with a huge veterinary bill. What follows is the proportioning of blame to others by the various parties. The new owner now claims that the breeder of the puppy is to blame because the breeder sold them a sick puppy. They also consult their own veterinary surgeon about the matter and expect them to support their theory that the breeder is to blame. They start with an academic debate of the incubation period of the respective infectious causes of gastro enteritis. On the other hand, the breeder insists that the puppy was in perfect nick when it left their premises. The breeder also maintains that because none of its littermates have picked up the same problem, the puppy must have picked up the cause of the illness in their new home. The breeder will also contact his veterinary surgeon in an attempt to corroborate his version of the events. The latter reminds the new owner that the incubation period of for instance parvoviral enteritis may be as short as 2-3 days. At this point, potentially four parties are now involved and dragged into this dispute! Everyone involved tries to distance themselves from blame.

13.6.3. Dispute regarding defects that become evident post sale
The new owner is in agreement that the puppy was in good health at the time of sale. After some time however, sometimes as long as a year or later, the dog develops a condition which requires veterinary attention. It comes to the new owner's attention this condition might indeed be a genetic fault. Examples are hip dysplasia, elbow dysplasia and dozens more. The new owner now claims that the breeder of the puppy is to blame because it had a "latent genetic defect" and should be held accountable. In response, the breeder claims that they only breed from hip dysplasia free stock and that environmental influence like incorrect nutrition and exercise might very well have been the cause in this case. Again, the two veterinary surgeons are drawn into this dispute.

13.6.4. Dispute regarding suitability for breeding post sale
The breeder sells a puppy of "breeding quality" to another breeder or prospective breeder, specifically for breeding purposes. Because the puppy came with a "title" and perhaps a premium price tag, the new owner has higher expectations than normal of this puppy. If it then becomes evident, albeit totally unforeseen or impossible to predict, that this puppy is not fit for breeding, a serious dispute arises. The new owner is very unhappy because they assumed that a puppy sold as a breeding animal should be guaranteed as free from genetic faults and fit for breeding. They feel that the extra money paid was like an "insurance policy" against these potential risks.

13.6.5. Outcome of these disputes
The outcome is always unpleasant. The new owners may claim damages. They may insist that the breeder replace the puppy or refund them. They may insist on being refunded and in addition claim all the veterinary expenses as well. Depending on the local laws governing livestock, these requests may be enforced or not. In most cases this won't be possible because usually there were no terms of sale. Although some diplomatic breeders may have the ability to pacify some of the new puppy owners, the end result is an unhappy owner who spreads the news of yet another transaction going awry with an "unscrupulous" dog breeder.

13.6.6. Solutions to these disputes
The breeder should first and foremost explain what it is they do to prevent possible problems in their breeding stock. If certain measures are not taken the breeder should say so to the new owner and put

that in writing as well. Secondly, despite preventative measures, they should communicate with the new owners the element of risk that remains unavoidable.

Lastly, the terms and conditions regarding this sale should be entrenched in a written contract. This document should spell out precisely the rights of all parties. A carefully worded standard contract should be compiled in accordance with the trade laws of the country. This is best achieved with the assistance of a legal entity. The contract should also clearly outline the fact that breeders cannot take responsibility for a latent defect. For the purposes of the contract, a latent defect is defined as a defect/condition/disease or syndrome which may or may not be present within the genes of the puppy at the time of sale or may have infected the puppy at the time of sale but has not manifested itself yet, and may do so later. In case of a puppy, both the breeder and the new owner may be totally unaware of such defect but such defect may very well surface later. It is also good practice to advise that the new owner must present the puppy to his/her own veterinary surgeon within a given period (usually 3 days or less) to examine the puppy and alert the breeder immediately if there is a problem. This is very important because the breeder's veterinary surgeon may have overlooked something and also because some new owners may be suspicious of the breeder's veterinary surgeon's abilities and partiality.

This contract should determine what course of actions should be taken in case of various eventualities. It is generally advised that all guarantees, if any, expire within a week or so post sale and that any guarantees only include value paid for the puppy and not any other expenses which may have been incurred. Breeders should not undertake to pay veterinary expenses because there may be no ceiling to these fees. Whatever is decided upon, breeders should make sure that the obligations of all parties are clearly stated within a written agreement.

Breeders should think twice to replace puppies. This is because history often proves that a new owner with one complaint may have another about the replacement puppy as well. No breeder should still sell any puppy to anyone without some form of legal document.

Chapter 13 The Normal Neonate

Chapter 14

Neonatal Disease

The neonatal period in dogs is not as well defined in the literature as it is in humans. It could be fair to define the neonatal period starting at birth until 8 weeks of age. This is because at that stage the organ functions have matured and more closely resemble adult function. For the purposes of this discussion, the puppy's development is divided in three separate phases. The first is the first 3 weeks of life, second from 3 weeks to weaning (around 6-8 weeks) and third from 8 weeks till adulthood. This is done because as a rule, many conditions present themselves in these distinct age groups. It is however true that slight overlap is possible.

Canine neonatology and paediatrics are respectively the fields of study involving conditions of the neonate and conditions of the puppy before adulthood (puberty). These fields of study are neglected in veterinary science. As a result, veterinary surgeons are generally poorly equipped to deal with sick neonates. Furthermore, disease in the puppy especially below 3 weeks of age can be very frustrating. This is because even when the breeder recognises the early symptoms of disease, their veterinary surgeon is usually unable to change fatal outcome irrespective of their interventions. The breeders' frustration is further exacerbated by the veterinary surgeons' inability to diagnose accurately and propose preventative strategies. Furthermore, post mortems and exhaustive tests may be unrewarding, leaving the breeder with more veterinary costs, more dead puppies and still no answers. Also, lack of experience on behalf of the veterinary surgeon results in their reluctance to encourage breeders to present puppies in the first place. For these reasons, breeders may have become despondent and fail to consult veterinary surgeons regarding sick puppies. This unfortunate state of affairs is counterproductive as it does not improve skill in care of sick puppies and creates the incorrect perception by breeders that nothing can be done in any case. Some breeders have also become "used to" an unacceptably high percentage of puppy losses.

Despite all these difficulties, veterinary surgeons and breeders should realise that it is in their interest to present and examine as many as possible sick, dying and dead puppies for the establishment of accurate diagnoses. In the hands of progressive veterinary surgeons, this more enthusiastic approach leads to higher success rates in diagnoses and survival rates but most importantly, proposing of preventative protocols.

It is important that breeders realise the effect of early intervention on outcome in case of neonatal disease. In the case of adults the time interval from the start of first clinical signs of disease until death may in some cases be in the order of days. In stark contrast to this, in many cases in neonates, this period may be in the order of hours. This is because neonates, relative to adults, have low energy reserves, lower resistance to disease, poor thermoregulation, poor resistance to dehydration and generally poor ability to maintain homeostasis in adverse conditions. Sick puppies should therefore be treated as soon as possible.

Dead puppies presented for post mortem examination should preferably be presented on the day of death and kept cool on ice in the interim or kept in refrigeration. They should not be frozen as this spoils the opportunity to perform a post mortem and some laboratory tests on them.

Chapter 14 Neonatal Disease

14.1. Therapeutic principles in puppies

Irrespective of cause of disease, the therapeutic principles in all these puppies remain the same. In neonates, the veterinary surgeon must address hypoxia, hypoglycaemia, hypothermia and hydration using the paediatric treatment principles. These principles are to:

- Ensure delivery of oxygen
- Administer energy in form of glucose solution
- Provide heat
- Administer balanced electrolyte fluids to correct hydration status

The doses of therapeutic agents should be tailored to suit the neonate's metabolism. Fluids and drugs can be administered orally but in cases where the puppy is in shock the fluids should be administered intravenously in the jugular vein, intraperitoneally (in the abdominal cavity) or subcutaneously.

To the breeder it is important to make sure that the temperature of the puppy is normal before milk replacers are fed to the puppies. This is because at a lower temperature, the enzyme systems are not as active, the peristaltic movements of the gut halts (termed ileus) and the puppies are left incapable of digesting the milk. This leads to fermentation, bloating and later regurgitation and aspiration on follow up feeds. It is a good idea for breeders to have at hand an electrolyte solution containing some glucose which they can administer orally to sick puppies. This mixture should be heated to body temperature before administration.

14.2. Neonatal disease and conditions in puppies from birth to 3 weeks of age

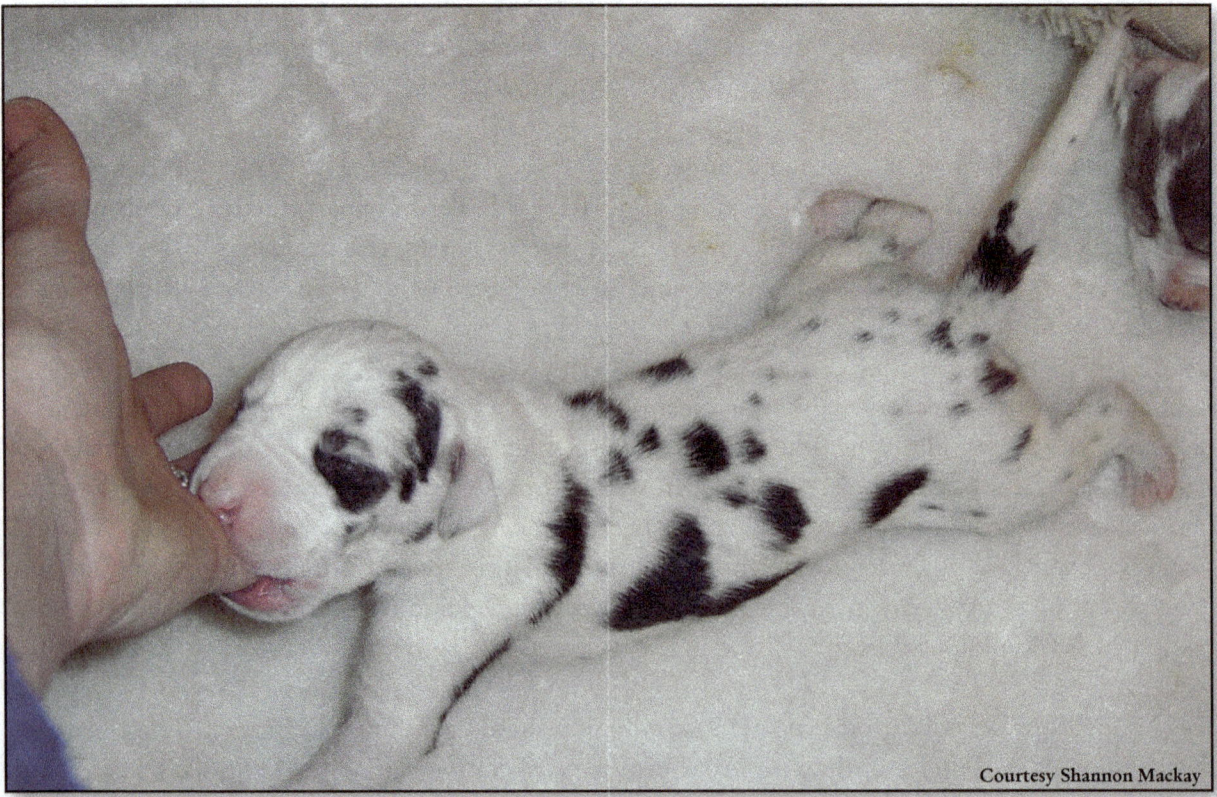

Courtesy Shannon Mackay

Testing puppy's suckling reflex

There are a host of conditions which are lumped together under this heading. This is because to the breeder all these conditions appear to be "one syndrome". In young neonates, irrespective of cause, all the puppies show the same symptoms. The clinical signs of sick puppies under 3 weeks of age are generally poor suckling reflex, weight loss, slight diarrhoea, bloating, slight cyanosis of mucous membranes and tummy skin (turning bluish) and continuous crying of puppies. The bloat probably accounts for the apparent display of abdominal pain when handled.

It is also important to realise that a compromised puppy, bigger or smaller than its littermates, irrespective of cause, will have difficulty in competing for feeding space on the dam's teats. Also they may have poor sucking or no sucking ability and therefore intervention via tube feeding is indicated. Maternal neglect is usually pronounced and deliberate in weak puppies' calling for intervention.

14.2.1. Low birth-mass puppies

Low birth-mass puppies should be identified at birth. Puppies which were of normal birth weight can appear to look smaller in comparison to its littermates at 5 days of age, due to failure to gain weight. Low birth-mass puppies have decreased ability to breathe and maintain metabolic function. They are also more susceptible to infection, hypothermia, hypoglycaemia and generally have a decreased chance for survival. These compromised puppies usually die within the first few days after birth. There is usually a spread of birth weights in big litters, but puppies weighing 25% below average for the breed are considered low birth-mass. There are many causes for low birth-mass. In very large litters, limited uterine space and placental insufficiency may lead to impaired nutrition of the foetus. Herpesvirus infection may also be a contributing factor in susceptible bitches. In some species, the critical birth-mass below which an individual neonate cannot or is very unlikely to survive, irrespective of intervention, has been established. These values are not known for dog breeds. The significance of this discussion is that if a puppy died which was suspected to have been a low birth-mass puppy, the cost of diagnostic work ups are probably not warranted because it is less likely to give conclusive answers. Due to their poor prognosis, some breeders elect to euthanize them early on. This is different from cases where entire litters are affected or apparently normal puppies abruptly die. In these cases proper work ups and interventions are more likely to be fruitful.

14.2.2. Weak puppies

Weak puppies are discussed separately from the others because if the weakness is the only clinical sign in absence of other pathology, it may be easily reversed using the general paediatric principles of intervention. The puppy may have become temporarily hypoglycaemic or hypothermic and if corrected the puppy quickly regains strength, and its suckling reflex. The main cause for weak puppies is

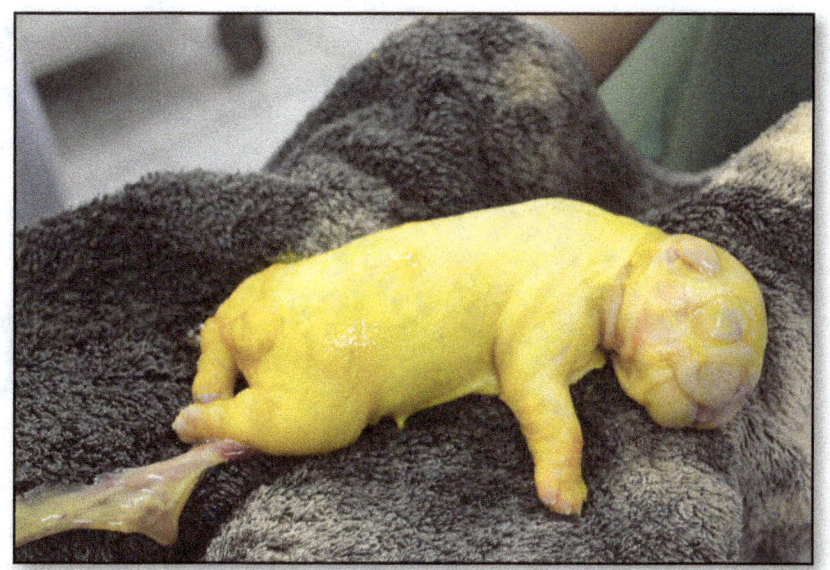

Meconium staining of puppy due to dystocia

dystocia and prolonged birth. Unfortunately a number of these puppies will develop respiratory infections due to the aspiration of meconium prior to birth.

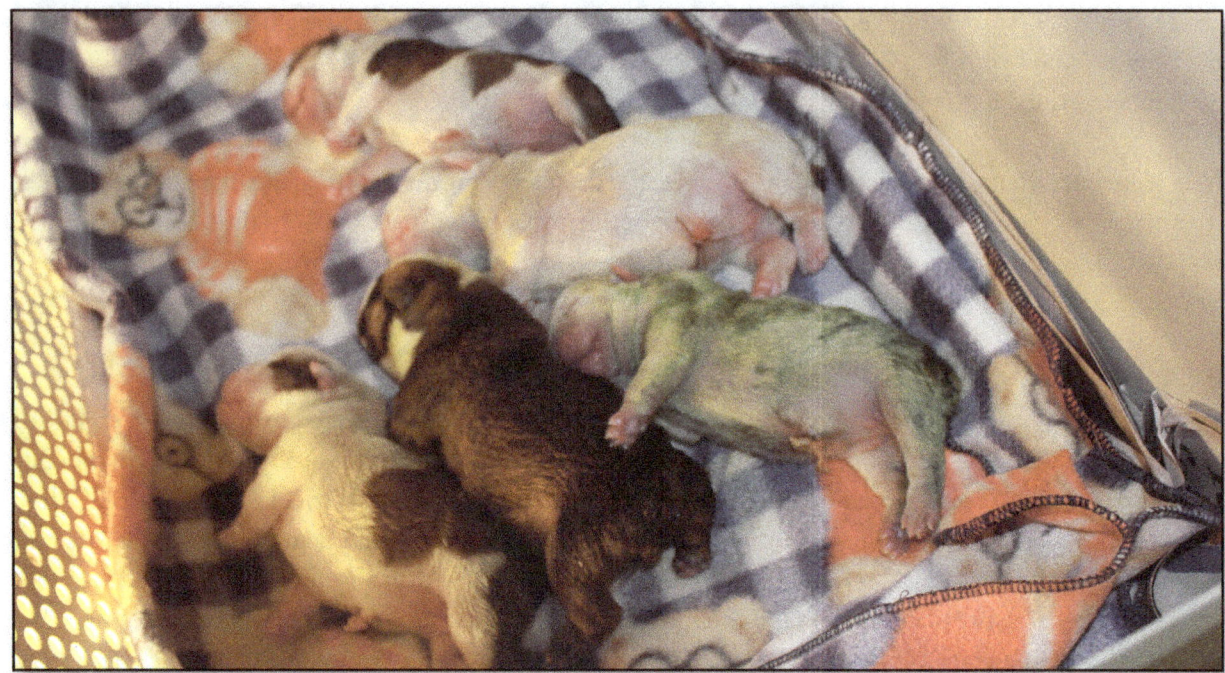

New-born puppies delivered by caesarean section. Note the green (uteroverdin) stained puppy and note also that its muzzle's colour is bluish whilst the other puppies are a healthy pink

Dams or their owners neglecting to remove meconium from puppies may lead to bacterial growth on new-born leading to neonatal dermatitis.

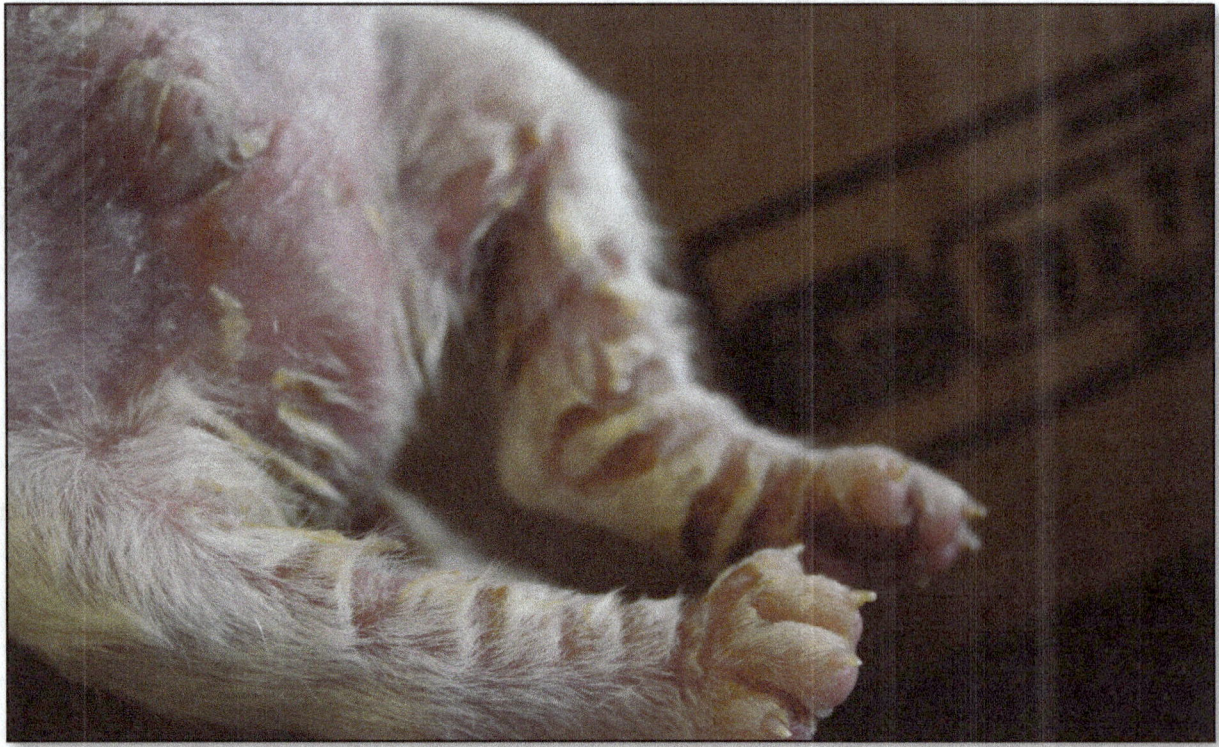

Neonatal dermatitis

Maternal neglect and poor mothering may lead to trauma to the puppy and weakness. There is the common notion that a dam has the ability to identify underlying problems with puppies and therefore selectively neglect those individuals hence deliberate neglect. Breeders should not fully trust this "instinctive ability" as many puppies which turn out perfectly normal can be saved from this neglect.

When the weakness is a result of another underlying, yet unidentified cause, the recovery will not be that prompt. In these cases the underlying cause must be identified and addressed as discussed under other headings.

14.2.3. Neonatal septicaemia

Puppies have immature immune systems during the first 2 weeks of life, making them very vulnerable to infections. Colostrum deprived puppies are at an even increased risk for infections at this age. Puppies which were subject to a difficult birth, or were exposed to chilling are also at increased risk. The incidence of septicaemia also increases in puppies of dams suffering from urogenital or mammary gland infections. The value of clean whelping quarters and the cleansing of bitches have previously been discussed and may help prevent infections. It is very likely that once the first puppy presents with the symptoms others will soon follow. Neonatal septicaemia is caused when the blood is invaded by bacteria which cause an infection in all the organ systems and blood. The layman term is blood poisoning. The bacteria may enter the body through the umbilical cord but entry through other routes is also possible. Umbilical hygiene soon after birth cannot be overemphasized. Omphalitis is infection of the umbilical site and is characterised by redness and wetness of the umbilical area. This may progress and spread to cause septicaemia. The source of the bacteria may be the environment or the dam. In addition to the normal clinical signs of illness in puppies, septicaemic puppies may show respiratory distress from fluid build-up in lungs.

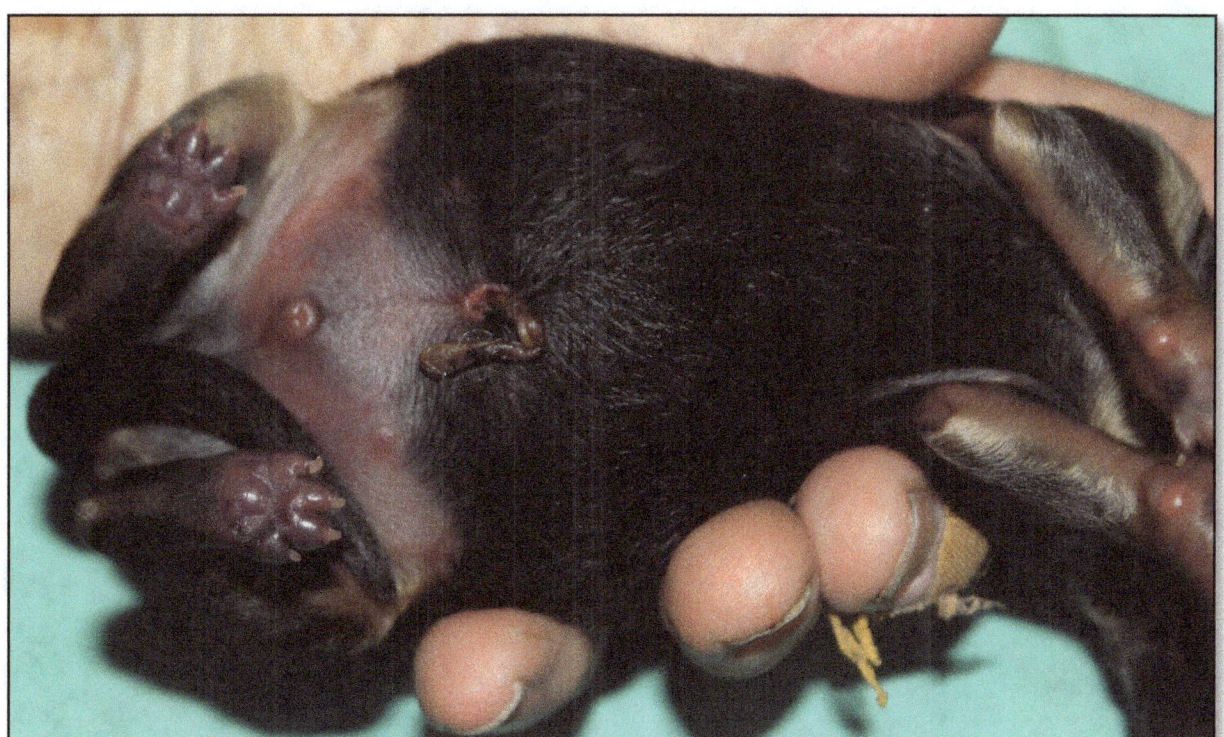

Septicaemic puppy, note the purple discolouration of the abdomen

Broad spectrum treatment which includes the gram negative spectrum is indicated in these cases. However, treatment of advanced cases is usually futile as they die within 2 days. Appropriate antibiotic therapy of litter mates showing either no symptoms or early symptoms may help prevent further losses.

Neonatal tetanus is a very rare cause of death in puppies. Despite the occasional typical case (tetanic spams) seen by veterinary surgeons and breeders in puppies at the age of 3-5 days (younger than the 6-8 days in humans), it has not been well documented in the dog. The few cases the author has seen have all originated from warmer climates and premises where other livestock (especially horses and cattle) are kept.

14.2.4. Colic puppies

Colic refers to abdominal pain caused by accumulation of gas in the intestinal tract. The gas build-up may be caused by the milk formula or by gut stasis. Stasis of the gut may be the result of any number of diseases. Eventually all sick puppies will show some extent of abdominal distension and colic.

Unlike babies, colic in puppies may be fatal and is difficult to treat. It may be argued that it is the underlying cause of the colic that will be the cause of death. It is however also true that those puppies which were previously perfectly normal and received milk replacer may develop colic and die. Inferior commercial milk replacers and inappropriate homemade milk replacers are more likely to cause colic but even the very best formulas may still cause bloat. Increasing the fat percentage appears to reduce the fermentative capacity of the milk and reduce incidence of bloat in the hands of the author.

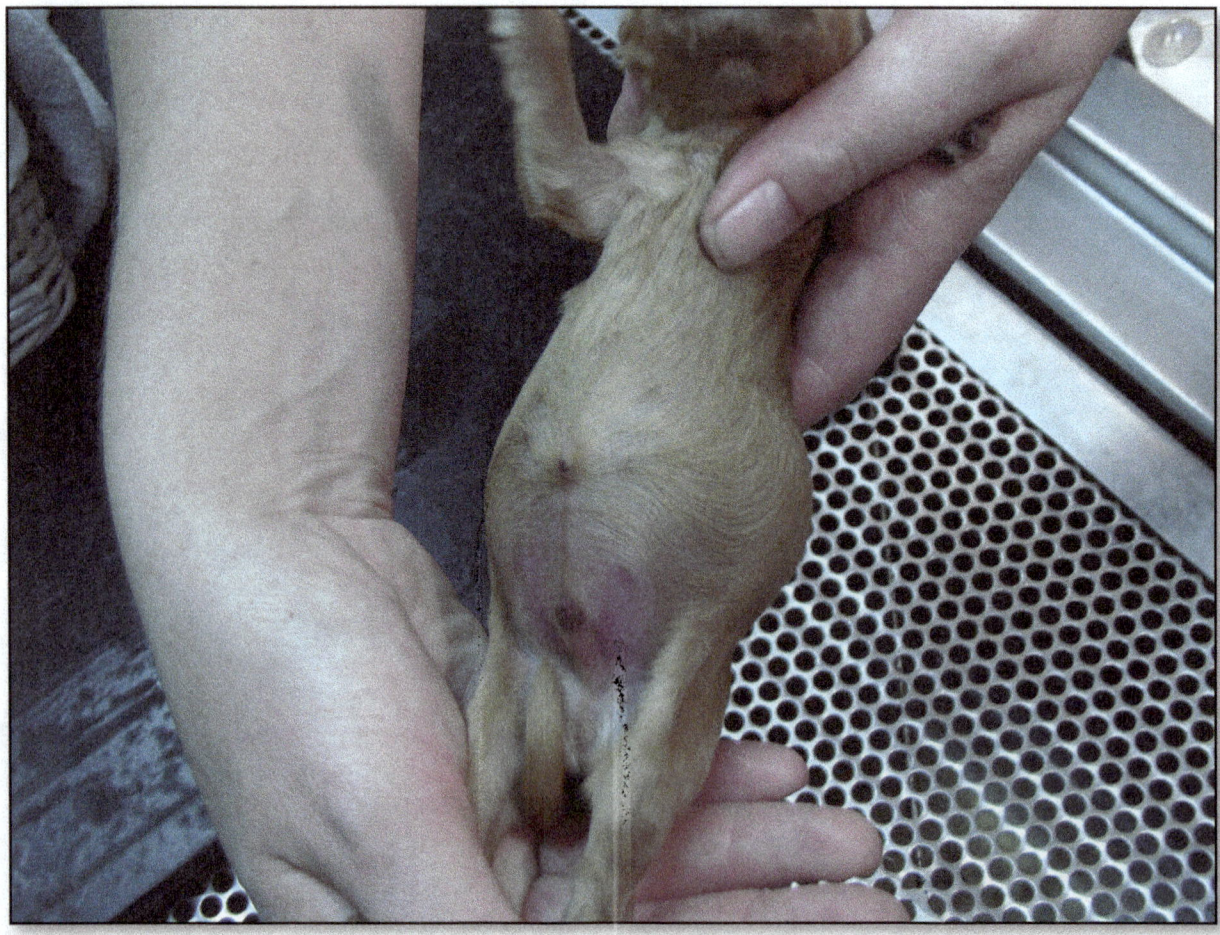

Bloated puppy

At the first signs of colic, the milk formula can be withheld for one meal and a 5% glucose/electrolyte fluid can be fed orally. At the next meal the formula (best quality possible) should be used and its fat percentage be slightly increased as explained and mixed 50:50 with the glucose mix. The following meals the puppies can be fed the enriched milk formula only. The puppies can also be treated with antispasmodics, drugs to induce gut motility as well as prebiotics.

14.2.5. Toxic milk syndrome

Toxic milk syndrome is a poorly defined syndrome recognised in puppies nursing on a bitch which is presumed to secrete toxins in her milk as a result of an infection of the uterus or mammary glands. Signs suggesting toxic milk syndrome are if all the puppies in the litter show illness simultaneously and if the bitch has a low grade fever and is not eating that well. There need not be clear evidence of infection in the bitch externally. The puppies will bloat, cry, show diarrhoea and strain continuously.

The suspicion of toxic milk syndrome can be confirmed if the puppies are removed from the bitch and show an immediate recovery. The bitch should also be treated. Once the bitch has fully recovered, it may be considered to reintroduce the puppies. Care must be taken to use drugs which are safe for the puppies. Unfortunately, in most of the cases the removal of the puppies combined with the illness in the dam may have affected her milk production completely or partly and continued supplementation of the puppies may be required.

In some cases the uterus infection may be so stubborn that it requires either long term therapy or even sterilisation in bitches not intended for further breeding. Clearly in these cases, hand rearing is the only option. Toxic milk syndrome is fatal in puppies which are not removed from the dam.

14.2.6. Congenital abnormalities

It is by no means the intention of this book to cover all the possible congenital abnormalities in all the breeds. Only a few of the more common abnormalities are mentioned. There are good books available on the congenital defects of the dog in breed context. It is of importance that breeders familiarise themselves with the more common abnormalities in their breed. If they notice an abnormality in a puppy which is unfamiliar to them, it is recommended that they present it to their veterinary surgeon to at least get an indication of what it could be. This allows the breeder to put a name to the abnormalities for record keeping purposes. The significance is that when breeders get repeat occurrences of abnormalities, this may alert them to possible genetic problems.

a) Cranial clefts

Cranial clefts (also known as open heads) is a condition known to dog breeders characterised by a skull which has not closed properly during embryonic development and the resultant puppy is born with a cleft in its skull with the brains frequently protruding from this cleft. The eyes also seem to pop out of the skull. These puppies are mostly alive at birth. This defect seems to be part of the midline closure defects like spina bifida, hemi vertebrae and cleft palates. Cranial clefts appear to be reported more often in the Bull Terrier breed but the author has photographic evidence of this defect in numerous small and large breeds.

The condition is well documented in humans, laboratory animals and pigs. The condition in humans has been linked to folic acid metabolism and in animals to folic acid and manganese metabolism. It is not necessarily a diet deficient in manganese or folic acid that is implicated but rather a deficit in folic acid

Chapter 14 Neonatal Disease

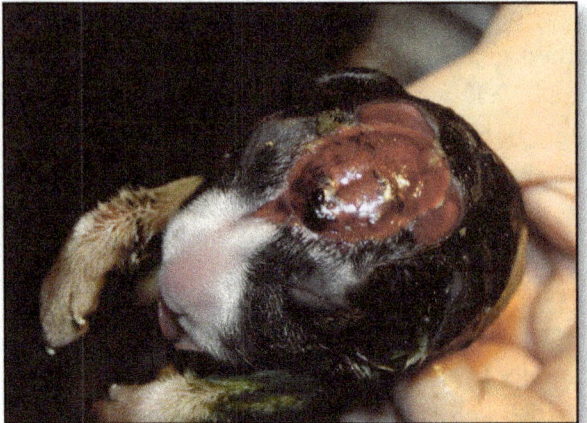
Bull Terrier puppy with cranial cleft

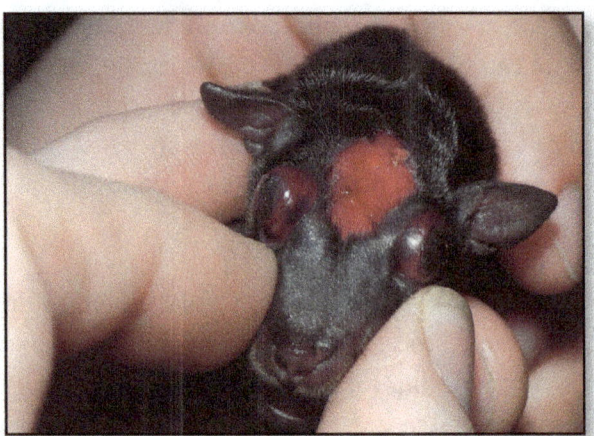
Cranial cleft in Miniature Pinscher

metabolism which increases the requirement of both folic acid and manganese. It is speculated that this defect folic acid metabolism is hereditary.

It is not known whether the defect seen in dogs is primary a hereditary defect as is hemi vertebrae or whether a defective folic acid metabolism is involved. There is no scientific evidence to support whether folic acid supplementation can indeed prevent cranial clefts in dogs. We do know however that moderate supplementation of folic acid cannot harm the pregnant bitch.

More research is obviously required regarding this mysterious syndrome. To the sceptics, it is true that the condition exists albeit rare (photographic evidence is available) and it occurs in dogs fed a balanced diet that are not suspected to be deficient in any nutrient whatsoever.

b) Cleft Palate/Cleft Lip Complex

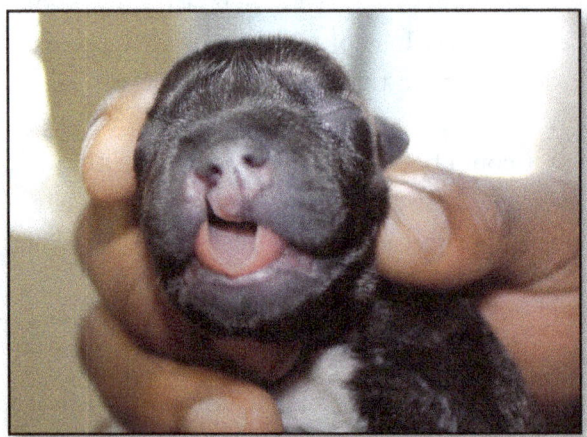
Harelip

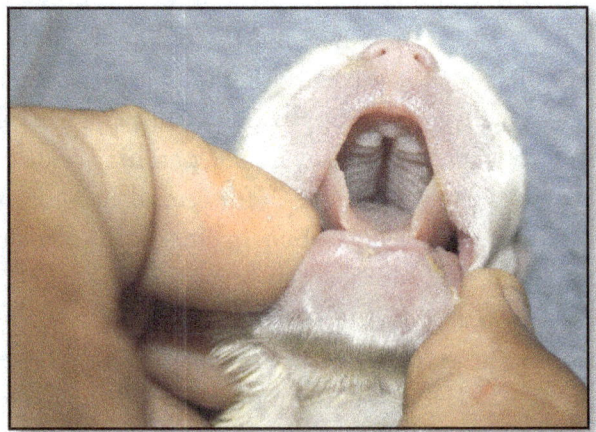
Split palate

Harelip and split palate (cleft lips and/or palates) are two conditions which result from failure of the maxillary buds to fuse in the canine foetus at around midterm-pregnancy.

Cleft of the lower lip is rare and usually occurs on the midline. Clefts of the upper lip are usually just off the midline nend usually unilateral. They may or may not be associated with clefts of the palate as well. The most common defect however is the split palate on its own.

Chapter 14 Neonatal Disease

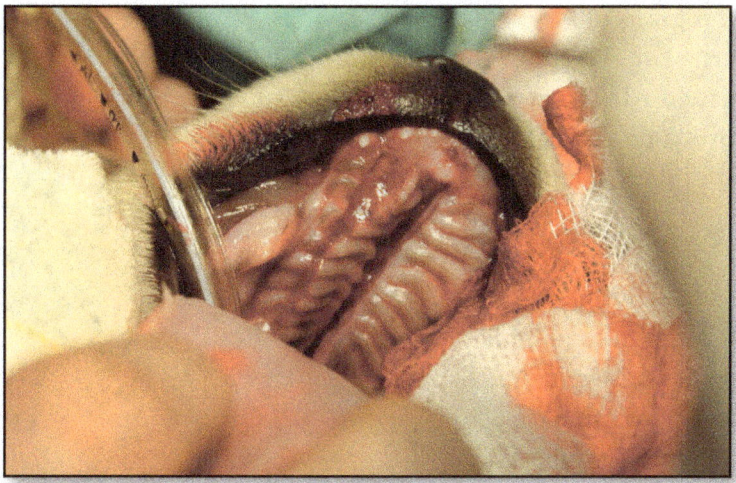
Split palate clearly visible

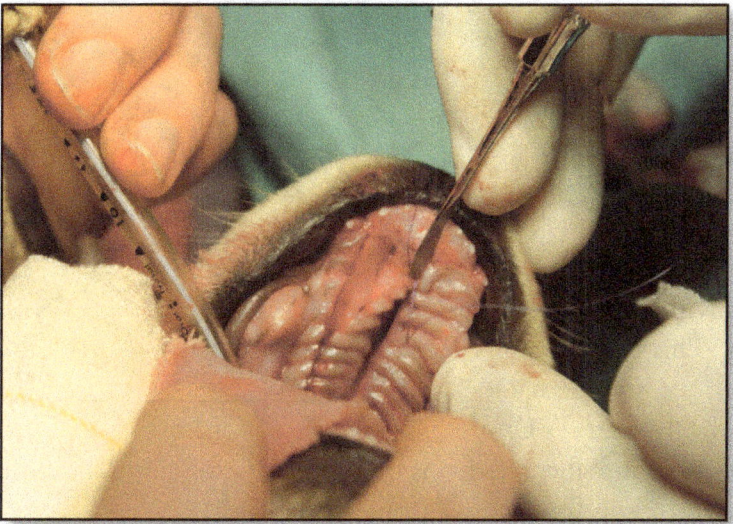
Hard palate is being resected

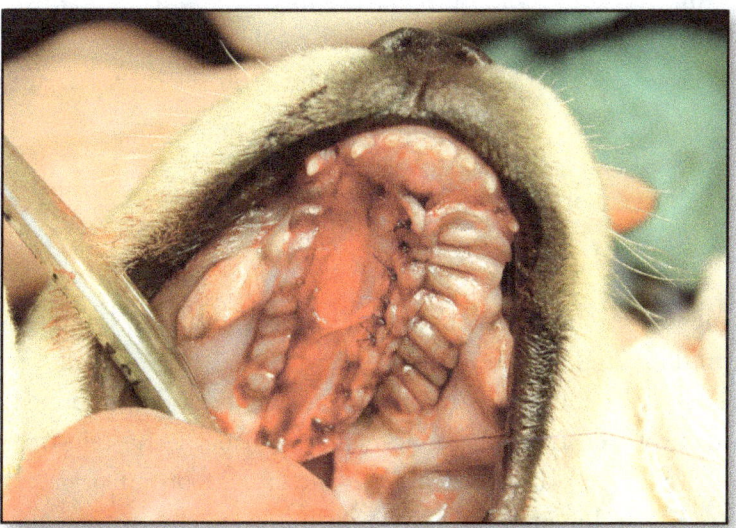
The flap is almost complete to close the defect. Images are shown to illustrate that it is possible to surgically correct cleft palates albeit tricky surgery

Distinct breed incidences have been reported but this abnormality may occur at a low frequency in most breeds. In some cases, sporadic instances are due merely to accidents of development at the embryo stage. However, if a number of cases recur in the same strain or breed, a genetic basis should be suspected. Brachycephalic breeds can have up to a 30% risk factor. A specific gene has been identified that controls this event and plays a crucial role in the folate cycle. Work is in progress to identify a specific marker so carriers can be detected. Although the primary aetiology (cause) is thought to be hereditary, drug or chemical exposure, mechanical interferences with the foetus and some viral infections during pregnancy have also been implicated. In humans the maternal supplementation of folate very specifically during the first month of pregnancy reduces the risk of cleft palates in children of predisposed woman by up to 50%. Studies in Boston Terriers and French Bulldogs have shown the same. It is therefore justified to supplement folate in at-risk breeds at doses of around 5 mg folic acid per day from around mating till last quarter of pregnancy. Some breeders wish to continue till near parturition. The puppy born with a split palate is easily identified as milk pours from its nose whilst attempting to suckle and it soon loses weight and fades. This condition can in some cases be surgically corrected when the puppy is weaned (after extensive tube feeding). It is advised that this puppy be sterilized and certainly not bred from.

Chapter 14 Neonatal Disease

c) Hernia of the umbilicus or inguinal regions

A hernia is a failure of the muscular part of the abdominal wall to close but the skin overlying it is closed. When this happens it allows abdominal content to protrude through the defect in the abdominal wall and become visible as a bubble or lump of tissue underneath the skin.

In case of an umbilical hernia, it is failure of the umbilical ring to close. The hernia is expressed as a soft lump in the middle of the abdomen. Umbilical hernias may vary in size from a few millimetres to a few centimetres. Some may extend up into the diaphragm. The incidence in the general population is low but it may vary between breeds and blood lines. This observation is highly suggestive of an underlying genetic role. Very often the breeder will blame the bitch for having pulled the umbilicus and torn the muscular wall leading to the hernia. In cases where the puppies were delivered by caesarean section the breeder may suspect that the veterinary surgeon may have pulled on the umbilical cord leading to the tearing and formation of a hernia. This is not true.

It is true that some small hernias may "seal off" with a piece of omentum (net of fat in abdomen) and will never show any clinical sign associated with the hernia. This has led many breeders to believe that delayed closure of the umbilicus does happen in some dogs. The latter is probably untrue. Until

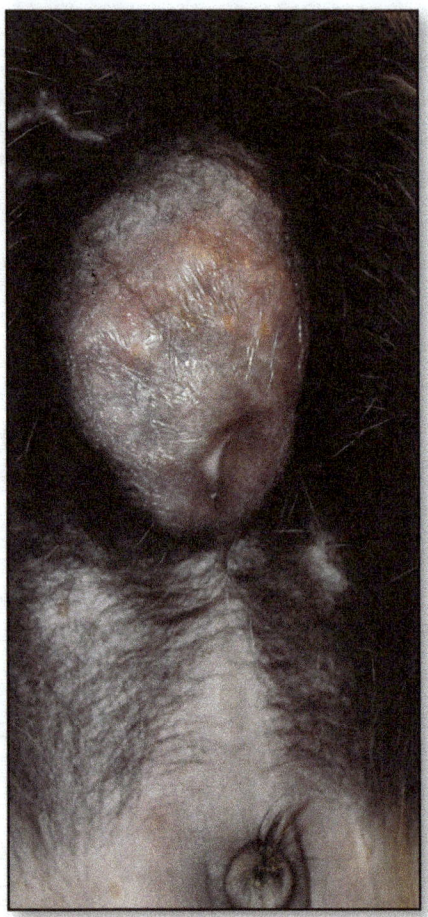

Very large umbilical hernia that stretches almost to the chest

proven otherwise, it is safer to assume that an umbilical hernia is of genetic origin. Hernias can be readily surgically corrected but excessive scarring is frequently encountered.

Inguinal hernias are hernias of the inguinal ring. This is the region between the hind legs where the thigh and abdomen meet. The inguinal ring is a slit in the musculature in this region. If the ring is too lax it allows abdominal content (usually fat and intestine) to protrude through the muscle and become visible under the skin in that region. It is potentially fatal and requires early surgical correction.

In both cases the correct thing to do is not to breed with affected animals and select against this defect.

d) Omphalocoels and gastroschisis

Omphalocoels and gastroschisis refers to incomplete closure of the abdominal wall and skin, stretching over a large distance on the abdominal midline and unlike umbilical hernias, are not restricted to the area surrounding the umbilicus. In both these conditions the defect in the abdominal muscular wall and skin allows abdominal organs to protrude from the abdomen. It is usually the intestines which are protruding but liver and other organs may also be visible. If the extra-abdominal viscera (abdominal contents) are not covered by peritoneal membrane, the condition is termed gastroschisis and if it is, it is termed omphalocoel.

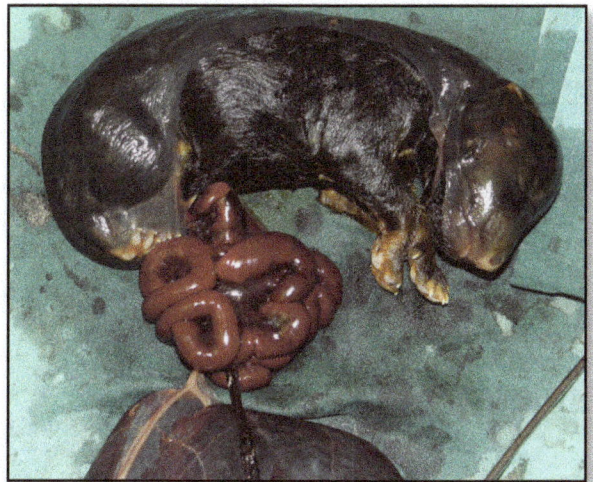
Gastroschisis

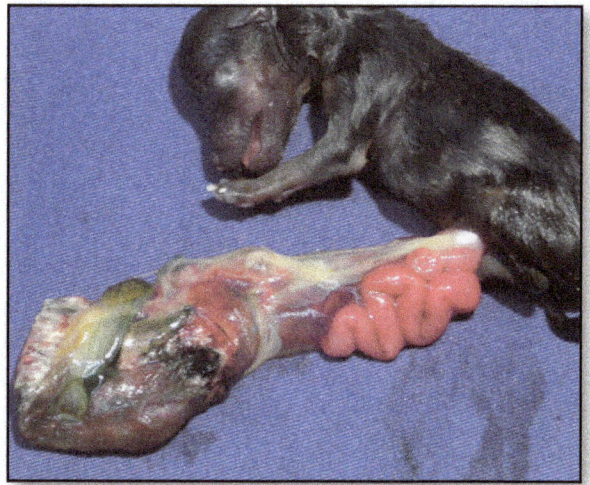
Omphalocoel

The latter is of academic interest only. What is of practical interest is that this defect may occur in any breed and may be of genetic origin.

Breeders may suspect that the bitch caused the defect following birth. As with umbilical hernias, they may also suspect that the veterinary surgeon may have caused it by excessive traction on the umbilical cord during delivery by caesarean section. Affected puppies should be euthanized.

e) Congenital hydrocephalus

Hydrocephalus is the abnormal accumulation of fluid in the ventricular system inside the brain. There are numerous causes of hydrocephalus and it may be congenital or acquired. Congenital hydrocephalus is by far the most common and toy and brachycephalic breeds are most commonly affected. In some breeds a hereditary origin is suspected. Hydrocephalus can easily be diagnosed by virtue of the greatly enlarged head of the puppy relative to the rest of its body. The skull may also appear dome shaped. The dome may appear to have a soft spot where no skull bone can be felt. This is referred to as a fontanel. It is however important to note that some toy breeds (mainly Chihuahuas) may have open fontanels and this may be perfectly normal in them. Unlike children, puppies of most breeds are not born with fontanels. Also, unlike children, in breeds where the puppies are born with an open fontanel, it does not close in time and remains a permanent feature of the dog in adulthood. Lastly, it appears that breeds in which open fontanels is a normal feature, are predisposed to hydrocephalus.

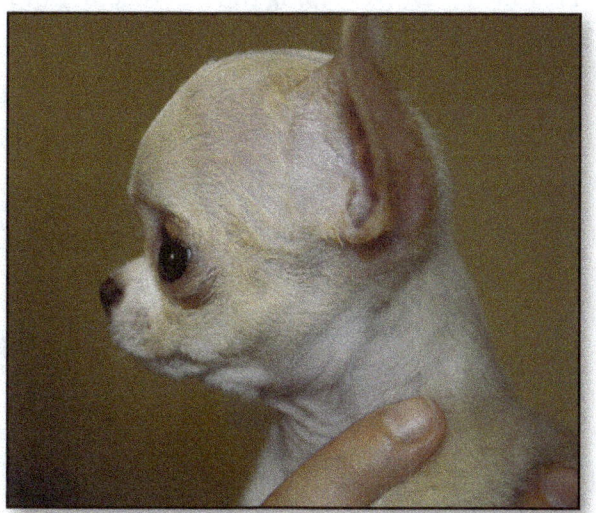
Hydrocephalus in puppy

Puppies suffering from hydrocephalus may be either symptomless or show an array of neurological signs varying from retardation, epilepsy, loss of balance and many other signs. It is usually advised that these puppies are euthanized.

f) Swimmer puppies

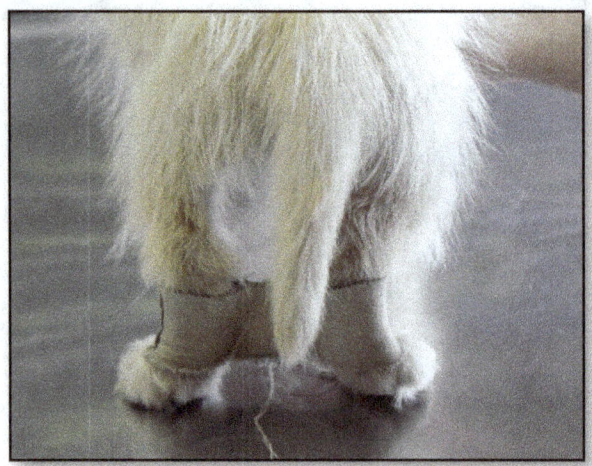
Bandaging together puppies legs affected by swimmer pup syndrome (hind legs)

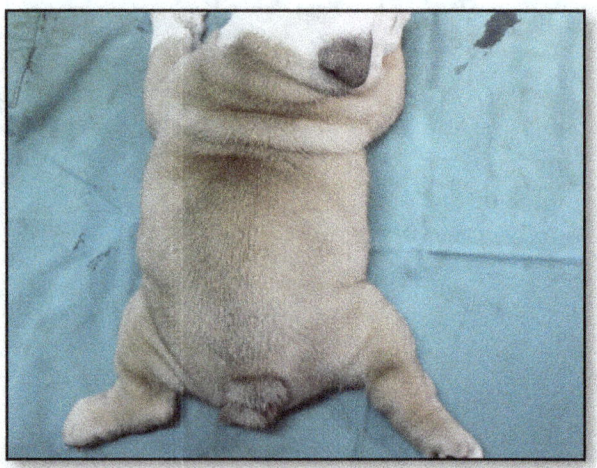
Swimmers pup

Swimmer puppies are ones that have their limbs spread out sideways. They are unable to stand or walk. The cause is unknown but hereditary factors may be involved. Swimmers may occur in litters of any breed, although medium to large breeds are overrepresented. Environmental factors include slippery surfaces, excessive milk consumption, limited crawling and walking space or opportunity. Treatment involves taping the legs together (hobbling) and providing a non-slip surface to walk on. Severely affected puppies which do not respond to treatment may have to be euthanized.

g) Limb defects at birth

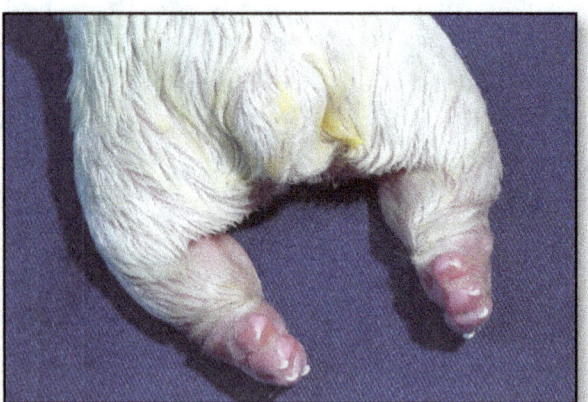
Limb defect in newborn

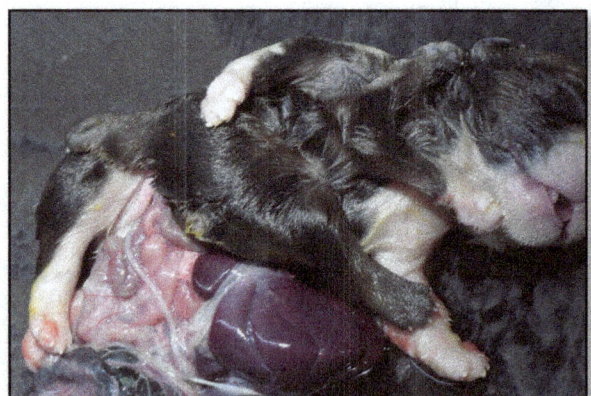
Polydactyly meaning abnomal amount of feet associated with other defects in this puppy delivered by caesarean section

There are numerous defects of puppies born with deviation of limbs in any direction. Some are ascribed to developmental defects due to "positioning" or limited space in the uterus. Whatever the causes, many of these defects may spontaneously resolve before weaning age and such puppies should be given the benefit of time. Abnormal number of limbs has also been reported as a rare congenital defect named polymelia.

Chapter 14 Neonatal Disease

h) Pectus excavatum (flat chest)

This is a congenital malformation of the sternum and ribcage causing flattening of the chest. Some flat chested puppies are swimmers as well. These puppies may show respiratory or cardiovascular symptoms or be asymptomatic. As with swimmers, they will first be noted around 3-4 weeks of age. Severely affected puppies may have to be euthanized.

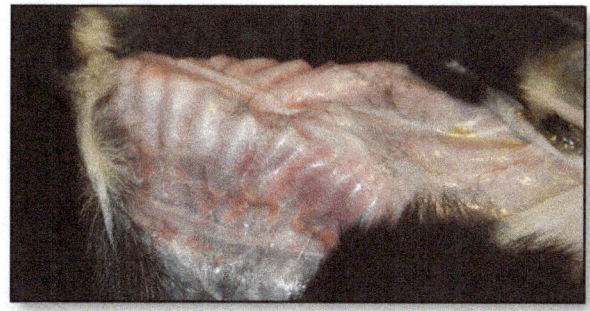
Flat chest in puppy

i) Hydrops foetalis (anasarca puppies, oedematous puppies, walrus puppies, jelly puppy, water puppy)

This condition has numerous synonyms. It is a condition where the puppy has massive water accumulation present underneath the skin and this is clearly visible at birth. Most of these puppies are too big to allow for natural birth and have to be delivered by caesarean section. The exact cause remains unknown but a genetic cause is suspected. These puppies can easily be detected on ultrasound and will predict a caesarean section. Some mildly affected puppies may survive with careful nursing. Most of these puppies however, die within minutes after birth due to breathing difficulties caused by fluids on the lungs. The condition is by far the most common in Bulldogs but can occur in almost all other breeds.

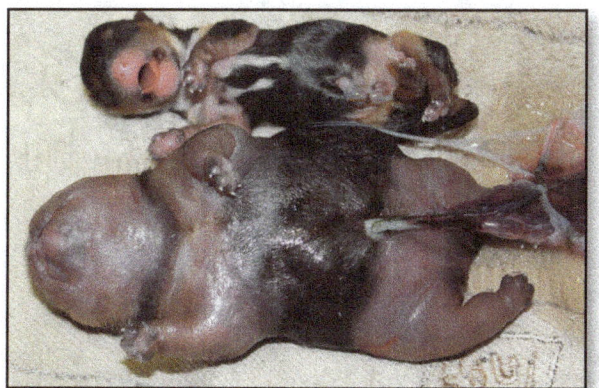
Yorkie puppy with anasarca

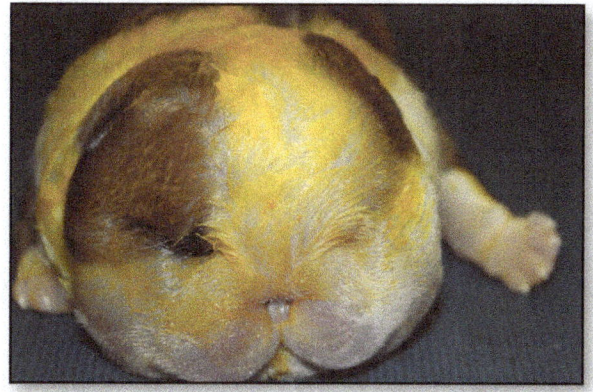
Bulldog pup suffering from anasarca

14.2.7. Fading puppy syndrome

This "condition" is aptly dealt with last under this heading. The fading puppy syndrome is a layman term breeders use to describe puppies which were apparently born healthy, but within a few days of birth fail to thrive, become weak and die. Once dead, fading puppies usually have no clear discernible cause identifiable on post-mortem examination. This syndrome should not be considered a diagnosis or condition. The lack of knowledge of the true causes of most neonatal illnesses or death has led to this collective term. It is probable that any number of undiagnosed conditions may cause the syndrome. As mentioned before, irrespective of the initial cause of illness in these puppies, the clinical signs will end up being similar in all cases. These symptoms are; a puppy which gets weaker, loses weight, cries and dies. These puppies may have; an underlying infectious cause, suffered from shortcomings in animal husbandry, been subjected to traumatic cause or have congenital defects. This syndrome has very little significance, except for the fact that if breeders are plagued with an unacceptably high percentage of "fading puppies", they should in consultation with their veterinary surgeon start looking for the underlying cause. More research is required on this important subject.

14.3. Neonatal disease and conditions in puppies from 3 weeks of age till weaning

14.3.1. Neonatal opthalmia (opthalmitis neonatorum)

Neonatal opthalmia is a condition where the puppy develops build-up of puss behind its eyelids before they have even opened. The breeder may notice that the eyelids are bulging or that they have partially been opened with some puss emerging from them. In some cases the only clinical sign may be eyelids which appear pussy and are stuck to each other. It is thought to be caused by bacterial infection. It may occur in one or both eyes and generally when one puppy presents with the first signs it is highly probable that more if not the entire litter may develop it soon. The eyelids should be gently forced open and the eyes washed out with an appropriate eye wash. Antibiotic therapy is indicated as well as antibiotic eye drops. When opening the eyelids early, the eyes should be protected using artificial tears for a week or so. It may be prudent to preventatively treat yet unaffected littermates with systemic antibiotics.

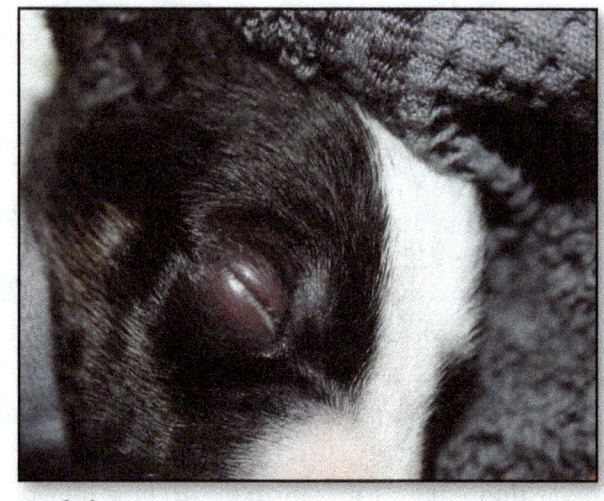
Opthalmia neonatorum

Response to treatment is generally good but permanent damage to the eyes or blindness is possible in cases where treatment was delayed.

14.3.2. Puppy strangles (juvenile cellulitis, juvenile pyoderma, submandibular abscesses)

Puppy strangles is a poorly understood condition which usually occurs at the age of 2-4 weeks. Puppies with strangles may show one or more of the following clinical signs; huge fluctuating swelling under their chin filled with puss, swollen submandibular glands (glands under chin), pustules on chin, muzzle or ears or abscesses in one or more joints. The treatment involves lancing the abscesses combined with corticosteroid therapy. Despite the fact that most of these abscesses appear to be sterile, antibiotic therapy combined with corticosteroids makes perfect sense in these cases to prevent secondary infections. The fact that frequently more than one puppy in the litter is affected, suggests some infectious cause despite failure to isolate infectious organisms in most of these cases. Polyarthritis is sometimes associated with the sub-mandibular abscesses. Some anecdotal evidence suggests that preventative treatment with antibiotics and steroids for litter mates of puppies with puppy strangles is helpful. Treatment of affected puppies is mostly successful. In contrast, untreated cases frequently die.

14.3.3. White scours

White scours is a very apt name given to a form of diarrhoea seen in puppies 2-4 weeks of age that are still nursing. Unlike dogs, it is a well-recognised condition in domestic livestock. The condition is characterised by the sudden onset of profuse white diarrhoea (semi congealed) without mucus or blood. Based on bacterial culture of stool and response to treatment using gram negative spectrum antibiotics, gram negative bacteria such as *Escherichia coli* and others are suspected. Use of antibiotics and rehydration fluids usually quickly resolves the problem. Preventative antibiotics in yet unaffected puppies is advised. Colostrum deprivation is also suspected to play a role.

14.3.4. Infectious juvenile pneumonia

This condition is often associated with large breeding kennels which host a large number of susceptible puppies at any given time. Typically these puppies will be 3-5 weeks but puppies as young as 1 week or as old as 7 weeks may be involved. Initially the condition will spread to puppies of similar age (seldom young adults and older). Initially, the condition appears benign and frequently a mild tracheobronchitis (Kennel Cough) is suspected. Later it becomes evident that the condition is poorly responsive to treatment and the dogs develop a full blown pneumonia and sinusitis with puss running from their noses. The exact cause is not known but is probably multifactorial including colostrum deprivation, chilling, herpesvirus infection, bordetellosis and other kennel cough infectious agents. Although some puppies may survive following treatment, many may resume coughing after apparent recovery. Many of the affected puppies are euthanized due to failure to respond to treatment and expense of the protracted treatment. Attempts at controlling an outbreak should include isolation of affected individuals, improving ventilation, raising environmental temperature and treatment of in contact littermates and litters. Including a Bordetella vaccine in your vaccination regimen (particularly breeding dams) may help prevention of the condition if bordetella is involved.

14.3.5. Hypoglycaemia in toy breeds

Hypoglycaemia means a low glucose (blood sugar) level. Glucose is the basic form of energy which the body uses for all its functions. It is formed following digestion of foods and is stored in the form of glycogen in liver and muscle. Newborns have very little fat and glycogen reserves. They also lack the metabolic capacity to generate glucose from precursors. Therefore neonates that are milk deprived for a couple of hours may develop hypoglycaemia. In contrast to the neonate, most puppies at post weaning age that are eating well and in good condition have adequate ability to quickly mobilise glucose from their stores and replenish these stores from food ingested. However, some puppies of the toy breeds appear to retain infantile glucose metabolism. As a result, they have a limited storage capacity of glucose and may very quickly develop hypoglycaemia if they skip as little as one meal or if they develop the mildest of illnesses. Most of these puppies will become less prone to hypoglycaemia when reaching adulthood but they never really fully outgrow it. Smaller individuals within the breed which struggle to maintain a good condition appear to be at increased risk. Hypoglycaemic puppies will only appear lethargic at first but later develop poor coordination, balance loss, seizures, opisthotonus (pulling back of head and neck) and finally coma and death.

Breeders whom specialise in breeding of the so called "teacup" sized dogs are familiar with the risk of hypoglycaemia in their puppies. To avoid this they normally advise their new owners to feed the puppies (3-4) small meals per day and always keep a glucose solution at hand for emergency use.

14.4. Neonatal disease and conditions in puppies from weaning onwards

The stress associated with weaning has already been discussed in 13.5. Stress combined with infectious agents may path the way for a great number of conditions which in isolation would otherwise not have caused a problem at all.

14.4.1. Concept of erosive and multifactorial disease

An erosive disease is a disease which seldom seriously affects the animal on its own but needs many other factors or agents to simultaneously impact on the animal in order to cause more serious disease. For the purpose of explaining these concepts, worm infection (verminosis) and coccidiosis will be used. In puppies for instance, the mere presence of coccidia in the stool will have little effect on the well-being of the puppies. Neither will a mild worm infection. If the puppies are however stressed due to any number of the following; insufficient milk intake, weaning stress, cold weather, crowding and poor hygienic conditions, then the host animal will become somewhat immune compromised and the worm burden increases or coccidian oocyst counts in stool increase. Under these circumstances the gut wall becomes compromised and other protozoa (spirochaetes for instance) which are normally ordinary commensals become pathogenic and the damaged gut may become secondarily infected with bacteria as well. These agents (worms, coccidia, spirochaetes and nonspecific bacteria) now together cause an enteric disease characterised by maldigestion and malabsorption seen as diarrhoea with sometimes blood specs on it. Typically these puppies may have a stunted growth, eat poorly, be thin and be poor doers. Often the diet is erroneously blamed for this condition and diarrhoea in these puppies. Clearly these puppies are now even more immune-compromised. Therefore, even a small infective dose of an enterovirus (for instance parvovirus) or Giardia or both are needed to cause an absolutely devastating parvovirus or giardia outbreak. In this example, both the coccidia and worms had an erosive effect on the host and together with other adverse influences; a so called multifactorial disease complex was created. Many other combinations of infection may under these circumstances synergistically cause severe disease. Individually however they would not have had a serious impact. It is important that both the breeder and their veterinary surgeon understand the concept of multifactorial disease. Failure to recognise its existence leads to failure to control certain diseases. The prevention of multifactorial disease lies in anticipating it, knowledge of contributing factors, knowledge of identity of participating infectious agents and employment of routine preventative measures and therapies against a multitude of infectious agents. Addressing hygienic matters also reduces risk.

14.4.2. Impact of crowding on disease

Although any condition or disease may afflict dog populations of any size, there tends to be an exponential increase in the number of problems directly associated with the size of a breeding colony. This happens not only because the stress factors increase in number and intensity but also because crowded conditions favour organisms which can potentially cause disease. For the purposes of this discussion a large breeding population is four active breeding bitches or more. In kennels dogs tend to be kennelled to avoid fighting (particularly the males of most breeds). More dogs are kept per surface unit and there is closer contact between these individuals. Hygienic conditions are more difficult to maintain. There occurs an increase in pathogen build-up in the environment e.g. viruses, bacteria, worms, protozoa and fungi. The re-infestation rate of mentioned pathogens which we wish to control is much higher. There is also evidence to support that, crowding increases the ability of pathogens to induce disease via various mechanisms. In crowded situations the impact of carrier animals (carrying disease but not showing it themselves) is more significant. In actively breeding kennels, there is a continuous supply of more susceptible individuals in the form of new-born puppies. The end result is that pathogens which would otherwise be normal commensals (harmless residents) now become part of disease syndromes. Also the protection of dogs against the various diseases in kennels needs more complex measures than is the case in household situations with individually kept dogs.

14.4.3. Non-specific diarrhoea at weaning age

Diarrhoea is the most common complaint by new owners in recently sold puppies. In addition to the nutritional diarrhoea at weaning due to diet change already discussed in 13.5, nonspecific diarrhoea may act as a source of irritation to breeders. In these cases no specific cause of the diarrhoea can be established. In most cases this diarrhoea will be self-limiting and spontaneously disappear as mysteriously at it came. In some cases however, bacterial overgrowth of the small intestine may be diagnosed. Bacterial overgrowth may also have been induced by the breeders' or new owners' attempts at self-treatment using various antibiotics. Specific intestinal prescription diets for diarrhoeic puppies combined with probiotics and colostrum based therapies may help speed up recovery. In stubborn cases or cases where the diarrhoea is associated with vomiting, more serious causes should be suspected and veterinary attendance sought.

14.4.4. Canine parvovirus

Canine parvovirus is the most common cause of serious enteritis in young dogs. It is a highly contagious disease which occurs worldwide. It remains a serious problem in recently sold puppies and in breeding kennels. Most breeders have either heard of this dreaded disease known as "canine parvovirus" or may have had the misfortune of having lost puppies to it. Parvovirus infection is also known as "cat flu" in some countries, but this is a misnomer, as cats have little to do with the virus. The disease is characterised by lethargy, anorexia, vomition, severe diarrhoea, dehydration and death if not treated promptly.

Treatment involves lengthy hospitalisation including intensive fluid and antibiotic therapy. Other causes of gastro-enteritis may mimic parvovirus infection. Corona virus is commonly touted as culprit but plays a minimal role and may only be of importance if associated with parvovirus. It is important for the breeder to realise that parvovirus infection in a breeding kennel may present in a much more severe form as opposed to individual puppies which fall ill after sale at the new owner's home. Puppies of breeders whom have several litters of similar age simultaneously are at increased risk of a serious outbreak, with increased mortalities. This is because the parvovirus may start spreading from one puppy to the next and from one litter to the next despite hygienic measures and isolation.

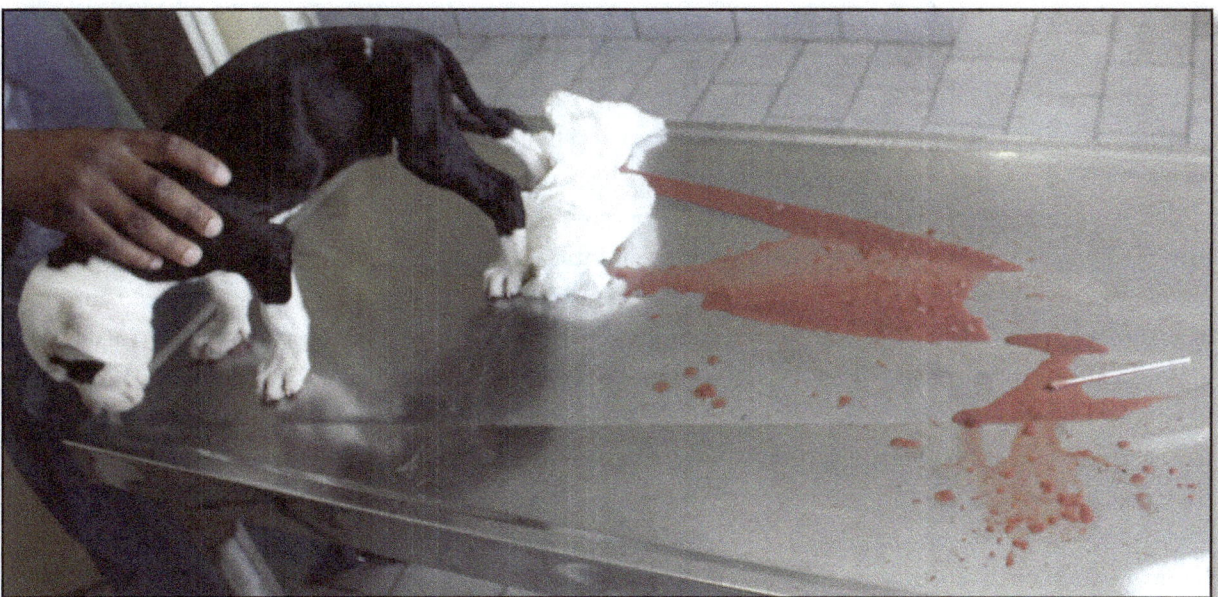

Typical parvoviral associated diarrhoea

Chapter 14 Neonatal Disease

What follows is an outbreak of parvovirus in the breeding kennel and a disaster in the making. During an outbreak of parvovirus infection in breeding establishments, a large number of puppies excrete virulent virus in unusually high numbers, resulting in very high doses of virus available to infect new susceptible puppies. This, in combination with stress factors associated with overcrowding, may explain the observation that the severity of parvovirus associated gastro-enteritis and mortality in breeding kennels, despite treatment, is far greater than that encountered in general practice using the same treatment protocol. Intensive treatment of an infected puppy will usually be successful in about 80% of cases when small numbers are involved. However, in contrast to this, only 20% of puppies may survive despite the same treatment in cases of a parvovirus outbreak. Unfortunately, the cost of treatment may surpass the value of the puppy and hence some breeders and owners may elect to euthanize affected puppies.

In addition, the age of affected puppies tend to be older (7-10 weeks) in pet homes than those of affected puppies in breeding kennels (5-7 weeks). Parvovirus is ubiquitous, hardy and may persist for long periods of time in the environment. Large breeding concerns have continuous movement of both animals and people on their premises. These cannot be considered closed isolated kennels. The implication is that the introduction of problems like verminosis, coccidiosis and other causes of gastro-enteritis cannot be adequately controlled.

Keeping a closed kennel and maintaining hygiene are good principles which will decrease risk but certainly not eliminate it all together. Living with the threat of parvovirus may be a source of huge frustration to some breeders. This is because strict isolation and hygienic measures do not always adequately protect against the onslaught of parvovirus. This virus is so ubiquitous that it somehow slips into the kennel. Although direct transmission from dog to dog and indirect transmission via virus carried on shoes, clothing and hands are the most likely routes of transmission, fomite transmission of parvovirus is speculated to also be possible. Fomite transmission is where an infectious agent is carried on dust and other particulate matter in the air. This may explain why parvovirus associated enteritis is more common following the windy season in some countries. Another frustrating observation by breeders is the inexplicable occurrence of parvovirus in one kennel whereas the other remains unaffected despite the fact that the former may have superior management and hygiene. One explanation for this phenomenon may be the concept of herd immunity. The herd in this context refers to huge populations of dogs which reside in a geographic area. In areas where herd immunity has been achieved (when the percentage of vaccinated dogs exceeds 50%) this immunity will diminish the circulating virulent virus in that area and help protect many of the unvaccinated animals (domestic and wild) which are susceptible to the disease in question or unprotected animals (puppies which have not completed their vaccination program). This phenomenon may help explain why one breeder consistently reports great success in control of parvovirus and others fail in contaminated environments using identical vaccination protocols. Geographic pockets where herd immunity against parvovirus has been achieved are generally areas where cultural perceptions favour vaccination and other veterinary expenses on dogs. Breeders finding themselves in such geographic pocket where herd immunity is achieved, erroneously hold the view that they have the "correct recipe" to control parvovirus. If these breeders however, sometime and somehow, introduce parvovirus in their kennel, they will experience the full brunt of parvovirus.

It has been speculated that certain breeds are at higher risk for parvovirus infection than others. Although Rottweilers, American Pit Bull Terriers, Doberman Pinschers and German Shepherd

Dogs and some other breeds are reputedly at increased risk, breeders of other breeds should fully understand that, in case of a serious outbreak, parvovirus does not discriminate against breed. Under these circumstances all young susceptible puppies, irrespective of breed are likely to be equally affected.

The cornerstone of prevention of parvovirus infection in young dogs remains vaccination, but this has many shortcomings which require explanation. Puppies acquire immunity from their dam through ingestion of colostrum. If the dam was adequately vaccinated against parvovirus, this colostrum will contain antibodies against parvovirus. If not, the puppies will be susceptible to parvovirus almost immediately after birth. These antibodies protect the puppies against parvovirus for a period which varies for the first 6-10 weeks of life. However, the same antibodies may prevent response to vaccination. Scientists refer to this phenomenon as the interference of maternally derived antibodies with vaccination.

Therefore numerous vaccinations, 3-4 weeks apart may be required to adequately immunise a puppy. This has some important implications. This phenomenon leaves the puppy vulnerable to parvovirus from the age of about 6-11 weeks, also called the window of susceptibility.

Early studies following the emergence of parvovirus demonstrated significant interference by maternally-derived antibody to vaccination of puppies. This observation has aided to advance the practice of accepting 6 weeks as the earliest age of vaccination against parvovirus. However considering that parvovirus may affect puppies in breeding kennels at a younger age, it thus follows that it may be prudent to vaccinate puppies in infected breeding kennels at 4-5 weeks of age, rather than the standard 6 weeks in order to shorten the window of susceptibility. Early vaccination (4-5 weeks) against parvovirus is viable and recommended under these circumstances. Special parvovirus vaccines (so called high titre vaccines) registered for this purpose are available in most countries and are effective even in puppies with high levels of maternally-derived antibodies.

Veterinary surgeons acting as consultants to large-scale breeders are well aware of the significance of parvovirus infections as a constant threat to susceptible dogs, resulting in high morbidity and mortality. They should acquaint themselves with the use of these vaccines and breeders at risk should enquire about them. These vaccines may save many puppies' lives.

As explained, puppies appear to be at their most vulnerable at around 6-11 weeks. This corresponds with the time that puppies are weaned, vaccinated, dewormed, relocated and exposed to the new owner's environment and other pets. This is a very stressful period in a puppy's life. It should therefore come as no surprise that recently sold puppies frequently become infected with parvovirus. This also explains why some breeders and many owners of newly acquired puppies erroneously hold the view that the parvovirus vaccination caused parvovirus rather than prevent it. All that indeed happened in the above scenario was that the puppy still had enough antibodies in its bloodstream to prevent a proper response to the vaccine but not enough to prevent infection from exposure to the real parvovirus as soon as it left the breeders premises.

Puppies which fall ill soon after sale are a source of frustration to the breeder. This is because the new owners in these cases are likely to claim that the puppy left the breeder already ill or incubating the disease. The incubation period of a disease refers to the period that lapses between exposure of

Chapter 14 Neonatal Disease

the puppy to an infectious agent and the onset of symptoms of the disease caused by the infectious agent. In case of parvovirus, the incubation period may be as short as 2-3 days or as long as 10 days. Breeders whom consistently have problems with parvovirus soon after sale should also consider earlier vaccination. Due to the myriad of problems which newly sold puppies experience and the frustration it brings to the breeder, some breeders elect to sell puppies way after this vulnerable age. In these cases the breeders take care of adaptation to new food, almost complete their deworming and vaccination programs and sells them at the age of approximately 11 weeks. This practice may not be practical for the larger breeder who will run out of space and hands to care for these puppies. This also exposes the breeder to increased risk of disease outbreak other than parvovirus.

With regards to adult dogs, annual boosting against parvovirus is the norm. There are however vaccines which last longer in dogs which require boosting every third year only. For the time being, every third year vaccination or longer is not recommended in actively breeding bitches. This is because a dam may lose a significant portion of her antibody levels at sequential pregnancies with large litters, which may compromise her ability to adequately protect future litters against infectious disease. It is therefore suggested that, at least in active breeding bitches, annual vaccination against the core diseases not be abandoned until further research suggests that this is safe.

There are small animal vaccines registered for use in pregnant and lactating dogs and they may be used if the bitch requires her annual booster whilst pregnant. The deliberate vaccination of pregnant bitches 2-3 weeks before whelping in addition to annual boosters is practiced by some breeders and advised by some veterinary surgeons to ensure good colostral immunity. This practice has no value in bitches which are vaccinated annually.

Breeders whom have experienced parvovirus are quick to suspect that vaccine failure may have been the cause or indeed that the vaccine actually caused the problem in the first place. Vaccine failure may be defined as the inability of the vaccine to result in a protective immune response in the vaccinated animal. Although faulty vaccines have been reported, this is very rare indeed. It is true that some individual dogs may be poor responders to vaccines and fail to acquire immunity. If vaccine failure is suspected, large numbers of cases are expected to be involved and serological studies (studies of antibody levels following vaccination) are indicated and should be requested. Emergence of new parvovirus strains against which current vaccines do not protect is also a potential threat.

Parvovirus is a common nosocomial (hospital acquired) disease. This has important implications for the breeder. Any animal hospital with the best intentions and management, may act as sources of infection to admitted patients. For this reason, extreme care should be taken in veterinary facilities to prevent transmission of disease to puppies when presented for vaccinations. When puppies are however admitted for any ailment, inadvertent transmission of nosocomial disease may be unavoidable. In these cases it is advised that the puppy either remains in the veterinary facility, boarding facility or at the very least, in the quarantine facility of the breeder until it has completed all of its vaccinations. It may also be homed straight from the veterinary surgeon to its new home where risk of disease spread is minimal. The surest way to trigger a parvovirus outbreak in a breeding kennel is to introduce a puppy shedding parvovirus from elsewhere. Translocated puppies are stressed, immune-compromised, more susceptible and thus more likely to, firstly become infected and secondly, shed sufficient virus to infect others.

In summary, it is strongly recommended that current vaccination guidelines for puppies and dogs be followed according to region. In high risk situations, earlier vaccination than the accepted norm, at 4 weeks, should be considered. Reduction, but not complete elimination of parvovirus-induced disease in large breeding kennels or in highly contaminated environments is a realistic expectation using this approach. The control of other pathogens in breeding kennels which act as immune-compromising factors may both aid in prevention of infectious disease and further reduce severity of disease and favour treatment outcome in puppies originating from breeding colonies.

14.4.5. Nosocomial (hospital-acquired) disease

Often an owner or breeder will object to an animal being hospitalised due to the possibility of a hospital-acquired disease. Usually with adult animals, this objection is not founded. This is because adult dogs which are fully vaccinated are very unlikely to contract infectious disease. In contrast, with puppies the risk of hospital acquired disease is real. This may leave the breeder with a dilemma. Leave the puppy at home and it is not treated properly and dies or infects other puppies anyway. Take it in the hospital and there is a small but real risk that it picks up another disease and brings it home. For this reason in puppies younger than 3 months, it is often advised that the hospitalised puppy is quarantined for a period of 2 weeks following hospital discharge. This quarantine may be at the hospital, at an isolated area at the breeder or at another location where there are no breeding activities and other puppies at risk.

14.4.6. Canine coccidiosis

Many species of coccidia infect the intestinal tract of dogs. Although finding evidence of this parasite in the faeces is very common, disease caused by coccidiosis on its own is not. Infection usually is asymptomatic and self-limiting in puppies. In multifactorial circumstances, coccidiosis may become a clinical entity. The most common clinical signs then are severe diarrhoea (sometimes bloody or semisolid stool with slime and blood on it), weight loss and dehydration. Canine coccidiosis may be primary and in exceptional cases have fatal consequences. Usually, coccidiosis is associated with other infectious agents e.g. spirochetes; worms; Giardia, immunosuppression, and acts as an erosive disease as well as an opportunistic pathogen, always waiting to cause disease in the presence of a precipitating cause. The source of infection is usually the pregnant bitch which infects the puppies soon after birth. Typically the bitch will start excreting coccidia oocysts from 2 weeks before labour until 2 weeks or later after whelping. The coccidia infection in the bitch is usually asymptomatic and their only significance is as a source of infection to the puppies. Special therapeutic agents were designed for the control of coccidiosis in other species and these are also effective in its control in dogs. These anti-coccidial drugs may be administered to the bitch 2 weeks before labour (and 5 days later again) and again 2 weeks after whelping (and 5 days later again) in order to control coccidia oocyst shedding, reduce environmental load and prevent spread to the puppies. The puppies may be treated at 2 weeks (and 5 days later again), and at 6 weeks (and 5 days later again). These drugs appear to be safe during pregnancy but the responsibility for the use thereof lies with the prescribing veterinary surgeon. This is because these drugs are not registered for use in dogs. Sanitation is important, especially in kennels where large numbers of animals are housed. Faeces should be removed frequently. Faecal contamination of feed and water should be prevented. Runs, cages, and utensils should be disinfected daily. Excessive wet conditions (due to cleaning or weather), with extended periods where all surfaces are moist, seem to favour survival of the pathogen. Desiccation and ultraviolet light radiation (from sunlight) are effective in the control of many pathogens.

14.4.7. Giardiasis

Giardiasis is the disease caused by *Giardia lamblia* which is an organism found in the intestinal tract of many animals. Transmission occurs via oral contact with organisms in faeces of infected individuals. In dogs it is more common in kennels. Stress may result in higher parasite counts in the faeces and increased severity of disease. It may also be part of an erosive multi factorial disease complex. The clinical signs may vary from subclinical disease (not visible) to very severe enteritis, inappetence and weight loss. Giardia, given the opportunity via stressors, has the potential for a severe outbreak of gastro enteritis in both young and adult dogs. The best way to confirm giardiasis is to submit faeces samples of various dogs for examination.

Giardia is susceptible to most disinfectants and to desiccation. Allowing the kennels to dry and avoidance of pooling of water helps a great deal in reducing the environmental load of the organism and risk of reinfection. Effective treatment is available but may need to be administered for up to 10 days and must be administered to all affected dogs and in contact dogs. In some countries a vaccine is available but this control measure should not be fully relied upon and should be used in conjunction with other control measures.

14.4.8. Ringworm (dermatophytosis)

Dermatophytes are fungi which grow on skin and hair of many animals including man. Fungi produce spores which are the infective vesicles (eggs) and means by which the fungi translocate from one animal to the next. This transmission may occur following direct contact between animals or indirectly via spores which become airborne. Spores may remain viable in the environment for up to 18 months. Puppies and young adults are more susceptible. Immunocompromised animals and animals suffering from other skin conditions may also be at increased risk of ringworm infection. Although warm weather and high humidity may predispose animals in warm climates, these conditions can also prevail in colder climates where animals are kept indoors.

In the dog, ringworm normally has classical presentation, namely a round area on the skin which may be slightly raised and appear hairless. The lesions may be focal or multifocal and heal from the centre, enlarging peripherally. Ringworm may in some cases itch and become infected with bacteria as well.

The discussion of ringworm is not only important because it has the potential of reaching outbreak proportions in breeding kennels but also because it may wreak havoc in the home of the new owners. Puppies sold with an existing ringworm lesion or from stock currently infected are bound to develop a lesion soon after sale. They may also infect the new owner's other pets and or the people in the household. This may lead to serious discontent and complaints. Therefore breeders whom have the misfortune of ringworm infection in their puppies should strongly consider keeping the puppies back until they have the outbreak under control. The incubation period of ringworm is 1-3 weeks. The implication is that puppies might have to be kept back for at least this period (3 weeks). Topical treatments may lessen the spore load but are often ineffective in treating the deeper ringworm lesions. Treatment with oral medication for 30-40 days may be required. If it is impractical to keep the puppies back for so long, puppies may be sent to their new homes provided it is with full knowledge of the condition and appropriate instructions for treatment. This should consist of systemic treatment which typically involves oral intake of tablets for 30 days as well as topical treatments (medicinal shampoos and creams) to aid in curing of lesions but mainly to reduce risk of spread to humans and other pets by reducing spores on the skin.

In cases where the breeder experiences continued re-emergence of the ringworm in new puppies they should attempt to either identify carrier animals in their breeding stock or treat all the in-contact animals on the premises whether they appear infected or not irrespective of age. They may also consider treating the environment using disinfectants known to be effective against fungal spores.

14.4.9. Encephalitozoon

Encephalitozoon cuniculi is a widespread infection of rabbits and occasionally of rodents and dogs caused by a protozoan (microscopic organism). The condition is rare in dogs but nevertheless requires mention because it is more likely to be diagnosed in dog kennels as opposed to pet homes. The disease may be spread from rabbits or rodents via their urine to the dog and thereafter from dog to dog. Once infected, the dog may be totally asymptomatic but shed spores of this disease (microsporidia) into its urine for extended periods. They may ultimately shed the infection and demonstrate antibodies in their blood against the disease for variable periods. Other animals acquire the infection by the oronasal (mouth and nose) route, when an animal licks/sniffs the spore-infected urine of another animal. This disease is not venereally transmissible. There is generally a low potential for an Encephalitozoon outbreak but this may occur in unsanitary conditions. Infected dogs, irrespective of what age they were infected at, will usually show no clinical signs. Only puppies from infected dams will normally develop clinical signs. The puppies acquire the infection as foetuses in utero (when inside the uterus). In these cases the pregnancy and birth progresses normally and the clinical signs manifest in the puppies. In highly exceptional cases, immune-compromised nursing puppies may acquire the infection soon after birth. The age of manifestation varies and may be as early as 3-4 weeks of age or as late as 12 months. The normal age at manifestation is usually around 3 months of age. This may be a frustrating condition to the breeder as at that stage, the puppies are usually with their new owners.

The clinical signs are failing to thrive, depression, weight loss, ataxia (unsteady gait), head tilt, head swaying, blindness, hind quarter paresis and seizures.

The parasite mainly affects the brain, eyes and urinary tract, causing encephalitis, cataracts, kidney failure and death in all affected individuals.

An accurate diagnosis can be made by post mortem and histopathologic demonstration of the organism in the organs. In the live animal a diagnosis can be made on urinalysis as well as blood tests. There is no treatment for infected dogs and no vaccine to prevent it. Studies show that between 8-38% of dogs have been infected. This high prevalence of antibodies in dogs indicates that the parasite is a lot more common than the low incidence of confirmed clinical signs seem to suggest. This is probably because clinical disease only seems to occur after the small window when bitches are pregnant and transplacentally infect their offspring. This also explains its significance in breeding kennels.

There is absolutely no need to euthanize a dam or in-contact dog which has produced puppies which died from Encephalitozoon. A bitch which has had one litter affected with Encephalitozoon is unlikely to subsequently produce another infected litter. Generally in a kennel, only isolated cases will emerge. The spores are very sensitive to most disinfectants and simple sanitary principles will usually adequately control the problem.

Keeping bitches away from the general dog population during pregnancy and preventing contamination of drinking water and dog foods with rodent urine may also aid in its prevention. Dog breeders should preferably not keep pet rodents or rabbits in the vicinity of the dog breeding kennels and should adequately control pest rodents. *Encephalitozoon cuniculi* is also a potential zoonoses but human infection is very rare.

Chapter 15

Routine Preventative Health Measures

Breeders whom have had a brush with the horrific clinical signs of distemper or the devastating losses of entire litters to parvovirus, need no convincing that they should attempt everything available to them to try prevent these and other dread diseases. Unfortunately, disease control in a breeding kennel is complex. Breeders whom are by nature perfectionists may get very despondent if their "perfect disease prevention protocol" is strictly adhered to and they still fail.

There are two inherent problems with the latter concept. Firstly, there is no perfect disease control protocol which works under all circumstances. Secondly, it might be considered arrogant to even expect that we are able to suddenly eradicate all pathogens which have over millennia adapted to their host (dogs). Breeders should also remember that these diseases do indeed evolve in response to efforts to control them. Disease control should therefore be viewed as tactical warfare, against very cunning enemies. This book has already alluded to the multifactorial nature of disease and the role that stressors and erosive diseases play in manifestation of disease in kennels. Controlling the large number of diseases in kennels require, a thorough understanding of these individual diseases, of how they interact and how to reduce their impact. A mature approach to disease control involves the understanding that in some cases total eradication of the disease or condition is a realistic expectation whereas in others only reduction of impact, morbidity, mortality and severity is possible. It is however important to never give up and always maintain high hygienic standards.

All breeders should employ routine preventative health measures discussed in detail with their veterinary surgeon. Breeders cannot simply adopt verbatim the health program of one of their "breeder friend's" from a different area, state or country. This is because the program must make local sense and address diseases which are locally relevant. The disease prevention program should also be in a state of flux as new vaccines, medicines and information on disease control becomes available to breeders. The routine preventative health measures include vaccination, deworming, controlling external parasites, disinfection and maintaining general hygiene.

15.1. Choosing a veterinary practice

Giving that this chapter deals with routine preventative measures, it is prudent that the choice of veterinary practice is discussed. As may be noticed, reference is made to veterinary practice rather than veterinary surgeon. This is because a specific veterinary surgeon may not always be available and the team and collective ability at a veterinary practice should be regarded more important than one individual. This does not mean that breeders will discard personal preferences. It is imperative that the breeder irrespective of scale identify a veterinary practice to assist with disease control and many other aspects of breeding management. This decision by the breeder shall rest upon individual preference and ability of the practice to service the breeder adequately.

Some veterinary surgeons remark of their dismay in dealing with breeders. In fact, very few veterinary surgeons have the temperament to deal with breeders in the long term and their relationship is in many cases strained or soured. This stems from various factors relating to both parties. Veterinary

Chapter 15 Routine Preventative Health Measures

surgeons on their part may be; insensitive to the breeder's needs, be too sensitive to criticism themselves, not be equipped to deal with breeder requirements, be agitated by demanding breeders, not prepared to learn from breeders or anyone else, not be up to date with current information and become irate when breeders spot this. Lastly, many veterinary surgeons feel that servicing breeders is not financially rewarding due to their demands for excessive discounting.

Breeders on their part may be unforgiving if their "perfect veterinary surgeon" blunders, stress their usual veterinary surgeon if they cannot be at the practice all the time, often make a statistic of a single observation, have a problem distinguishing facts from fiction or, may sometimes exhibit paranoia by suspecting that their veterinary surgeon is in cahoots with another breeder. Last but not least, many veterinary practices feel that breeders often do not keep track of the normal going rates of veterinary expenses and become unappreciative of the discounted prices offered to them.

Because veterinary science has become a very specialised field, breeders may elect to choose more than one practice depending on the individual skills and field of specialisation available to them. A breeder may for instance see one practice for surgical matters, another for diagnosis of medical problems and yet another for reproductive issues. As a rule of thumb, practices which are larger and are dedicated to companion animals are in most cases better equipped and more experienced in servicing breeders and dealing with their often challenging cases. On the other hand, some breeders prefer the individual attention they receive from, in some instances, very dedicated and up to date veterinary surgeons in smaller practices. Whatever the final choice, it is crucial that breeders have available to them a dedicated veterinary surgeon to assist them in disease prevention and cure.

15.2. Control of diseases preventable by vaccination

The cornerstone of prevention of infectious diseases in young dogs remains vaccination. Considering the fact that the risk profile for disease in a breeding kennel is considerably higher than those experienced in a pet home, the vaccination program which the breeders' veterinary surgeon proposes

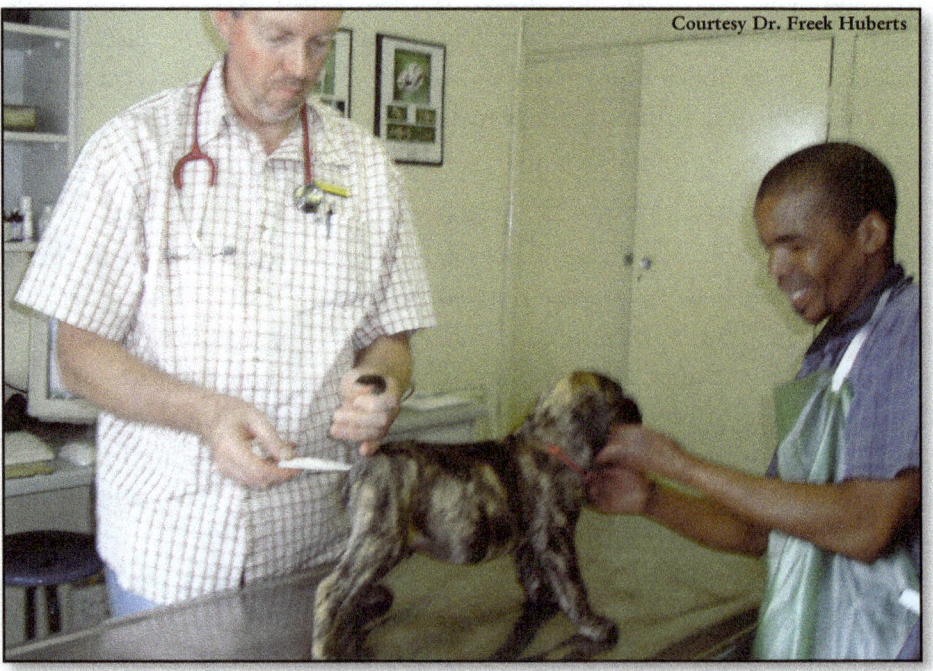

Veterinary check at vaccination

might differ from the one they recommend for ordinary pet homes. Based on the ubiquitous nature (worldwide distribution) of some diseases, they are considered core diseases against which all dogs should be vaccinated. These diseases are canine distemper virus, canine parvovirus, canine adenovirus-2 and rabies virus. Although the latter is not present in all countries it is still considered core because of the serious nature of the disease and risk of cross border spread. With specific reference to rabies, the breeders should consult their veterinary surgeons regarding local rules and regulations and vaccination recommendations. Although not classically considered core, Para-influenza virus is part of the kennel cough causing infectious agents and vaccination against it is considered highly recommended in kennel situations. Likewise, vaccinating against Bordetella bronchiseptica is optional. This vaccine should be seriously considered by most if not all breeders, particularly in areas where it appears to be a risk or history dictates its use.

Vaccines against Leptospirosis and *Borrelia burgdefori* (lyme disease) are considered optional and may be indicated if considered geographically relevant. Some other antigens in vaccines are considered as "not generally recommended" because of limited efficacy, limited relevance or both. Ultimately, the final decision on what vaccination protocol should be followed, is made by the breeder following a risk benefit assessment discussion with their veterinary surgeon. In this assessment a number of factors should be considered. Large breeding concerns have continuous movement of both animals and people on their premises. Breeders may visit other breeders and veterinary premises which are both high risk environments. Another factor is the concept of "herd immunity" or absence of disease in different geographic pockets. If for instance a breeder resides in an area where vaccination compliance is very high then the entire "herd" of dogs will collectively be immune and disease incidence is likely to be rare. This lack of disease may instil a false sense of security erroneously leading them to believe that their vaccination program is working. Breeders under these circumstances may suddenly find themselves victim of an outbreak of disease. Proof of success of a vaccination program can only be assumed if there has been disease challenge.

Most vaccines are combination vaccines (protect against several diseases). Also, these combinations may contain core and optional diseases and may also differ depending on vaccine manufacturer. This may complicate the vaccination program somewhat and may result in diseases included not really considered essential.

The specific choice of vaccine brand (manufacturer) may be of less significance than is generally perceived to be the case by some veterinary surgeons and breeders. This is because registration standards for all these products ensure that quality products enter the marketplace. In most circumstances, where control of disease in a small population is the objective, the conventional 6, 9 and 12 week (or minor variation thereof) core vaccination protocol is recommended. This recommendation is generally accepted and followed worldwide. Similarly, most vaccine manufacturers also recommend the use of their vaccines according to the 6-9-12 week approach. At the very least, new puppy owners should be advised to follow this program. In addition, only in high risk environments and dog breeding colonies, vaccination at 4 weeks of age using a single antigen CPV vaccine registered for this purpose should be considered. Some veterinary surgeons may advocate the last of the puppy vaccinations be at 14-16 weeks of age. This recommendation is speculated to stem from the observation that in some instances, confirmed parvovirus cases do indeed occur in puppies having already received the recommended three vaccinations at 12 weeks of age. In these cases a thorough investigation is indicated to elucidate the reason for the vaccine failure.

15.3. Should breeders annually vaccinate all their dogs?

During the early days of disease control using vaccines, annual revaccination was generally recommended. This stemmed from the observation that not all dogs were fully protected by these vaccines and that studies revealed that they had a limited duration of immunity. Since those early years there have been significant advances in biotechnology. There is also a school of thought that annual vaccination constitutes "over-stimulation" of the immune system. This, they propose, may indeed be contributing to amongst others auto-immune conditions e.g. inflammatory bowel disease, immune mediated arthritis and others. Others argue that the link between vaccine induced diseases and vaccinations is not adequately proven and that the risk of vaccination is far less than risk of not vaccinating. The truth is that most veterinary surgeons see a lot more problems in unvaccinated animals versus those that were "over-vaccinated". The aim is to vaccinate adequately to prevent infectious disease and repeat vaccinations at intervals before the dogs lose the immunity from previous vaccination without leaving a gap where they may be susceptible. The fact however remains that vaccination should not be considered an innocuous procedure and may in some instances have harmful consequences. As a result there is a strong move towards minimal intervention with regards to vaccination. Breeders are becoming increasingly aware of this trend and may demand such an approach by their veterinary surgeons. Hence the concept of extended intervals between vaccinations was born. Many duration of immunity studies are on-going and manufacturers are licensing their products for extended periods (3-5 years) and advisory boards are recommending prolonged intervals between vaccinations. It is however important to strictly follow manufacturer recommendations. Some veterinary surgeons recommend discontinuing vaccinating dogs at an age where they consider their patients to be geriatric (normally 10 years of age or above). Breeders are only to practice this if there is scientific proof to corroborate this approach and that the vaccine used is licensed for that purpose and the appropriate duration of immunity is indicated by the manufacturer. It has to be conclusively proven that the decline of immunity in older animals, termed immunosenescence, does not leave the dog unprotected in advancing age without vaccination. The above argument pertains to dogs kept as pets.

In breeding kennels, annual vaccination is recommended for all dogs unless the vaccine used is licensed for extended vaccination protocols for all the diseases the breeder wishes protection against. As mentioned before, the risk profile of a breeder is entirely different and veterinary consultants to large commercial breeders mostly recommend annual vaccination against core diseases.

15.4. Strategic vaccination

Strategic vaccination refers to vaccination based on results of antibody titre tests. This involves drawing a blood sample of the dog in question and sending it for an antibody titre test. If the antibody levels are adequate (above minimum protective levels) then the dog is deemed safe for the disease the antibody protects against only, and vaccination is postponed until the next year. If one wanted to check for all the core diseases, one would have to test for each individual disease separately. Owners of dogs wishing to do this would be obliged to pay for these titre tests and pay another fee for the vaccination fee should revaccination be advised. Clearly most dog owners will simply choose the less expensive way to simply have the animal revaccinated annually. Most dog owners find strategic vaccination protocols prohibitively expensive and thus it is usually only employed to monitor response to vaccines in large dog populations or if vaccine failure is suspected and investigated.

15.5. Vaccinating breeding bitches

Historically the vaccination of pregnant animals has been advised against. This is in part due to the paucity of data concerning vaccine safety and efficacy during pregnancy. The practice of vaccinating pregnant bitches as routine may be questioned. When the immunity of the dog is unknown however, the risk of maternal, foetal and neonatal infection must be weighed against risk of vaccination. There are small animal vaccines registered for use in pregnant and lactating dogs and there is no harm in using them. The deliberate vaccination of pregnant bitches 2-3 weeks before whelp is practiced by some breeders and advised by some veterinary surgeons to ensure good colostral immunity. This practice is not harmful providing safe vaccines are used but has no value in bitches which are vaccinated annually. The question is whether it is necessary to vaccinate a bitch annually with a vaccine even if the vaccine is registered for use every 3 years. The answer to this question requires special consideration. Bitches lose antibodies in the colostrum every time they start a new lactation and at subsequent lactations the immune system may need to be boosted in order to ensure adequate levels of antibodies in the colostrum. It is speculated that failure to vaccinate breeding bitches annually may compromise her ability to adequately protect future litters against infectious disease. It is therefore highly recommended that at least in active breeding bitches, annual vaccination against the core diseases cannot be abandoned until further research suggests and proves otherwise.

15.6. What about rabies vaccination?

Rabies inoculation requires special mention. This is because breeders often export dogs abroad and then require certification for the puppy. The rules and regulations may differ both from the region the breeder resides in and the region the breeder wishes to send a dog to. The age of the puppy may also matter. Therefore breeders should consult their veterinary surgeon to correctly inform them about these, preferably well in advance of such exportation. In most areas, if the puppy is less than 3 months of age it may travel on the dam's vaccination records provided the bitch was vaccinated in the 11 months prior to the puppy's birth. Puppies older than 3 months must be vaccinated as soon as they turn 3 months old and may then travel exactly 30 days later. For this reason it may be important to keep the bitch's rabies inoculation current (annual vaccination) irrespective of local regulations or claims of extended duration of immunity.

15.7. Import and export regulations

Breeders should make sure that they make timeous inquiries regarding the rules, regulations and requirements for the import and export of livestock to various regions. These rules change from time to time and differ from country to country. These enquiries can be made to their veterinary surgeon or reputable pet travel company. Considerable testing, vaccination, treatments and time delays may apply depending on destination and country of origin. This may also be accompanied by considerable cost.

15.8. Routine veterinary check of puppies prior to sale

Although some breeders elect to vaccinate their puppies themselves or not vaccinate them at all, contending that veterinary expenses are prohibitive, most others take advantage of vaccination at their regular veterinary surgeon. These regular visits help them establish a rapport with their veterinary practice and helps them remain informed about current disease prevention and cure. The issuing of a vaccination certificate or booklet also instils confidence in new puppy owners that the puppy they purchased from the breeder was subject to; at least a basic health check, appropriately dewormed and

Chapter 15 Routine Preventative Health Measures

vaccinated. The minimum examination that a puppy is usually subject to on a "vaccination visit" is the temperature check, auscultation (listening with stethoscope) of heart and lung fields, visual inspection of mucous membranes, coat, skin, eyes, ears and mouth as well as taking of history of appetite and stool consistency. In some cases it may be possible to, at that stage, identify undescended testicles, gross skeletal abnormalities, some heart defects, misalignment of jaws, hernias as well as signs of illness and many other defects.

Chapter 16

Genetics for Dog Breeders

16.1. Foreword on genetics

Any book on dog breeding without an extensive chapter on genetics would simply be incomplete. Dog breeders should have some knowledge of genetic principles in order to better understand the reasoning behind selection with the ultimate goal of genetic improvement in mind. The intention of this section is not to educate the reader on the vast topic of dog genetics but to lay out information pertinent to the dog breeder making it easier to make informed decisions. It is important for breeders to take note of the fact that most conditions, diseases or "syndromes" may have a genetic (hereditary) component to it within a given breed. Study of the literature on these may be very confusing. This is because the literature is also not always clear on the mode of inheritance or cannot always quote heritability coefficients relating to a genetic or suspected genetic trait or defect. It is generally accepted however, that whenever a specific problem within a breed (or bloodlines within that breed), is being diagnosed more often than in other breeds (over represented in the breed), this specific trait should be considered heritable until proven otherwise. It is however also important to consider popularity of a breed when evaluating the true incidence of defects or conditions (genetic or otherwise) and comparing the incidence to other breeds. One notable example is the German Shepherd Dog breed. This breed is singled out because it is not only a very popular dog breed but also a very well-studied dog breed. This is owing to its popularity but also due to the fact that this breed is over represented in the service dog industry, an industry that frequently has both motive and resources to fully investigate and scientifically report defects and conditions. The result is that this breed may therefore be unfairly over-represented in all these reports, erroneously creating the impression that this breed is riddled with problems. Other well-studied breeds have to a lesser extent also fell victim to this "injustice". Responsible and ethical breeders are those that are sincere in their efforts to eradicate known and suspected adverse heritable traits in their breeds.

Poor understanding of genetic principles may frequently mislead breeders to make incorrect assumptions. Breeders are often tempted to give their own stud or bitch the benefit of doubt if some genetic problem has arisen in the offspring. Breeders in this case would frequently remark that this specific defect had never been detected in their lines and therefore must originate from the stud or vice versa. This rhetoric would even be used in cases where the mode of inheritance for the defect in question clearly indicates that both parents carried the defective gene. This attitude towards reality is not always a malicious attempt to deceive others, but frequently inspired by ignorance of the mode of inheritance or a state of denial. Whatever the motive, it does not further the interests of the breed or the breeders. In defence of breeders, it needs to be mentioned that today still very many conditions considered heritable have unknown modes of inheritance or have yet unproven heritability. At least for the conditions in which the heritability is proven to be of genetic origin, strong selection against carriers is encouraged in most cases.

What follows is a detailed explanation of terminology, genetic principles and concepts and modes of inheritance. This is specifically for those wishing to understand current genetic advances and more specifically for those individuals involved in genetic counselling and breed advancement interest groups. The vast majority of breeders will however benefit more from the section "practical genetics for dog breeders". This latter section will help explain how all this information can be of practical use.

16.2. Introductory terminology

16.2.1. Congenital
Relates to a condition which is present at birth. This may be as a result of either heredity or environmental influences.

16.2.2. Heritable (hereditary, inherited)
Relates to a condition or trait (quality, characteristic or predisposition) that is capable of being passed from one generation to the next.

16.2.3. Genetics
Genetics is the scientific study of heredity, understanding how organisms transmit biochemical, anatomical and behavioural traits from parents to offspring.

16.2.4. Genetic disorder
Refers to a pathological condition caused by an absent or defective gene or by a chromosomal aberration. It is also known under many other names e.g. hereditary disease, inherited disorder, genetic disease, genetic abnormality and more.

16.2.5. Genomics
The genome is the entirety of an organism's hereditary information which in the case of mammals is encoded in its DNA. Genomics is the discipline that concerns itself with the study of the genome. In production animals it is being employed to select superior stock. Genomics is therefore likely to play a role in companion animals in the future. This will however require the data collection on objective parameters collected on a statistically significant number of dogs. Once this has been achieved, it may be possible to improve our selection methods based on genotypes rather than phenotypes.

16.2.6. Genotype (what the animal has within its genes)
This is in short what the animal produces. Genotype may be more important than what the dog looks like. The genotypes are determined by the genes and the trait (physical, physiological, biochemical, or behavioural) they produce is the phenotype (what the animal looks like). Phenotype in many instances may however also be influenced by environmental factors.

16.2.7. Genes, alleles and locus
In the simplest terms, genes are the units of heredity present on the chromosomes like beads on a string and hold the information in DNA to build and maintain their cells and pass genetic traits to offspring.

In more detail a gene is the region of DNA capable of being transcribed to produce a functional RNA molecule. They are the DNA regions which encode proteins. They come in different variants called alleles. When there are more than two alleles at a locus, greater number of genotypes and phenotypes are possible.

The position of the gene (or all alleles for any particular gene) along a chromosome is called the locus of the gene. In higher organisms, each cell contains two copies of each type of chromosome. Such organisms, in which chromosomes are present in pairs, are called diploid. In each pair of chromosomes, one member is inherited from the mother through the egg and the other inherited from the father through the sperm. Since the chromosomes are present twice in the body cells and once in the germ cells, it follows that, the genes are present twice in the individual (one gene on each chromosome) but singly in the germ cells (gamete). In genetics this fundamental principle of segregation means that an organism possesses two alleles which code for a trait and these two alleles will separate in equal proportions when sex cells (sperm or egg) are formed.

At every locus, therefore, diploid organisms contain two alleles, one each at corresponding positions in the maternal and paternal chromosomes. When two gametes unite at fertilization a zygote (fertilised egg) is formed which will ultimately develop in a new organism (puppy).

16.2.8. Chromosomes

Chromosomes are structures where the DNA molecule stores biological information, and are made up of tightly packed double strands of nucleotides. The nucleotides itself are made up of complementary G–C or A–T base pairs, these being pairings of the bases adenine (A), guanine (G), cytosine (C), and thymine (T). It is convenient to refer to each nucleotide by the first letter of the name of its base: A, G, C, and T. Why this is useful to know is that the protein coding information that are a sequence of bases within nucleotides, ultimately specifies the amino acid sequence of proteins an organism will make and where and when the protein synthesis will occur.

There are two types of chromosomes, autosomes and sex chromosomes. For instance, domestic dogs have a total of 78 chromosomes (2 sex chromosomes, the well-known X (female) and Y (male) chromosomes and 38 pairs of autosomes = 78).

16.2.9. Genetic testing

The nucleotide sequence is the genetic sequence that is tested for in detection of diseases by geneticists and seen in some of the Polymerase Chain Reaction (PCR) reports that breeders often receive from laboratories. The PCR is a laboratory technique which allows the amplification of a specific DNA region that lies between two regions of known DNA sequence. For example, the base sequence TACGGGGCCCT........TTAACCCGGTT will only pair with ATGCCCCGGGA......... AATTGGGCCAA. The tests therefore take advantage of the fundamental tenet that is the complementarity of bases on DNA's two strands, allowing for genetic information to be replicated in the organism. Practically, the sequence TACGGGGCCCT might be part of a sequence that makes a protein which causes an abnormal condition or may just be present close to it. In the lab, the molecular geneticists will artificially make the complimentary sequence ATGCCCCGGGA that in a laboratory machine will pick up its partner sequence (if present in the test sample submitted), giving a positive PCR result. This is passed on to the breeder as evidence of a positive result, be it presence of a hidden disease, coat colour or whatever trait or defect under investigation. Breeders are often confused by much of the terminology they come across within laboratories' genetic test result explanations. A term often seen is autosomal recessive. This is the simplest form of inheritance where a gene from a chromosome which is not X or Y is transmitted to the offspring. The condition is then seen only if both the stud and bitch carry this condition. If it is linked to X or Y chromosome, it is called sex-linked gene.

16.2.10. Homozygous and heterozygous

If the two alleles at a locus are identical, having the same nucleotide sequence along the DNA, the organism is said to be homozygous at the locus; if the two alleles at a locus are different, the organism is said to be heterozygous at the locus.

In genetics, the fundamental principle of segregation means that an organism possesses two alleles which code for a trait and these two alleles will separate in equal proportions when sex cells (sperm or egg) are formed. When at fertilization many identical alleles combine that organism will be homozygous at many loci. This means that a high degree of homozygosity has been achieved. Heterozygosity means the opposite.

16.2.11. Dominance, co-dominance and penetrance

Another principle of importance is that of dominance, where in the presence of two different alleles in a heterozygote, only the trait of the "dominant" allele is observed in the phenotype and the hidden or masked allele is termed "recessive".

The dominant genes are denoted by capitals and recessive genes by lower-case alphabet letters. For instance if the letter capital B refers to coat colour black and lower-case b refers to brown and black is dominant to brown then capital B would denote dominance of black over b recessive brown. BB would be homozygous dominant black, Bb heterozygous black and bb recessive homozygous brown. In this example the dog with BB would be black and only produce black, Bb would also be black but potentially produce brown if combined with another Bb or a bb and finally bb crossed with bb would produce brown only.

Incomplete dominance is where the heterozygote exhibits a phenotype that is an intermediate between the homozygote phenotypes.

When the offspring exhibits traits of both parental homozygotes it is called co-dominance. The percentage of offspring having a particular genotype that exhibit the expected phenotype, is termed penetrance. When other genes and the environment affect the phenotype, incomplete penetrance may be the result on the phenotype. Genes can interact with each other also, genetic interaction refers to such interaction between genes at different loci which can mask or suppress the expression of other genes, producing unpredictable modifications to phenotypic ratios.

The genes on the X and Y sex chromosomes in animals determine sex-linked characteristics, whereas sex-influenced characteristics are encoded by autosomal genes but are expressed more readily in either male or female.

16.2.12. Developmental anomaly (defect)

This refers to any congenital defect which results from interference with the normal growth and differentiation of the foetus. Developmental anomalies can arise at any stage of embryonic development and may vary greatly in type and severity. Developmental anomalies may be caused by a wide variety of factors, including genetic mutations, chromosomal aberrations, teratogenic agents and nutritional and other environmental factors. Although all developmental anomalies are present at birth, many are apparent but not all. Developmental anomalies involving organs may not become evident until days, weeks, or even years after birth. Developmental anomalies are normally not heritable.

16.2.13. Heritability and heritability coefficient

Heritability refers to the extent to which a trait may be inherited from one generation to the next. This extent or degree of heritability for a trait is measured in the heritability coefficient. At best these heritability coefficients are estimates. This can vary between 0 and 1. High heritability coefficients mean the likelihood of the trait being inherited from one generation to the next is high whereas with traits with low heritability coefficients, the chances are less.

The heritability coefficient of traits has very important practical implications for breeders. For instance, if the heritability coefficient of a particular trait is low and the importance of that trait is minor compared to other traits a breeder wishes to eliminate, the breeder may elect to ignore this trait until more serious defects have been weeded out of the genetic pool.

16.2.14. Mutation

Mutations are changes to the nucleotide sequence of the genetic material of an organism. Mutations can occur when errors creep in during cell division. Mutations may be induced when rapidly dividing cells are exposed to UV light, radiation, mutagenic chemicals and certain viruses or may occur spontaneously. If the mutation is contained within the reproductive cells, it can be passed on to its offspring. Depending on how the mutation has altered the gene, it may either be detrimental or beneficial to the health of the organism.

16.3. Hybridisation

Hybridisation refers to crossing of organisms across the species barrier. For instance in the genus Canidae, a dog crossing with a coyote would result in hybrid offspring. The crossing of different breeds within the dog species would however result in a mixed breed or mongrel. Members of the dog genus Canis; wolves, coyotes, dogs, red wolf, dingoes and the golden jackal species all have 78 chromosomes arranged in 39 pairs and can all interbreed to produce fertile offspring whereas they cannot interbreed with members of less closely related jackal species (74 chromosomes) and also not with any fox species like red fox (38 chromosomes), the raccoon dog (42 chromosomes), Fennec fox (64 chromosomes) and other fox species many with varying chromosome numbers. Despite a total absence of scientific evidence and genetically confirmed cases of hybrids of dogs with foxes and black-backed and side-striped jackal, anecdotal evidence of such alleged hybrids is common. Photographic evidence of such hybrids exists and is certainly in some cases very compelling. Also, "tame" male foxes and jackal habituated with similar size bitches of various dog breeds have been witnessed to mate and these bitches are in some cases alleged to have born live hybrids. Despite this, most scientist agree that such claims are very unlikely because of genetic differences between the dog and the fox.

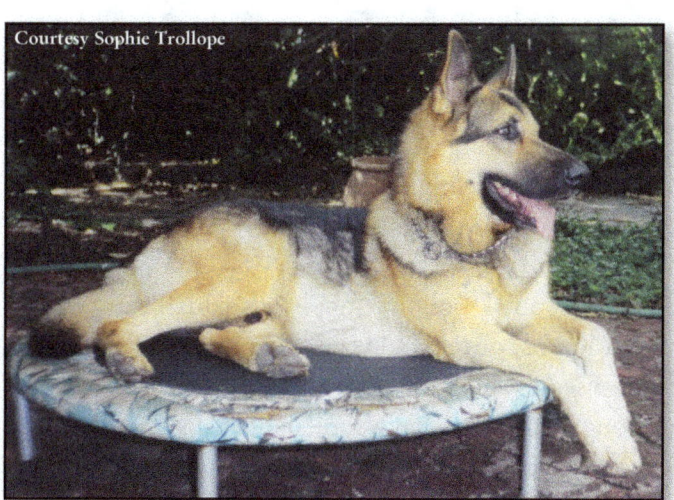

Wolf cross dog hybrid also called wolf dog. This particular specimen is a hybrid (German Shepherd dog and wolf) crossed back to a German Shepherd dog, resulting in a 12.5% wolf: 87.5 % GSD hybrid. Such "diluted" hybrids may show little resemblance to a wolf.

Chapter 16 Genetics for Dog Breeders

The number of chromosomes contained in the genetic makeup in part explains ability to hybridize and produce fertile offspring but in other species there are exceptions. It is not fully understood why African wild dogs which also have 78 chromosomes cannot hybridize with dogs and this may indicate the presence of other unknown factors influencing hybridization in this species. Although the African Wild Dog has 78 chromosomes, it is considered distinct enough to be placed in its own genus.

The motive for creating canine hybrids varies from wanting to improve domestic dogs, satisfying curiosity to creating an exotic pet for commercial purposes. Hybrids in any species will always remain controversial. Hybridization threatens native populations of Dingoes and Ethiopian wolves (the most endangered canid). It is very possible that in the latter species, such hybrids will overwhelm the populations and the original species may go extinct. This is not so much because of direct human intervention but more because feral dog populations are so well adapted and successfully compete with their wild canid counterparts and successfully cross with them. The control of feral dogs in these areas is therefore of utmost importance to preserve the original population.

16.4. Mixed breeds

A breed is not a separate species but a group within the species which has been selected for specific genes which are responsible for the expression of very specific traits. These may be traits like coat type or colour or other anatomical traits. This group of animals which looks similar is then referred to as a breed. If one were to cross one breed with another the result is a mixed breed. Mixed breeds may vary much in appearance with a continuum of looks from the dam to the sire with litter mates looking very different. Mixed breeds may have both good and bad genes from their purebred parents. Mixed breeds may have the advantage of what is called hybrid vigour, or heterosis. Hybrid vigour may indeed increase fertility and the F1 (first generation offspring) may be superior to the better of the two parents. Hybrid vigour may indeed depress effects of inbreeding but the genetic basis of heterosis has been debated for long without an emerging consensus. Mixed breeds are often referred to as being less prone to disease and heritable conditions. Whilst this may be true for the F1 generations, this is not likely for follow up generations. This is because the mixed breeds have all the problems their parents have but they may be temporarily masked in the F 1 generation because of dominance. Indeed if their heritage is from several breeds they may have increased likelihood of genetic faults. Mixed breeds which have been selected over many generations, for instance in hunting communities which are not known to seek veterinary attention, do lose a large percentage of dogs to disease. Therefore through this natural selection for disease resistance, the resulting offspring is certainly less prone to disease than the average purebred. This results not from hybrid vigour but from plain natural selection by breeding only from survivors from infectious disease (Distemper and tick borne diseases).

Mixed breeds can indeed benefit from being rid of autosomal recessive mutations which exist within one breed if the other breed does not have the mutation of concern. On the other hand, mixed breeds often exhibit the same predisposition to infectious diseases and complex heritable conditions like hip and elbow dysplasia. Evidence suggests that, although such dogs have similar propensity to become infected with infectious diseases, the result of the selection process alluded to earlier means that their mortality rates are significantly lower.

It can however not be disputed that many mixed breeds (also called crossbreeds mutts or mongrels) adopted from pounds make the most wonderful companions or even working dogs. From a genetic point of view they are however so varied, making selection for and against traits pointless.

16.5. Designer dogs

A designer dog is a cross between two purebred dogs from different breeds which forms a true hybrid between the two purebred parents from different breeds. In some cases more than two breeds may contribute to the genetic "design" of the designer dog. They may be first generation in which case they stem from two or more purebreds or second and subsequent generations stemming from other designer dogs. Designer dogs are named according to the contributing breed names. For instance the very popular Labrador cross Poodle is named the Labradoodle. Considering the number of breeds there are, there are a very large number of possibilities of designer dogs. In some countries there has been somewhat of a craze regarding the demand for designer dogs. By virtue of the hybridisation and thus the creation of heterozygosity, it is to be expected that dissimilar phenotypes may result. For this reason, puppies in the same litter may look quite different. Time will tell where the designer dog road will lead and whether the fad will pass or crystallise as recognised pure breeds. Designer dogs differ from mixed breeds in that in the former the contributing ancestors are purebred and known.

16.6. Polygenic inheritance and complex conditions

Polygenic inheritance refers to the inheritance of a phenotypic characteristic which varies in degree and can be attributed to the interactions between two or more genes and their environment. In most cases polygenic disorders require a number of genes to combine and cross a threshold to produce a so called threshold trait.

Defects caused by polygenetic mode of inheritance are complex. It becomes even more complex if there is an interaction between these genes and the environment. Most tests for polygenetic traits can detect certain mutations which tend to increase the risk of developing the associated condition, but cannot predict with certainty whether a dog will become clinically affected or not. Hip dysplasia is such a condition. Until tests become available that can accurately and reliably identify carriers for polygenetic inherited defects, breeders will remain reliant on eradication schemes based on testing parents and offspring for defects under investigation and selecting against affected individuals. Hip dysplasia eradication schemes are examples of such strategies against defects for which tests are not yet available.

Linked-marker based test: A type of genetic test which identifies a DNA sequence which is closely linked (lies close on the chromosome) to a defective gene, but not the actual defective gene (as usually it has not been identified yet). It should be kept in mind that as the paired maternal and paternal chromosomes exchange material during fertilisation, an unintended cross-over can occur between a linked-marker and a defective gene leading to erroneous results. If this occurs, puppies of such a dog might inherit this portion of the chromosome and might also show false results.

Direct mutation-based test: This type of test identifies a specific mutation in the DNA of the defective gene. The majority of these tests identify simple Mendelian disease-causing (versus susceptibility) genes. There are no false results with this type of test, except when the error is due to a human cause. Direct mutation-based genetic tests for simple (one-gene) genetic disorders are the easiest to understand. For recessive diseases, the results are normal (homozygous for the normal gene), carrier (heterozygous; one copy of the normal and defective gene), and affected (homozygous for the defective gene). Therefore, with any genetic test one must understand what is being tested for, how it relates to the disease, and how to properly use the results of that test.

Chapter 16 Genetics for Dog Breeders

16.7. Genetics of dog breeds

The sequencing of the canine genome has moved canine genetics to the forefront of research in animal genetic disorders and traits. Understanding causative mutations at the DNA level and making available tests for breeders to detect crippling disorders before they become apparent in the puppies has proven to be critical for scientific breeding. The Online Mendelian Inheritance in Animals (OMIA), an expanding catalogue of inherited disorders, other (single-locus) traits and genes, currently lists 222 known traits/disorders for dogs, of which 155 have had the key mutation identified. This is work in progress and more are being identified. Of the 587 total traits of interest, over 303 are potential models for human disease. Earlier trends in canine genetics and breeding research have primarily focused on mode of inheritance of genetic disorders.

Recent years have also seen increasing number of studies focused on the polygenic or quantitative mode of inheritance for conditions such as hip and elbow dysplasia, heart defects and deafness. The genetic basis of behavioural traits in dogs is an on-going area of research, where researchers have to unravel the environmental effects from genetic effects.

Selection decisions made by dog breeders are most often based on the breed characteristics which are well-defined but with little knowledge of the genetics of these traits. It is now suspected that such selection has over decades lead to some breeds ending up with a high proportion of undesirable genetic traits, while still producing the desired breed phenotype. Examples have been that selection for coat colour unintentionally selected for deafness in some breeds whilst in others diligent phenotype-based selection has increased incidence of elbow dysplasia. It is the hope of the authors that this book will result in increased awareness of the tools available to canine genetics and lead to increasing the quest for access to DNA testing for genetic parameters.

16.8. Genetic theory & testing: a status check for the dog breeder

The background for the recommendations that follow in the next section should be considered in the well documented context that certain dog breeds (particularly breeds in countries where the gene pool may be very small) are already highly inbred. In these breeds, the breeders are cautioned that attempts to summarily weed out carriers would inevitably lead to more inbreeding. Special recommendations for these circumstances might differ from those offered to breeds and areas where the breed population is substantially larger. Progressive breed authorities should thus take local breed population sizes into account when formulating recommendations. An example is the scenario with Danish Bedlington terriers and the prevalence of copper toxicosis in this breed. The initial recommendation to exclusively breed only dogs tested negative was modified to include heterozygous carriers into the breeding population to decrease inbreeding. Such recommendation makes perfect sense in instances where accurate tests exist to prevent the breeding of affected puppies and where accurate selection based on these reliable tests can ultimately completely eliminate the genetic disorder from the dog breed without losing to much genetic diversity and enabling breeders to limit inbreeding in the process.

A historical background leading to this section is useful for the breeder to understand how the current situation came about. By the beginning of the 1900's, the reproductive isolation of breeds accelerated as stud books closed. The various breeds therefore became genetically substantially different from each other and showed little intra-breed genetic variation. The within breed genetic character of each breed has been defined and set in permanence over the past few hundred years by targeted inbreeding and selection.

The mating strategy commonly followed by breeders, for practical reasons, is that a single male is used for siring a large number of offspring. This is the start of breed creation that has been proven to be the stage where maximum genetic diversity has been lost, where the founders (sires) of breeds were intensively selected and inbred for multiple generations.

Current genetic testing using advanced techniques has split various dog breeds into different groups of dogs. Depending on the authors dogs may be grouped as ancient/Spitz dogs, toy breeds, working dogs, herding dogs, sight hounds, mastiff-like dogs, retrievers, small terriers, spaniels and scent hounds or other classifications.

While the above background has lead us to 400 plus breeds (and still growing in numbers), the other facet of dog breed genetics is that the inter-breed genetic differentiation now explains between 27 to 30% of all variations which exists between dogs. Very usefully for geneticists, this means that it is possible to use genetic markers with statistically acceptable variability to determine a dog's breed membership. The section that follows later on 'breed identification services' elaborates on this.

The ability to identify genetic susceptibilities by DNA testing and to use these for disease diagnosis, guidance of treatment and breeding strategies, will become more and more important for veterinary medicine and is likely to be increasingly incorporated into breeding recommendations and genetic counselling.

The advance of the canine genetic and linkage maps later progressed towards the sequencing of the entire dog genome. The technologies that lead to these developments aided the process of finding disease mutations. Previous to this, scientists would make an educated guess on what might be the potential genes contributing to a specific condition, most often comparing the function of known genes that were in a similar area in humans or laboratory mice.

Recent advances have involved using massive parallel gene sequencing methods which use arrays of single nucleotide polymorphisms (SNPs), reducing the time and effort required to detect mutations.

Current studies on complex conditions involve screening of extensive databases which are already in place by advanced genetic mutation/variation detection techniques. The contact with breeders is usually through the veterinary interface, direct appeal via mass media and, increasingly nowadays, through social media such as Facebook and dedicated breeding society webpages and forums. Once a clinical condition has been defined and inheritance model inferred, the next objective is to detect the basal frequency of carriers of this mutation. Breeders and veterinary surgeons are then contacted and samples of blood or cheek cells are collected (buccal swabs) for this purpose. The end result is then to report the distribution by sex, age, geographical origin and variety.

16.9. Genetic testing: practical considerations for the dog breeder

Understanding and applying the genetic tests is what this section is all about. Significant progress has been made regarding genetic testing. More and more tests for deleterious and non-deleterious conditions are becoming available. Most of these tests are for simple inherited conditions which have a recessive mode of inheritance. These are conditions which occur as a result of mutations which cause the loss of function of a biologically important single gene, where inheritance of the faulty gene from both parents causes the dog to become clinically affected or exhibit the trait. If they get the mutated gene from the one parent, the dog will not be affected but be a carrier.

Chapter 16 Genetics for Dog Breeders

Tests for dominant mutations are more complex in that they detect mutations which cause gain of function of a gene leading to disease. In such instances, dogs with one or two copies of the mutation will develop the condition whereas dogs which are clear of the mutation will remain healthy and not be carriers. Certain cases might be of incomplete penetrance, where not all dogs with the dominant mutation will develop the disease but in these cases the dog is still a carrier.

Complex conditions such as hip and elbow dysplasia are a result of mutations in multiple genes and are complicated because there is interaction between genes and the environment which may both influence the presence of the defect and severity of it. In such instances, certain isolated mutations tend to increase the risk of developing the associated condition, but cannot predict with certainty whether a dog will become clinically affected.

An example is the test for the mutation associated with hyperuricosuria (HUU) in the Russian black terrier, the bulldog, the large Munsterlander and the Dalmatian. Though the carrier dog's chances of developing urinary stones are high, it is known that some dogs may have two copies of the mutation and still remain clinically free of the condition. This is possibly due to effects of additional mutations and possibly modifying environmental factors. As the breeder can very well appreciate, interpreting the results of such tests requires a combination of careful understanding of your dog's pedigree and continuing clinical evaluations from your veterinary surgeon.

It must be reiterated that with the documented scenario regarding high levels of inbreeding within certain breeds in the background, the general advice with respect to breeding out recessive mutations is to be very careful in eliminating all carriers from the gene pool.

For this to happen, the breeder/society must follow a policy based on the genetic make-up of the breed and the number of carriers present. If carriers are to be retained in the breeding pool, this policy can be controlled as long as they are mated to dogs tested clear of the mutation. The resultant puppies will turn out to be 50% carriers and 50% clear. This involves diligent administration from the breeders and the society involved. The benefit is that the policy will ensure retention of sufficient genetic diversity and does not dramatically increase inbreeding levels.

With respect to dominant mutations which lead to severe disease, unless the breed is already impacted by severe inbreeding, carriers should be eliminated at the earliest opportunity from the gene pool, as all carriers reaching the appropriate age eventually develop the disease or condition. For the sake of animal welfare, the testing and elimination by sterilisation or euthanasia (in severe conditions) should therefore occur before they are used for breeding. This is particularly important in situations where the condition in question might only manifest late in life. This author's opinion is that animal welfare rather than breed protection should take precedence in these circumstances.

With respect to the constantly evolving market on genetic testing, breeders through their breed associations, are advised to follow a logical and sensible approach to what this new test really means to the advancement of their breed. The best way to achieve this is for the breed association to mandate a breed specialist group to investigate the merits of the new test. This specialist group should consist of mainly breeders, veterinary surgeons and geneticists familiar with the breed and animal breeding in general. Ideally, any new test on offer should have been peer-reviewed and published. The information for the breeder should include whether DNA test is a mutation-based or a linkage

Chapter 16 Genetics for Dog Breeders

test, and if it is a linkage test what the estimated error rate is. Excluding human error, a well-designed mutation-based test is 100 per cent accurate.

Linkage based tests on the other hand are tests for changes in DNA markers close to the gene causing the mutation and may be influenced by genetic recombination. It is therefore important that the error rate is known. The laboratory should reveal if the mutation being tested for is recessive or dominant. The associated risks to dogs with different genotypes of developing clinical disease should be clearly detailed and preferably published. If it is incompletely penetrant, it should be documented. Individual breeders should not concern themselves so much with these details but the breeding authorities and specialist groups appointed to make breeding recommendations, certainly should.

Since it is probable that various dominant mutations can lead to genetically distinct forms of the same disease in the same breed, it is pertinent that information on this is available so that breeders can appreciate their dog's risk of developing a disease even if it receives a clear DNA test result.

Other information that is of use is knowledge of the genetic frequency of the mutation within the breed and the geographical area of its prevalence. It is also useful if specialist groups tasked with making breeding recommendations could collaborate with genetic testing laboratories on the frequency of a specific mutation within a breed as a whole or at least from a specific geographic location, so that they can make breeding recommendations which are locally relevant. Another factor to consider when doing this is to first get an estimate of what percentage of purebred dogs of the breed in question are tested for the mutation of interest. This is because if too few dogs are being tested the power of the test is low. Secondly, making available results from genetic testing should be done on a percentage base without breaching confidentiality agreements by revealing dog or owner details and their results without their consent. Even though individually affected dogs cannot be identified from this, strong trends within the breed regarding a trait can be identified and guide breed specialists.

16.9.1. Testing for coat colour traits

As our knowledge has grown on genetics of coat colouring in dogs, there has been growing interest in detecting coat colour genes. Genetic laboratories have been offering tests for hidden colours in the sire and dam which have the potential to show up in offspring. A breeder can thus test the parents for potential of litters to show, for example, colours like fawn, sable, tawny, tan point, tricolour or recessive black in the puppies.

Tests for the genes which act on the pathways which produce the two major pigments, phaeomelanin and eumelanin, or affect the distribution of those pigments form the majority of coat colour tests.

Tests for the coat colour include testing for variants of the MC1-R gene, TYRP1 gene, K Locus, A (agouti) locus, D locus and M locus.

16.9.2. Testing for coat colour, length and type

More recently, tests have been made available to detect variants of the FGF5 gene which is responsible for whether a dog has a long coat (rough or fluffy), or a short (smooth) coat. Tests offered detect carriers of the hidden "long coat" allele. Some laboratories also offer tests to detect for "woolly" long coat.

Chapter 16 Genetics for Dog Breeders

Tests for curly coat are also offered by laboratories, where in breeds where variations are noted, dogs can be tested to see if they carry curly or non-curly versions of the KRT71 gene which determines curliness. Tests for furnishings (referring to the longer moustache and eyebrows seen in dogs with wire-hair) are available, where the breeder of wirehaired breeds can test for presence of carriers of the recessive unfurnished trait.

16.10. Breeding strategies for the management of genetic disorders

The severity of the defect tested for, percentage of affected individuals in the breed, size of the genetic pool and lastly presence of other genetic defects will all determine what the 'breeder community' genetic breeding advice will ultimately be and how the new tests are best interpreted. For most breeders, this approach is likely to yield better results opposed to breeders individually making these complex decisions.

With respect to severe defects caused by dominant mutations, carriers should be eliminated from the gene pool at the earliest opportunity. Depending on severity and nature of the defect, the affected dog may be sterilised to prevent further breeding or if the defect justifies it, for the benefit of dog's welfare, even euthanized. However, with respect to defects caused by dominant mutations which are of less importance, it could be considered to continue breeding from affected individuals and mate them as far as possible to non-carriers. This may be of value in carrier dogs otherwise highly prized for superior qualities and also in situations where there is a limited genetic pool for that breed in the specific location.

16.11. Selection in practice

16.11.1. Science or art

Selection of dogs rests not only upon science as this text so far has implicated but also on wisdom and experience accumulated by breeders over many years. Some may compare ability to select and combine good parents for planned litters to an art. Science and this "art" should complement each other in this process. The reason why there will still for a long time to come, be a strong element of art in dog breeding is because the phenotype of dogs is varied, breeders will have different "tastes" and not everyone will have the same interpretation of the breed standard. Most breeders will have their own personal preference of what they perceive to be valued traits in their breed. Most will try to harmonise these preferences with the breed standard but they will have their own unique interpretation of the breed standard which may become recognizable within that breeder's "bloodlines". This is then sometimes referred to as a "style" but this style should still conform to the breed standard and be close enough to still be considered true to "breed type". Provided this selection for aesthetic and or competition favoured aspects does not adversely affect the health of that breed, this practice should be considered good for the breed. It ensures genetic variability. Within the breeder fraternity, many are considered to be "kennel blind". This refers to breeders failing to recognise sometimes even obvious health problems in their own stock whilst in some cases being very critical about the faults in other breeders' dogs, akin to a mothers love for her children and blaming other's kids for negatively influencing hers. Likewise, the affection breeders have for their own dogs is perfectly normal but this should not blind them to the faults of their stock or to the merits of others. The aspects these breeders often fail to recognise may relate to conformation, behavioural traits or genetic disease. Kennel blind breeders are not necessarily deliberately dishonest. More often than not their passion, energy and love impair their objectivity.

When selecting, breeders should avoid being sticklers for the one trait at the expense or detriment of overall conformity to breed type. Some breeders wish to ignore pedigrees in the selection of their future breeding stock and select based on comparing puppies of one or similar generations to each other and keeping back the best ones. In doing so they totally ignore pedigrees, familial relationships and the quality of the ancestors. This selection method thus concentrates on phenotypic traits. Whilst this type of selection method does not necessarily result in great genetic progress, it certainly does not limit the genetic pool.

16.11.2. Inbreeding as genetic "tool"

It is important that breeders have a good grip on the concept of inbreeding. Inbreeding, by definition, means the mating of individuals which are more closely related to each other than is the case for the average of the population from which they come. Inbreeding is not just a man-made phenomenon but occurs naturally in many species as well. Wolves and various wild dogs may become intensely inbred because of isolation from other populations, overhunting or the all too common destruction of habitat and extermination of their prey.

Likewise in any dog breed there will be some extent of inbreeding. What indeed happens when animals are inbred is that they start looking more alike. This is because increased homozygosity is achieved in the offspring. Clearly this is how breeds were developed in the first place. All dog breeds have to some extent been inbred, the extent of which depends on location and dog breed population size. With continued inbreeding the genetic similarity increases progressively from one generation to the next. From this perspective, breeders would already deduce that some extent of inbreeding is required to make progress. This is why outstanding studs and bitches are selected for and used more than others, to genetically entrench (fix) the good characteristics of the parents in their offspring. When some extent of homozygosity has been achieved, as witnessed by having achieved uniformity

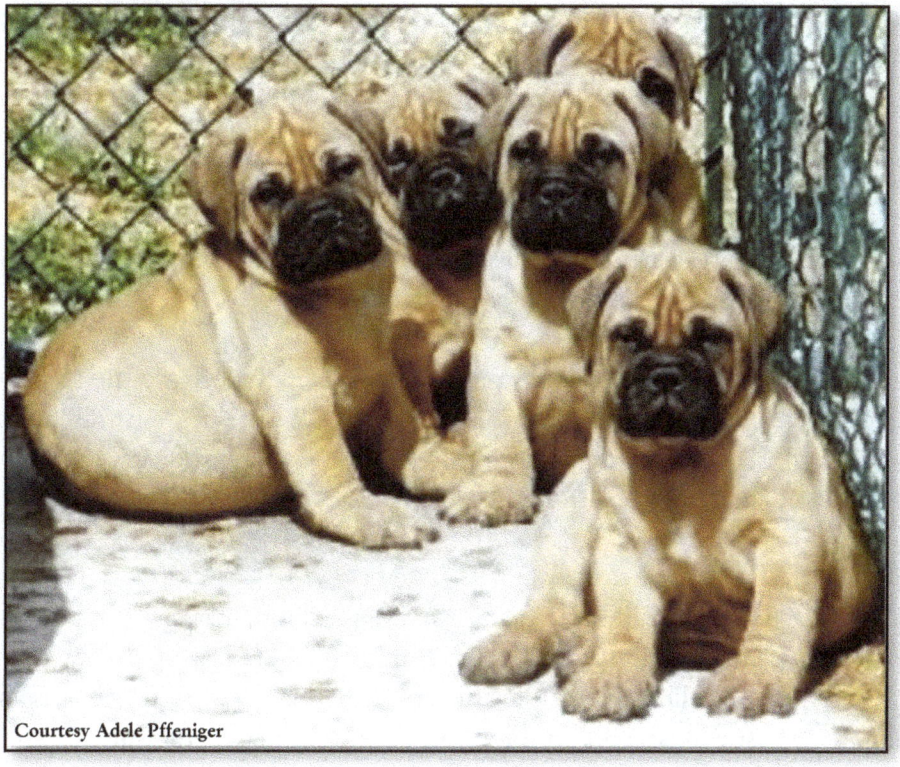

Linebred puppies looking alike

Chapter 16 Genetics for Dog Breeders

in the offspring and high degree of resemblance of offspring to both parents, then a line or breed line has been established. Hence if some extent of inbreeding is practiced it may be referred to as line breeding. Line breeding can be defined as a less intense form of inbreeding and is usually the result of concentrating the genes of a particular ancestor or group of closely related ancestors.

When line breeding is practiced and it is clear that there is a high degree of phenotypic resemblance between the offspring and ancestors, a "bloodline " has been established. Line bred dogs are more likely to breed true.

This means that they produce offspring which possess many of the good qualities they have themselves. Prepotency is sometimes used by breeders as breeder "slang", synonymous to breeding true or having the ability to produce offspring bearing a strong resemblance to itself. The term prepotency is mostly used for studs.

It is very important for breeders to understand that mere selection of good, and mating good to good, will not always result in good in the progeny. This is because if the parents are too heterozygous, too many combinations are possible and the statistical chance of uniformity is much less than if line bred dogs of perhaps even lesser quality were combined. Achieving homozygosity using judicious inbreeding is therefore a must in the quest for progress to breed to and improve the standard.

Since the merits of inbreeding have been adequately discussed, it is prudent that the potential risks are discussed as well. The extent (intensity) of inbreeding is a subject of much debate. This is because too intense an inbreeding may reveal detrimental effects because of deleterious recessive genes combining. Most deleterious traits tend to be recessive. This can be easily explained. If a deleterious trait were dominant (and has a simple single gene mode of inheritance), it would be easily detected and the carriers selected against and rapidly eliminated from the breeding population. Conversely, recessive deleterious genes can hide for many generations in succession. At this point it is very important for the breeder to understand the following concept; inbreeding, irrespective of how intense cannot create a defective gene. What inbreeding can do however is to increase the likelihood of two complementing deleterious recessive genes combining, leading to the expression of the defect.

Inbreeding can also limit the genetic pool because popular studs may be overrepresented in stud registers and less popular studs used sparsely or not at all.

Lack of genetic diversity may have serious consequences. It may decrease the statistical chance of finding individuals within the inbred population that retain the genes to resist disease if new diseases emerge. A common consequence of intense inbreeding is decreased reproductive success characterised by low conception rates and increased mortality rates in the offspring.

16.11.3. Measurement of intensity of inbreeding

Inbreeding can be practiced as in full brother sister matings, sibling matings, doubling up on parents, half siblings and many more combinations. Inbreeding is measured using coefficient of inbreeding (inbreeding coefficient) also called Wright's coefficient. It may be expressed either as a percentage or as a proportion and is usually denoted by the term F. Inbreeding coefficient can be defined as the proportion of all variable gene pairs which are likely to be homozygous due to inheritance from ancestors common to the sire and dam. By studying the pedigree and relationships of prospective parents, the inbreeding coefficient of the potential litter can be calculated prospectively.

16.11.4. Outbreeding (outcrossing)

Outbreeding is the exact opposite of inbreeding. It decreases the possibility of likeness (homozygosity) because it introduces new genes into the gene pool and will therefore produce more variability in the offspring (heterozygosity). An advantage of outcrossing is that it greatly reduces the possibility of recessive deleterious genes combining, resulting in less affected individuals. However, because it does not reveal recessive genes it also makes it difficult for the breeder to eliminate them by selection.

16.12. DNA profiling services

Many institutions offer 'profiling' services for dogs. These laboratories can provide a profile certificate for dogs that may in some countries and breed societies be a requirement for registration. DNA Profiling also positively identifies dogs in the event that it is stolen or lost and subsequently recovered by another party. Profiling can be used to verify or exclude parentage whereby the DNA from dam, offspring and possible sires are compared.

16.13. Parentage testing services

An offshoot of the development of canine genetic markers is that parentage analysis has become routine practice for many breeders. Many breed societies mandate such testing to be done before they will accept the litter to the register. From DNA marker based parentage testing, it is possible to categorically include or exclude individuals as parents. If both parents are known, dogs which are suspected to be siblings can be tested against known progeny and if the tested individual has a DNA marker which is not present in parents it can be excluded as a sibling. Cost of these tests is decreasing as it becomes more commonplace to perform them.

Parentage testing has typically been employed to confirm parentage in cases of suspected mismatings or to resolve disputes regarding alleged parentage. It may be used to confirm parentage when frozen semen was used provided a sample or profile on the donor is available. It can positively confirm identity of imported breeding stock. It can confirm parentage of puppies in cases of multi-sire breedings. It may also be used when a natural mating was performed on a bitch which had already been inseminated with semen from another sire and certify identity of the sire when using artificial insemination.

The analysis involves sampling via a cheek swab or blood based sampling. Samples from the dam, puppy(s) and potential sires (in suspected multiple paternities) are used as templates in PCR reactions using pieces of DNA called primers which are DNA markers specific for dogs. These DNA markers (called microsatellites) are adapted to be run together (called multiplexing). It has been established that when ≥ 15 microsatellite markers were used, accuracy in excess of 99% was achieved.

In sire exclusion tests, the results are a comparison of allele sizes of the dam and puppy's DNA to identify the paternal allele in the puppy. The potential sire's results are then analysed for the presence of the detected 'unknown' alleles, leading to exclusion of sires which do not have the allele/s. Certain breeds have poor genetic variation and therefore do not generate the robustness required for such multiple exclusions. The breeder is therefore advised to consult with the testing service and get

Chapter 16 Genetics for Dog Breeders

information on the breed database available to the testing laboratory and the polymorphism of the genetic markers used for the tests for the breeds which are tested.

This type of technology may also assist to confirm breed heritage and identify frequently used sires. Work is in progress to improve these techniques and increase their accuracy, especially for breeds which are not fully represented in existing databases.

16.14. Breed identification services

16.14.1. Identification of purebred dogs

Laboratories worldwide have over the past years built up vast databases of purebred dogs in close collaboration with breed societies. The option exists to test a dog against the many patented 'genetic panels', comparing genetic patterns within a dog against the genetic signatures in the database of known purebred dogs.

From the laboratory's perspective, a purebred dog is defined when the sire and dam of the dog are members of a recognized breed and the ancestry consists of the same breed over many generations. Most laboratories differ on how many generations suffice to meet this criteria and it is proportional to the availability of a co-operating breed society and testing requirements. The breeder often has no choice but to follow the mandatory testing recommendations set forth by the breed society if their puppies have to be registered.

16.14.2. Identification of mixed breed dogs

Various laboratories have tests which proclaim to test a dog's ancestry. Depending on the laboratory chosen, the owner now has the option to test the ancestry of a mixed-breed dog by testing against up to 200 breeds (proprietary databases maintained by various laboratories worldwide). The resulting 'Ancestry Report' which reveals the dog's genetic background is expected to answer the owner's curiosity on the dog's 'mix' and help understand its natural tendencies and behaviour similar to the designer dog report. From the veterinary surgeon's perspective, it gives some insight into what to be looking for with respect to certain conditions or diseases they may otherwise have never expected.

16.15 List of currently identifiable breeds (2013)

Affenpinscher	Bearded Collie	Borzoi
Afghan Hound	Beauceron	Boston Terrier
Airedale Terrier	Bedlington Terrier	Bouvier Des Flanders
Akita	Belgian Malinois	Boxer
Alaskan Malamute	Belgian Sheepdog	Boykin Spaniel
American Water Spaniel	Belgian Tervuren	Briard
Anatolian Shepherd Dog	Bernese Mountain Dog	Brittany
Australian Cattle Dog	Bichon Frise	Brussels Griffon
Australian Kelpie	Black and Tan Coonhound	Bull Terrier
Australian Terrier	Black Russian Terrier	Bulldog
Basenji	Bloodhound	Bullmastiff
Basset Hound	Border Collie	Cairn Terrier
Beagle	Border Terrier	Canaan Dog

Chapter 16 Genetics for Dog Breeders

Cardigan Welsh Corgi	Harrier	Petit Basset Griffon Vendeen
Cavalier King Charles Spaniel	Havanese	Pharaoh Hound
Chesapeake Bay Retriever	Ibizan Hound	Pointer
Chihuahua	Irish Red and White Setter	Pomeranian
Chinese Crested	Irish Setter	Poodle
Chinese Shar-Pei	Irish Terrier	Portuguese Water Dog
Chinook	Irish Water Spaniel	Pug
Chow Chow	Irish Wolfhound	Puli
Clumber Spaniel	Italian Greyhound	Rhodesian Ridgeback
Cocker Spaniel	Italian Spinone	Rottweiler
Collie	Japanese Chin	Saint Bernard
Curly Coated Retriever	Japanese Shiba Inu	Saluki
Dachshund	Keeshond	Samoyed
Dalmatian	Kerry Blue Terrier	Schipperke
Dandie Dinmont Terrier	Komondor	Scottish Deerhound
Dobermann Pinscher	Kuvasz	Scottish Terrier
Dogue de Bordeaux	Labrador Retriever	Sealyham Terrier
English Cocker Spaniel	Lakeland Terrier	Shetland Sheepdog
English Foxhound	Leonberger	Shih Tzu
English Setter	Lhasa Apso	Siberian Husky
English Springer Spaniel	Lowchen	Skye Terrier
English Toy Spaniel	Maltese	Smooth Fox Terrier
Field Spaniel	Manchester Terrier	Soft Coated Wheaten Terrier
Finnish Spitz	Mastiff	Staffordshire Bull Terrier
Flat Coated Retriever	Miniature Bull Terrier	Standard Schnauzer
French Bulldog	Miniature Pinscher	Sussex Spaniel
German Shepherd Dog	Miniature Schnauzer	Tibetan Spaniel
German Shorthaired Pointer	Newfoundland	Tibetan Terrier
German Spitz	Norfolk Terrier	Toy Fox Terrier
German Wirehaired Pointer	Norwegian Elkhound	Vizsla
Giant Schnauzer	Norwich Terrier	Weimaraner
Glen of Imaal Terrier	Nova Scotia Duck Tolling Retriever	Welsh Springer Spaniel
Golden Retriever		Welsh Terrier
Gordon Setter	Old English Sheepdog	West Highland White Terrier
Great Dane	Otterhound	Whippet
Great Pyrenees	Papillon	Wire Fox Terrier
Greater Swiss Mountain Dog	Pekingese	Wirehaired Pointing Griffon
Greyhound	Pembroke Welsh Corgi	Yorkshire Terrier

16.16. Genetic testing and dog breeding the way forward

Dog breeds have been subjected to a selection process to get the best breed standard conformity. This process has caused direct and indirect influence on occurrence of certain conditions. An example of direct impact is the recent detection of a major duplication mutation recently found in the Chinese Shar-Pei breed. The selection for breed phenotype, the thickened wrinkled skin, resulted in a periodic fever syndrome (Shar-Pei fever syndrome) which was inadvertently selected for along with the skin phenotype. Increased expression of the relevant gene results in higher risks for fever. In these Shar-

Pei dogs, the persistent inflammation resulting from elevated expression often leads to amyloidosis and renal failure.

In cases such as the above and others, the breeder will quickly conclude that discussion on breeding strategies are often complicated when complex traits are involved, as well as traits which are a result of interactions between multiple genes, leading to difficulties in detection and 'breeding out'.

For many conditions which do not have a clearly identified causative gene or mutation, there is a tendency from laboratories / testing agencies to attribute risk profiles to alleles detected by linkage and develop genetic tests for such conditions. In such cases, testing for a given risk allele which is considered to provide the highest contribution to disease is thought to be most effective. This is a developing area and breeders are advised to wait and watch rather than to jump at the most recent test available for the most recent allele/variant detected.

In the absence of more concrete genetic testing developments for such traits, schemes like the current canine hip dysplasia scheme are the best available selection strategy against complex conditions. More recently however, it has been suggested that HD control programmes should not be based on phenotypic selection alone but that more emphasis should be placed upon estimated breeding values. Breeders have to be careful while interpreting DNA test results as clinically similar conditions can be caused by different mutations. An example is that various forms of progressive retinal atrophy (PRA) are known to affect many different breeds; currently around a dozen different mutations have been identified which cause PRA in specific breeds. Another example is the test for hereditary cataract, where the detection of the mutation in the gene HSF4 is only valid for the Staffordshire bull terrier, the French bulldog, the Boston terrier and the Australian shepherd dog, though the mutation exists in many other breeds.

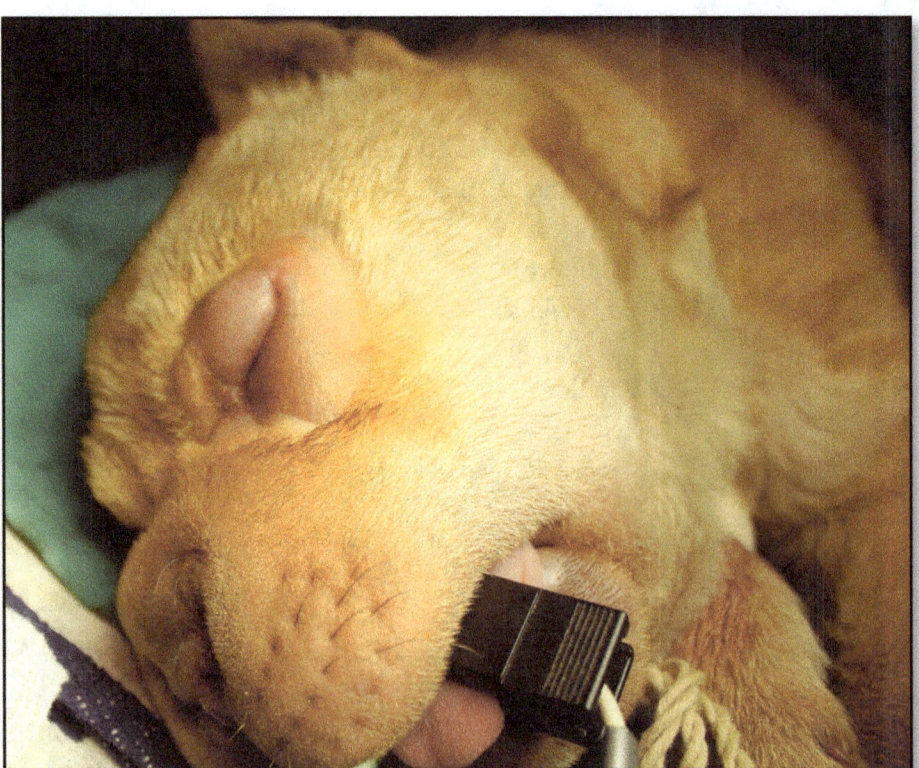

Entropion in a dog before surgery

Kennel Clubs and breeding societies around the world have started to be proactive in working with veterinary surgeons and breeders to encourage the stakeholders to recognise unwanted traits and avoid breeding from such dogs.

An example can be found in a recent Kennel Club of the UK policy in highlighting 15 breeds for targeted action. They include the Basset Hound, Bloodhound, Bulldog, Chow Chow, Clumber Spaniel, Dogue De Bordeaux, German Shepherd Dog, Mastiff, Neapolitan Mastiff, Pekingese, Shar-Pei, St Bernard, French Bulldog, Pug and Chinese Crested. Veterinary surgeons tasked with clinical evaluation of dogs at shows, are given clear guidelines on how to focus on clinical signs associated with pain or discomfort. For example, they will be looking for evidence of external eye disease (entropion, ectropion, and corneal damage), lameness, skin disorders (dermatitis) and breathing difficulty on moderate exercise.

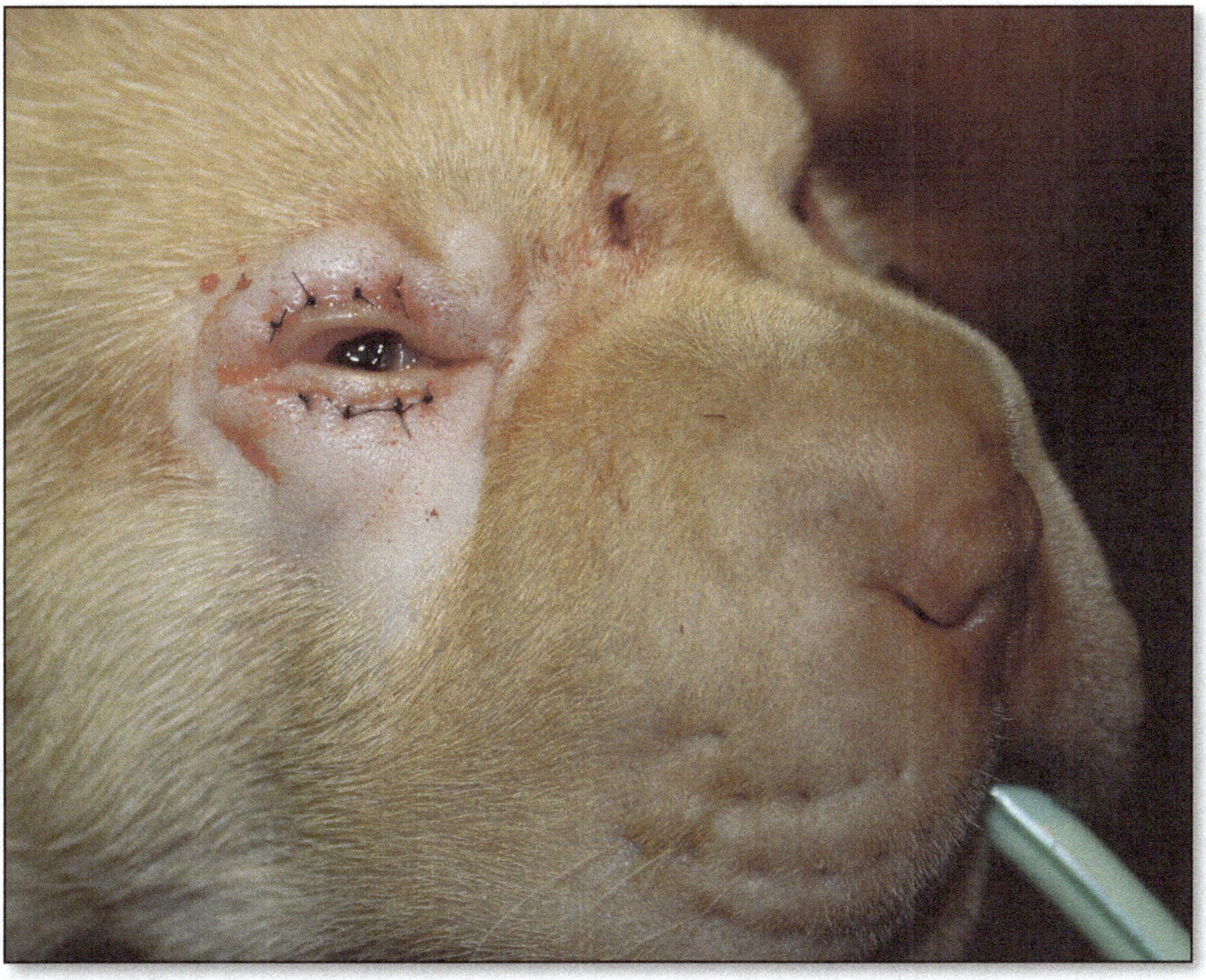

Entropion after surgery

Kennel Club of the UK Assured Breeder Scheme currently includes the following tests:
CEA (collie eye anomaly)
CLAD (canine leucocyte adhesion deficiency)
CSNB (congenital stationary night blindness)
CT (copper toxicosis)
Fuco (fucosidosis)

Chapter 16 Genetics for Dog Breeders

PRA (progressive retinal atrophy)
L2-HGA (L2-hydroxyglutaric aciduria)
vWD (von Willebrand disease)
Primary lens luxation (PLL)
Curly Coat and Dry Eye (CCDE) Syndrome in Cavalier King Charles Spaniels
Episodic Falling (EF) in Cavalier King Charles Spaniels (CKCS)

Close to 50 breeds have mandatory tests prescribed for registration and further 'recommended' tests in addition to the mandatory ones. This reflects the status of breed testing at the time of compiling this table in March 2013. The DNA testing recommendations set by the UK Kennel Club may be taken as the cutting edge of DNA testing based breeding advice.

The breeder is reminded that these recommendations are adding to the already stringent set of mandatory testing based on the breed in question, including hip and elbow scoring, elbow grading, eye testing (annual), gonioscopy, BAER testing (brainstem auditory evoked response) and various mandatory breed specific Club Schemes.

For a DNA testing based breed screening program to succeed, the test has to be reasonably priced, must be available for all breeders, and be repeatable and conservative. The aspect of a test being conservative refers to more complex conditions, where just the presence of the mutant gene does not mean that the dog is condemned. There should be absolute proof that the detected gene is not an incidental polymorphism and has the proven biological effect to cause disease.

The driver for breed testing and screening should ideally be the breeding community, not the registering authority or veterinary surgeons. The community of breeders have to be united in wanting to implement and actively network with registering bodies, the veterinary societies and testing laboratories to make such testing a reality. This type of activism is common in many Scandinavian countries.

In other countries, registering bodies are playing increasing roles in setting standards and what is acceptable and what not. The UK Kennel Club recently decreed that it will no longer register Merle Bulldogs, including any imported dogs due to the deleterious effect of the dominant merle gene. The appearance of this unnatural colour in dogs with two copies of the merle gene is related to an increased risk of developing impaired sight and hearing.

The implementation of a mandatory genetic test for a breed by the registering authority of the country usually takes the following route:

A high level panel of experts including the breeder representatives, veterinary surgeons, genetic specialists and registering authority set an arbitrary deadline for all new litters to be tested for a trait for which a DNA test is available. This usually follows a period of consultation and general discussion among all stakeholders.

An approved list of laboratories is kept by the registering authority and all breeders are directed to consult with the testing agency directly.

Chapter 16 Genetics for Dog Breeders

Test result copies are forwarded directly by the testing laboratory to the registering authority for logging onto the breed database.

The owner of the dog will be required to submit a copy of their dog's DNA test result if they wish to register their dog with the registering authority as a breeding dog (sire or dam).

Owners whom do not exhibit their dog's DNA test result are unable to take part in any activities organised by the national breed society and are excluded from a list of approved breeders.

16.17. Concept of genetic registries

It is in the interest of all purebred dogs, breeders, prospective breeders and purchasers of pet dogs that for the conditions for which there are available direct genetic tests, the test results be made available so that they can make informed decisions. Such information may be made available on request or become available to everyone by access to a freely available on-line database.

With regards to conditions where there is no direct genetic test available, the test results for phenotypically affected or carrier status could also be made available in open health database registries.

Open health database registries will remain a topic of discussion for some time still. This is because participation in these registries depends on the open truthful reporting of disorders. Many breeders fear that by participating they will be stigmatized and that dishonesty by others may thwart the concept. In time to come more consumers will become aware of genetic testing, breed improvement schemes and the role that genetic registries play in protecting their interests when buying puppies. When all these data bases are fully in place, informed consumers will be able make better informed decisions and have an insight into the risk involved in buying puppies.

16.18. DNA tests possible and offered by various laboratories worldwide

Breeders should note that this information is provided as a guide to expertise and does not mean that the indicated breed needs to be tested for the specific condition. Breeders wishing to have these tests performed should consult their local breeding authorities to find the providers of these genetic services. These services cost money and therefore awareness should be created that the purchase price of puppies and quality are linked.

BREED	CONDITION / COAT COLOUR
Afghan Hound	Canine Coat and Nose Colour
	Canine Mask Test
Airedale Terrier	Haemophilia B
	Factor V11 Deficiency
Azawakh	Lighter coat colour
Alaskan Malamute	Coat Length
Australian Cattle Dog	Progressive Retinal Atrophy (prcd-PRA)
	Primary Lens Luxation (PLL)
	Multi drug resistance (MDR1)
	Coat Colour Variations

235

Chapter 16 Genetics for Dog Breeders

Australian Shepherd	Collie Eye Anomaly (CEA) / choroidal hypoplasia (CH)
	Hereditary Cataract (HC-HSF4)
	Multi drug resistance (MDR1)
	Progressive Retinal Atrophy (prcd-PRA)
	Hyperuricosuria (HUU)
	Cobalamin Malabsorption (Methylmalonic Aciduria)
	Canine Coat and Nose Colour Bobtail gene
Australian Silky Terrier	Progressive Retinal Atrophy (prcd-PRA)
Australian Terrier	von Willebrand's disease
Basenji	Pyruvate Kinase (PK) Deficiency
	Fanconi Syndrome
Basset Hound	X-linked severe combined immunodeficiency (SCID)
	Thrombopathia
Beagle	Pyruvate Kinase Deficiency
	Factor VII Deficiency
	Musladin-Lueke Syndrome
	Neonatal Cerebellar Cortical Degeneration
Bedlington Terrier	Copper Toxicosis
	Copper Toxicosis, COMMD1
Belgian Shepherd	Canine Coat and Nose Colour
- Groenendael	Canine Coat and Nose Colour
- Laekenois	Canine Coat and Nose Colour
- Malinois	Canine Coat and Nose Colour
- Tervueren	Canine Coat and Nose Colour
	Lighter coat colour
Bernese Mountain Dog	von Willebrand's Disease Type 1
Border Collie	Collie Eye Anomaly (CEA) / choroidal hypoplasia (CH)
	Ceroid Lipofuscinosis
	Multi drug resistance (MDR1)
	Canine Cyclic Neutropenia
	Canine Coat and Nose Colour
	Coat Colour Gene Variations
	Trapped Neutrophil Syndrome (TNS)
Boston Terrier	Early onset, hereditary cataract (HC-HSF4)
Boxer	Degenerative Myelopathy
Briard	Congenital Stationary Night Blindness (CSNB)
	Canine Coat and Nose Colour
Brittany	Canine Coat and Nose Colour
	Bobtail gene
Bulldog	Hyperuricosuria (HUU)
Bullmastiff	Dominant Progressive Retinal Atrophy
	Canine Multi-focal Retinopathy
Bull Terrier	Haemophilia B (Factor IX Deficiency)
Bull Terrier (Miniature)	Primary Lens Luxation (PLL)

Cairn Terrier	Globoid Cell Leukodystrophy
	Pyruvate Kinase Deficiency
	Haemophilia B
Cavalier King Charles Spaniel	Curly Coat / Dry Eye
	Episodic Falling Syndrome
Chihuahua (Long and Smooth)	Pyruvate Kinase Deficiency
	Coat length
Chinese Crested	Progressive Retinal Atrophy (prcd-PRA)
	Primary Lens Luxation (PLL)
Collie (Rough)	Collie Eye Anomaly (CEA)/choroidal hypoplasia (CH)
	Multi drug resistance (MDR1)
	Progressive Retinal Atrophy (rcd2)
	Canine Cyclic Neutropenia
	Canine Coat and Nose Colour
Collie (Smooth)	Collie Eye Anomaly (CEA)/choroidal hypoplasia (CH)
	Multi drug resistance (MDR1)
	Progressive Retinal Atrophy (rcd2)
	Canine Cyclic Neutropenia
	Canine Coat and Nose Colour
Coton De Tulear	Canine Multi-focal Retinopathy
	von Willebrand's Disease
	Type 1 Neonatal Ataxia
Dachshund	Narcolepsy
	Pyruvate Kinase Deficiency
	Canine Coat and Nose Colour
	Ceroid Lipofuscinosis
Dachshund (Miniature Longhaired)	Progressive Retinal Atrophy (cord1)
Dachshund (Miniature Smooth Haired)	Progressive Retinal Atrophy (cord1)
Dachshund (Miniature Wire Haired)	Progressive Retinal Atrophy (cord1)
	Progressive Retinal Atrophy CRD (NHPH4)
Dachshund (Wire Haired)	Progressive Retinal Atrophy CRD (NHPH4)
	Osteogenesis imperfecta
Dalmatian	Hyperuricosuria (HUU)
	Canine Coat and Nose Colour
	Yellow / brown coat
Deerhound	Factor VII Deficiency
Dobermann	Narcolepsy
	von Willebrand's Disease Type 1
	Canine Coat and Nose Colour
	Lighter coat colour
Dogue de Bordeaux	Canine Multi-focal Retinopathy
English Setter	Ceroid Lipofuscinosis
	Canine Coat and Nose Colour
Entlebucher Mountain Dog	Progressive Retinal Atrophy (prcd-PRA)
Finnish Lapphund	Progressive Retinal Atrophy (prcd-PRA)
Fox Terrier (Wire)	Primary Lens Luxation (PLL)

French Bulldog	Hereditary Cataract (HC-HSF4)
	Canine Coat and Nose Colour
	Canine Mask Test
German Longhaired Pointer	Canine Coat and Nose Colour
German Pinscher	von Willebrand's Disease
German Shepherd Dog	Mucopolysaccharidosis VII
	Pyuruvate Kinase Deficiency
	Multi drug resistance (MDR1)
	Degenerative Myelopathy
	Hyperuricosuria (HUU)
	Dwarfism
	Anal Furunculosis
	Canine Coat and Nose Colour
	Coat Length
German Shorthaired Pointer	Cone degeneration
	von Willebrand's Disease Type II
	Canine Coat and Nose Colour
German Wirehaired Pointer	Haemophilia B
	von Willebrand's Disease Type II
	Canine Coat and Nose Colour
Giant Schnauzer	Cobalamin Malabsorption (Methylmalonic Aciduria)
	Factor VII deficiency
	Hyperuricosuria (HUU)
	prcd-PRA
Glen of Imaal Terrier	Progressive Retinal Atrophy (crd-3)
Gordon Setter	Progressive Retinal Atrophy (rcd-4)
	Coat Colour Gene Variations
Great Dane	Canine Coat and Nose Colour
	Canine Mask Test
Greyhound	Greyhound neuropathy
	Canine Coat and Nose Colour
	Lighter coat colour
	Canine Mask Test
Hungarian Kuvasz	Progressive Retinal Atrophy (prcd-PRA)
Hungarian Vizsla	Coat length
Irish Red & White Setter	Canine Leucocyte Adhesion Deficiency (CLAD)
	Progressive Retinal Atrophy (rcd1)
	von Willebrand's disease
Irish Setter	Canine Leucocyte Adhesion Deficiency (CLAD)
	Progressive Retinal Atrophy (rcd1)
	Progressive Retinal Atrophy (rcd4)
Italian Spinone	Cerebellar Ataxia
Japanese Chin	Canine Coat and Nose Colour
Japanese Shiba Inu	Coat Length
Keeshond	Primary Hyperparathyroidism PHPT

Chapter 16 Genetics for Dog Breeders

Breed	Condition
Kerry Blue Terrier	von Willebrand's Disease Type I
	Factor XI Deficiency
Kooikerhondje	von Willebrand's Disease Type II
Lagotto Romagnolo	Juvenile epilepsy
Lancashire Heeler	Collie Eye Anomaly (CEA)/choroidal hypoplasia (CH)
	Primary Lens Luxation (PLL)
Large Munsterlander	Hyperuricosuria (HUU)
	Canine Coat and Nose Colour
	Black Hair Follicular Dysplasia
Leonberger	Leonberger Polyneuropathy (LPN1)
Lhasa Apso	Renal Dysplasia
	Haemophilia B
Lowchen	Canine Coat and Nose Colour
Manchester Terrier	von Willebrand's Disease, Type 1
Mastiff	Dominant Progressive Retinal Atrophy
	Canine Multi-focal Retinopathy
	Coat length
Miniature Schnauzer	Progressive Retinal Atrophy, Type A
	Myotonia congenital
	Mucopolysaccharidosis
Miniature Pinscher	Mucopolysaccharidosis VI
Newfoundland	Cystinuria
	Canine Coat and Nose Colour
	Coat Colour Gene Variations
Norwegian Elkhound	Progressive Retinal Atrophy (prcd-PRA)
Old English Sheepdog	Multi drug resistance (MDR1)
	Primary Ciliary Dyskinesia (PCD)
Otterhound	Glanzmann's Thrombasthenia Type 1
Papillion	Von Willebrand's Disease Type 1
	Progressive Retinal Atrophy (prcd-PRA)
Parson Russell Terrier	Late Onset Ataxia (LOA)
	Primary Lens Luxation (PLL)
	Hyperuricosuria (HUU)
Pointer	Canine Coat and Nose Colour
	Coat Colour Gene Variation
Polish Lowland Sheepdog	Bobtail gene
Pomeranian	Canine Coat and Nose Colour
	Hyperuricosuria (HUU)
Poodle (Miniature)	Progressive Retinal Atrophy (prcd-PRA)
	von Willebrand's Disease Type 1
	Canine Coat and Nose Colour
Poodle (Standard)	Neonatal Encephalopathy
	von Willebrand's Disease Type 1
	Degenerative Myelopathy
	Neonatal Encephalopathy with Seizures
	Canine Coat and Nose Colour

Chapter 16 Genetics for Dog Breeders

Poodle (Toy)	Progressive Retinal Atrophy (prcd-PRA)
	von Willebrand's Disease Type 1
	Canine Coat and Nose Colour
Portuguese Water Dog	Progressive Retinal Atrophy (prcd-PRA)
	GM1 gangliosidosis
	Canine Coat and Nose Colour
Pug	Canine Coat and Nose Colour
	Pug Dog Encaphilitis (PDE)
Pyrenean Mountain Dog	Glanzmann's Thrombasthenia Type 1
	Canine Multi-focal Retinopathy
Retriever (Chesapeake Bay)	Progressive Retinal Atrophy (prcd-PRA)
	Degenerative Myelopathy
	Exercise Induced Collapse
Retriever (Curly Coated)	Glycogenosis (GSD) Type IIIa
	Exercise Induced Collapse
	Canine Coat and Nose Colour
Retriever (Flat Coated)	Canine Coat and Nose Colour
	Yellow / liver coat
Retriever (Golden)	Muscular Dystrophy
	Progressive Retinal Atrophy (prcd-PRA)
	Progressive Retinal Atrophy (GR_PRA1)
	Progressive Retinal Atrophy (GR_PRA2)
	Ichthyosis
Retriever (Labrador)	Cystinuria Narcolepsy
	Progressive Retinal Atrophy (prcd-PRA)
	Retinal Dyslasia/OSD
	Haemophilia B
	Labrador Myopathy (CNM)
	Exercise Induced Collapse
	Hyperuricosuria (HUU)
	Yellow / chocolate coat
	Canine Coat and Nose Colour
	Coat Colour Gene Variations
Retriever (Nova Scotia Duck Tolling)	Progressive Retinal Atrophy (prcd-PRA)
	Collie Eye Anomaly (CEA) / choroidal hypoplasia (CH)
Rhodesian Ridgeback	Degenerative Myelopathy
Rottweiler	Coat Length
Russian Black Terrier	Hyperuricosuria (HUU)
Samoyed	Progressive Retinal Atrophy X-linked
	Retinal Dyslasia/OSD
	Hereditary Nephritis
Schipperke	Progressive Retinal Atrophy (prcd-PRA)
	Mucopolysaccharidosis IIIB
	Coat Colour Gene Variation
	Bobtail gene
	Coat length

Breed	Condition
Scottish Terrier	von Willebrand's Disease Type III
	Coat Colour Gene Variation
Sealyham Terrier	Primary Lens Luxation (PLL)
Shar Pei	Canine Coat and Nose Colour
	Lighter coat colour
Shetland Sheepdog	von Willebrand's Disease Type III
	Collie Eye Anomaly (CEA)/choroidal hypoplasia (CH)
	Multi drug resistance (MDR1)
	Canine Coat and Nose Colour
Shih Tzu	Renal Dysplasia
Siberian Husky	Progressive Retinal Atrophy, X-linked
	GM1-gangliosidosis
Sloughi	Progressive Retinal Atrophy (rcd-1a)
Spaniel (American Cocker)	Progressive Retinal Atrophy (prcd-PRA)
	Phosphofructokinase (PFK) Deficiency
	Coat Colour Variations
Spaniel (Clumber)	Pyruvate Dehydrogenase Phosphatase Deficiency (PDP 1)
Spaniel (Cocker)	Progressive Retinal Atrophy (prcd-PRA)
	Phosphofructokinase (PFK) Deficiency
	Familial Nephropathy
	Canine Coat and Nose Colour
Spaniel (English Springer)	Fucosidosis
	Phosphofructokinase (PFK) Deficiency
	PRA – cord1
	Canine Coat and Nose Colour
Spaniel (Field)	Canine Coat and Nose Colour
Spaniel (Sussex)	Pyruvate Dehydrogenase Phosphatase Deficiency (PDP 1)
Spanish Water Dog	Progressive Retinal Atrophy (prcd-PRA)
	Bobtail gene
Staffordshire Bull Terrier	Hydroxyglutaric acidurea, L-2-HGA
	Hereditary cataract , HC-HSF4
	Canine Coat and Nose Colour
Swedish Lapphund	Progressive Retinal Atrophy (prcd-PRA)
Swedish Vallhund	Bobtail gene
Tibetan Terrier	Primary Lens Luxation (PLL)
	Neuronal Ceroid Lipofuscinosis (NCL)
	Progressive Retinal Atrophy (rcd4)
	Coat colour
Weimaraner	Hyperuricosuria (HUU) Coat Length
Welsh Corgi (Cardigan)	Progressive Retinal Atrophy (rcd-3)
	X-linked severe combined immunodeficiency (SCID)
	Degenerative Myelopathy
	Canine Coat and Nose Colour
	Coat Length

Chapter 16 Genetics for Dog Breeders

Welsh Corgi (Pembroke)	von Willebrand's Disease TypeI
	Severe combined immunodeficiency (SCID)
	Degenerative Myelopathy
	Coat length
Welsh Terrier	Primary Lens Luxation (PLL)
West Highland White Terrier	Pyruvate Kinase (PK) Deficiency
	Globoid Cell Leukodystrophy
Whippet Collie	Eye Anomaly (CEA)/choroidal hypoplasia (CH)
	Canine Multidrug Sensitivity Test (MDR1)
	Canine Coat and Nose Colour
	Lighter coat colour
	Canine Mask Test
Yorkshire Terrier	Progressive Retinal Atrophy (prcd-PRA)
	Primary Lens Luxation (PLL)

16.19. Genetic counselling

Genetic counselling to the breeder involves giving recommendations on which dogs to combine to result in offspring with the minimum statistical chance of defects whilst maintaining genetic diversity of the population. Genetic counselling thus ultimately decreases the number of defect carriers as well. It is the ethical responsibility and obligation of all breeders to make use of all tools available to them to improve the genetic health of puppies they breed. Genetic counselling may vary vastly depending on whether the mode of inheritance concerning a defect is known, and whether a test is available to separate normal dogs from carriers and affected dogs. It is very important to realize that the size of the breed pool, genetic diversity, incidence of other more serious defects and access to superior stock may play a central role in what breeding recommendations to make. As a general rule breeders of breeds with a small genetic pool and lack of access to new blood are limited regarding selection intensity and number of selection criteria they can afford to look at simultaneously. However, irrespective of the size of the genetic pool, breeders must not only consider the results of a single test but should consider all other traits such as general health issues, conformation to breed, temperament, working ability and many others in the final decision whether to breed the dog or not.

What follows is a number of frequent genetic dilemmas (frequently asked questions) that breeders encounter and the recommended breeding strategies to solve them.

16.19.1. Breeding recommendations for dogs carrying known recessive genes for which there is a test available

In this situation the answer is rather simple. The breeder should have his brood stock tested for the genetic defect and will then get a result stating normalcy, carrier or affected. It then makes sense to breed quality carriers to normal-testing dogs and replacing them with quality normal-testing offspring. Doing this, the bloodline with its good traits is preserved, genetic diversity is maintained and ultimately, the defect is eliminated from the breed. Breeders may elect to sterilize carriers which are not considered top quality. Clearly, breeders will only be able to afford to do this if they have access to normal testing dogs and their genetic pool is both large and diverse.

16.19.2. Breeding recommendations for dogs carrying known dominant genes

Affected breeding dogs should be replaced with normal dogs whether related or not. As with the recessive genes defect situation, theoretically the breeder can effectively eliminate these genes from their brood stock without losing genetic diversity within a few generations.

16.19.3. In the above cases, what does the breeder do with affected dogs?

This will depend on the severity of the defect. In debilitating defects it may be best to euthanize the dog. With less severe defects, some breeders elect to sterilize the dog and either keep it as a pet or rehome it to caring owners with full knowledge of the defect and its implications.

16.19.4. Breeding recommendations for conditions for which there are no tests for carriers

In these cases the breeder must perform a risk analysis. High risk dogs are dogs which have either produced affected offspring, have an affected parent, siblings or ancestors. These high risk dogs should then only be bred to lower risk dogs. By repeating this process of continually using lower risk dogs the incidence of the defect will decrease. Participation in breed improvement schemes and open health databases clearly help breeders in this regard as well as do studying pedigrees of planned matings. Unfortunately, selection against quality dogs based on subjective risk assessment excludes normal quality dogs from the genetic pool. In many cases however that is the price we have to pay for genetic progress until tests become available allowing identification of carriers.

16.19.5. How much of the defect could have been influenced by the environment and how do they know its presence is not purely a fluke (an unpredictably expressed trait)?

The first step here would be to identify the exact nature and terminology of the defect or condition detected in consultation with experts in the field. Having a name for the defect usually answers all our questions as the mode of inheritance or suspect modes will usually be known to the scientific community. If that did not help, the second step is to determine whether this defect has been reported by breeders before and if so the breed prevalence. Finally, attempts must be made to trace the breeding back as many generations as possible and determine the prevalence of the defect or suspect defect within the line. The above line of investigation will reveal the level of breed-related genetic influence as compared to the environmental.

16.19.6. How can one determine if the defect is not purely environmental?

The investigation carried out as described above will partly reveal the answer. If there are no previously reports of this defect within this and related breeds or there is no history of the defect within your breeding line which is traceable, it is prudent to be cautious and make careful notes of the mating scenario/season/condition of the bitch and sire before proceeding to use the same combination again. If it is not seen again the breeder can assume that it is purely environmental. In these cases it is strongly advised that the breeder at least contact their veterinary surgeon regarding suspect defects so that they can make further enquiries if they do not know the condition either. In some cases breeders will ignore a first time occurrence of a suspect defect. This is perfectly acceptable but the breeders should at least make some notes on it as described. Further investigations would then definitely be warranted if another case of the same defect is noted.

16.19.7. What role does the environment play in complex conditions?

They are both very important but perhaps with the accent on the genetic component. Adverse conditions such as poor calcium balance; overfeeding and rapid growth during the critical stages in puppyhood can either cause expression of the dysplasia and or increase the severity thereof. In the absence of environmental adverse conditions the dog may or may not have shown the dysplasia. However, despite adverse nutritional influence during the critical growth stage of a puppy, the puppy without genetic predisposition will not show dysplasia because it does not have the predisposition to express it. The chapter on nutrition alludes to various nutritional aspects which may influence expression of dysplasia in dogs but besides those and controlled exercise, no other definite recommendations can be made to positively decrease the development of dysplasia in prone breeds.

16.19.8. Is it possible to determine if a genetic condition is 'caused' by the sire or dam only?

This all depends on the mode of inheritance of the defect. If the defect is a recessive disorder, then both parents are carriers for the defect. If the defect is a dominant genetic disorder then both or only one of the parents may be involved and carry the defect gene. If it is a known sex linked defect then it is definitely possible to know. If the condition is one which has a test to detect its presence, and if the DNA of both parents is available and is provided to the testing lab, it is possible to detect if both parents are carriers or is it coming from sire or dam. If the mode of inheritance is not known but the sire has a known line of litters which are defect free, the probability that the defect is in the dam used increases. If no prior information is available, the sire should be used with caution (based on severity of defect) and litters recorded carefully and the dam mated with another sire at the next available opportunity. It is always recommended that breed specialists with a good basic understanding of genetics be consulted regarding these questions. With regards to the more common defects, breeding recommendations are likely to already be in place as proposed by the breed authorities.

16.19.9. How do we manage sex-linked genes?

Here one follows the same recommendation as with the simple recessive defects but in addition normal males can always be used as they do not carry the defective gene. In sex linked inherited defects all affected males have carrier mothers and will produce only carrier daughters. Carrier mothers produce male offspring of which half are affected. Given all this information it should be easy to select against carriers and potential carriers and replace them with normal male offspring, siblings or ancestors.

16.19.10. If the inheritability of the trait (excepting a very serious defect) is very low, may we risk breeding with these dogs?

This is a very difficult judgement to make but an experienced breeder will usually make the call based on his judgement on how the defect is affecting the welfare of the dogs they are breeding. The nature of the defect plays a big role in making this judgement call and expert opinion should be solicited in all such cases to understand the potential nature of inheritance (is it sex linked, autosomal dominant.). The appearance of a heritable defect within a known breeding line which has no previous history is generally met with concern and a wait and watch approach is usually noted. If the same combination produces defects in a following litter an active selection strategy must be put in place. Repetition of a defect with an unknown heritability quotient must be treated on the side of positive animal welfare and future use of that combination terminated. Breeding these parents to unrelated dogs would be the next option. Clearly if more defects arise from such matings this should alarm the breeder to stop breeding from the guilty partners.

16.19.11. What does the breeder do if the defect is not very detrimental to the breed and they have other issues of greater importance in the breed which requires stringent selection?

Whether the defect impacts the welfare of the dog is a consensus decision, generally taken at the breed society level. The breeders in collaboration with veterinary experts are the best judges to determine the order of importance for a genetic condition. Complex conditions where the mode of inheritance in unknown are debated between the interested parties and a strategy decided upon. The cost to benefit analysis of these decisions is usually looked at from the welfare perspective of dogs. In some breeds there are so many serious defects which still require selection against which it may be quite acceptable to ignore the more innocent defects. There are many examples which may differ from breed to breed. If a specific breed for instance suffers from a very high incidence of hip dysplasia; elbow dysplasia, epilepsy as well as vaginal fold hyperplasia, the latter may be temporarily ignored altogether until the others have been vastly reduced. Overzealous selection against a multitude of defects may either reduce the genetic pool to near non-existent, discourage breeders to participate in defect eradication schemes and indeed be counterproductive to genetic progress due to increased forced inbreeding.

16.20. Breeding recommendations summary

Any breed which has a showing standard is now expected to be inbred by the standards which determine inbreeding in domestic animals. Many dog breeds do in fact have an effective population size below the recommended minimum to maintain a rate of inbreeding that is sustainable. Application of appropriate breeding strategies can decrease the level of within-breed inbreeding. These strategies include reducing the degree of line breeding used, controlled use of popular sires to decrease their future impact on inbreeding, and using more individuals as sires and dams.

Breeding recommendations below should be part of a comprehensive breed health strategy, and should be inclusive of clear health and welfare objectives, broad in scope, evidence based, balanced and proportionate. They include the following:

1. Breeders should have a fundamental understanding of how line breeding impacts inbreeding levels within their kennel. They must be open to the possibility of out crossing at every potential opportunity.
2. Breeders should have a clear and coordinated focus to eliminate deleterious physical traits and reduce the incidence in inherited disorders.
3. Breeders should be aware of genetic factors which underlie complex genetic conditions, and be prepared to undertake veterinary testing for such conditions at the recommended time frames (e.g., hip dysplasia).
4. Breeders must coordinate and liaise with the registering authority to report and record health conditions and tackle existing conditions.
5. The possibility of maintaining an open health registry should be promoted, enabling research institutions and other interested stakeholders to participate in future advances.
6. Breeders should follow ethical mating and whelping practices, and should take caution not to overuse a 'popular sire'.
7. Breeders should engage with and enlist a team of researchers who are active in the area of determining and offering canine DNA testing. This will enable evidence based policies to be put in place and ensure that the most beneficial strategy is used.

Chapter 16 Genetics for Dog Breeders

Breeding recommendations are of no use unless and until a critical mass of breeders follow them. Open participation is essential and channels of communication must be open between the breeder, veterinary surgeon and registering authority, all directing potential dog owners to get the most up to date information and buy from approved breeders. This will go a long way in eliminating unethical puppy farms and should prevent such breeders from remaining in business.

Chapter 17

Internal Parasites (Endoparasites) of Dogs

Only the most common parasites are discussed.

17.1. Verminosis (worm infestation)

Verminosis refers to the infestation of an animal with worms. Worms are internal parasites and are one of the most common and sometimes most frustrating health problems which dog breeders may encounter. With the odd exception worms should be considered cosmopolitan. It is important for breeders to understand the lifecycle of worms in order to control them. Re-establishment of the worm infestation in kennel situations is common despite frequent deworming with worm remedies of known efficacy. Factors which aid in this re-establishment will be discussed.

17.2. Roundworms (*Toxacara canis* and other *Toxacara spp*)

Roundworms are the most common worms found in dogs. All these roundworm species have a direct lifecycle (therefore they have no secondary host) and all the stages of the worm are found in the gastro intestinal tract of the dog. *Toxacara canis* has a life cycle where the immature stages of the worm (larvae) migrate to the dog's organs and muscles. The adult stages (males and females) of the worms are found in the intestines of dogs. The females lay many thousand eggs per day which are excreted with the dog's faeces.

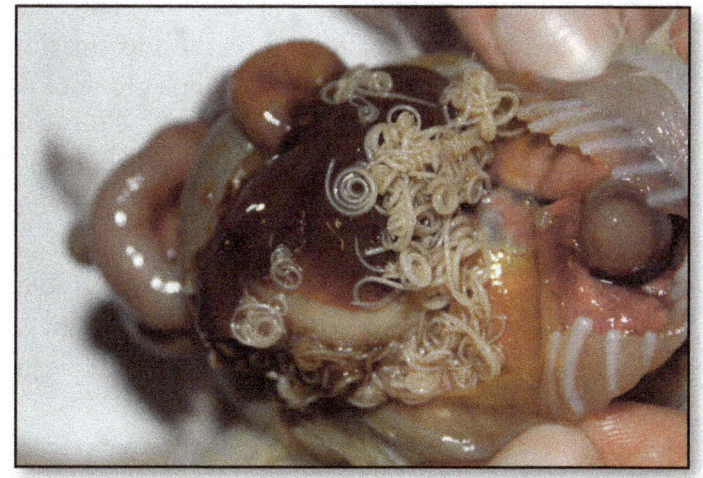

Post mortem of puppy with massive roundworm infestation

The first larval stage develops inside the egg, which can be ingested by other dogs or the same dog. When dogs are infested with roundworm, the larvae hatch from the eggs and migrate (travel) through the gut wall, enter the bloodstream and end up in the organs and muscles of the dogs. The larval stages can survive in the dog's muscles for over a year and remain dormant in these tissues. During pregnancy the larvae become reactivated/"awakened" and by around day 42 of pregnancy the larvae make their way through the placenta into the intestines of the puppies. This type of infestation is termed prenatal infection or transplacental infection. The puppies are therefore born with worm infections. The larvae can also be dormant in the mammary glands of the bitch. In late pregnancy the dormant larvae in the mammary glands become active and find their way into the bitch's milk and are ingested by puppies nursing on these bitches. Bitches can carry the dormant (somatic) worms in their tissues for many years perpetuating infections in their offspring. Generally the dormant larvae in the tissues are very resistant to single worm remedy treatment protocols, complicating worm control. This means that even if the breeder did deworm the pregnant bitch with an effective

Chapter 17 Internal Parasites (Endoparasites) of Dogs

dewormer, the worms in the bitch's gut may be controlled but not those worms that were "hiding" in the tissues. Excretion of the worm larvae into the milk starts within a few days after whelping and reaches a peak during the second week of lactation, before it gradually drops again. This mode of infection is termed trans-mammary or lactogenic transmission of worms from the dam to her puppies. The larvae develop into adults within 3-5 weeks and start producing eggs found in the faeces of the puppies. This results in 4 week old puppies being heavily infested with worms further contaminating their environment leading to a heavy worm burden in all in-contact animals.

Generally roundworm infestation will cause few clinical signs. With heavier worm burdens they may cause vomiting and diarrhoea. In very heavy infestations, worm associated pneumonia may occur as well as obstruction caused by the worms themselves. In very heavy worm burdens, the sudden worm-kill caused by administration of an effective dewormer can cause release of neurotoxins leading to nervous symptoms and convulsions in the puppies. The symptoms usually disappear within a day or two.

17.3. Hookworms (*Ancylostoma spp*)

Hookworms are common worms of dogs. Hookworms also have a direct lifecycle, thus worm eggs from infected dogs get passed in faeces and these eggs develop to free living larvae and infect other dogs again. Following hookworm infestation in bitches, larvae also migrate (travel) through the gut wall, enter the bloodstream and end up in the organs and muscles of the dogs. Again these larval stages can survive in the dog's muscles for years in the dormant (immobilised) stage. There is also lactogenic (via milk) transfer of worms from dam to puppies in hookworms but no prenatal infections can occur.

Hookworms are not only transferred by mouth, but can also penetrate the skin. Larvae of hookworms are very sensitive to desiccation and can only survive where there is sufficient dampness. High temperatures are also needed for larvae to become infectious. Hookworms flourish in areas with high rainfall and high temperatures. It is very difficult to control hookworms where puppies are raised on grass, because larvae survive easily in the wet warm grass. The larvae creep up the grass stems and will hook onto the puppies as they make contact with the grass and penetrate their skins.

Hookworm is more likely to result in clinical signs in dogs than do roundworms. The most obvious symptom of heavy hookworm infestation is anaemia, the degree of which depends on severity of infestation, nutritional status and age. Emaciation and weakening can also be seen. Puppies grow poorly, the coat becomes dull and loss of hair is visible. Upset stomachs are common and the faeces often have a slimy, bloody, jelly-like appearance. Deterioration of infected puppies may be very noticeable after weaning.

17.4. Common flea associated tapeworm (*Dipylidium caninum*)

The common dog tapeworm may be a problem in all parts of the world where its intermediate host thrives. Tapeworms have an indirect life cycle. They all need an intermediate host for completing their life cycle. The adult tapeworms which occur in the dog's intestines will release egg packets or tapeworm segments (proglottids) in the dog's faeces as the tapeworm grows. In the case of Dipylidium, these segments have the ability to move around for some time. During this movement, eggs are set free to the environment. The eggs will not infect the dog directly, but must be ingested by the intermediate host (flea or louse) first. An infectious bladder stage develops from the eggs in the intermediate host and only when the dog ingests the flea or louse accidently, will the adult tapeworm develop in the intestine of the dog.

Tapeworm infestations in adult dogs are not as deleterious to the host as are round- and hookworm infestations. In cases where young dogs are heavily infested, they show constant diarrhoea or constipation. Irritation of the skin around the anus, caused by the tapeworm segments, can cause dogs to scoot (drag their bottoms on the ground) and constantly lick the area around the anus. Since tapeworm infections are clearly seen by dog owners when the segments are sticking to the anal area and seen in the faeces, it has an actual "creepy" value and focuses the owner's attention on the dangers of worm infections. Without eliminating the flea, the Dipylidium tapeworm cannot be successfully controlled.

17.5. Whipworm (*Trichuris vulpis*)

Whipworm has a worldwide distribution. The eggs of whipworms are highly resistant and may survive in the environment for years. Dogs are infected by ingesting eggs from their environment. Whipworm infections may go unnoticed or result in diarrhoea with some mucus and blood. Whipworm may also be responsible for severe itching around the anus. Most but not all of routine deworming agents are effective against whipworm.

17.6. Other tape worms (*Taenia spp, Echinococcus spp*)

Dogs and many wild carnivores and in some cases, man, are the definitive host of these tape worms and harbour the adult worm in their small intestine. The intermediate hosts are domestic and wild herbivores, omnivores and primates. The dog (or other carnivore) may become infected by ingestion of the worm which is found in the meat or organs of the intermediate host. These worms are only of concern in situations where dogs have access to meat from domestic or wild species which are infected with the worm cyst in its tissues.

17.7. Treatment and control of worms in dogs

There is a wide range of worm remedies (dewormers) available for dogs. These medications are mostly broad-spectrum remedies, which are effective at treating most known worms in dogs. Breeders need be mindful that not all remedies sold are equally effective. Also, not all remedies are effective against all worm types and larval stages of the worms. This has very important implications for the successful control of worms in dog kennels.

It is well known that single treatment products are not highly effective in the treatment of larval stages of roundworm and hookworm. Research has shown that fenbendazole (the deworming remedy commonly used for sheep and cattle) is effective in killing the larval stages of *Toxacara canis* and *Ancylostoma spp*, which are dormant/reactivated in the muscles of the bitch and can infect the puppies either prenatally or lactogenically. To effectively prevent transmission of these worms from dams to their puppies it is advised that bitches should be treated daily with fenbendazole from day 40 of pregnancy up till 14 days after whelping at a dose of 50 mg per Kg body mass of the bitch.

17.7.1. Deworming program for dogs by ordinary pet owners

Worm control for ordinary pet owners whom have few dogs and do not breed is simple. Following the normal puppy deworming schedule, bi/tri-annual deworming is usually sufficient to keep their dogs worm free. It is recommended that all dogs and cats sharing the premises be dewormed by an effective broad spectrum deworming remedy simultaneously.

Chapter 17 Internal Parasites (Endoparasites) of Dogs

17.7.2. Deworming program for dogs in breeding kennels

Deworming in breeding kennels requires a different approach. Kennels usually have large numbers of adult dogs and puppies. If they are roaming freely and there is direct contact with most individuals within the breeding colony the risk for inter-dog worm transmission is increased. Breeders should deworm all puppies at 2, 4, 6 and 8 weeks. By around 8 weeks the puppy is likely to be with its new owners and henceforth deworming at each follow up inoculation is advised until 12 weeks. The early deworming will prevent the early worm infections transferred from the dam. The choice of deworming agent depends on area and availability. Breeders should save themselves the embarrassment of selling a puppy to a new owner, only to be reminded a couple of days later that the puppy was "riddled" with worms. It is important that breeders do not rely on deworming medication only to reduce worm infestations. Preventative practises are also just as important in the fight against worms. The most important method is to remove dog faeces regularly from the dog's environment and prevent accumulation of water which aids in worm egg and larvae survival. Provision of camps with cement floors is also very important. Grassy camps are more dog friendly, but nearly impossible to sterilise. As mentioned before, hookworms flourish mainly in the grass camps. Cement floors will drastically decrease the infestation of the environment.

Breeders wishing to prevent prenatal and lactogenic worm infestations in puppies may consider the fenbendazole treatment protocol. To some breeders this may be cumbersome and expensive. Therefore a shortened protocol is used by others involving fenbendazole treatment for only 10 days starting at around day 40 of pregnancy till day 50. Reactivated somatic larvae can only be controlled by these remedies when treated over extended periods and high doses. It is very important that the breeder be aware that these remedies do not work for dormant larvae in the tissues outside pregnancy or lactation. This is because the larvae only become susceptible to the worm remedy when pregnancy followed and lactation has reactivated them. Although research suggests that this treatment is safe for the embryos, breeders must realise that these medications are not registered for this use.

With regards to *Dipylidium*, using a broad spectrum dewormer and effective flea control is the only way to control this tape worm. With regards to the other tape worms the control is simple. It involves avoidance of feeding suspect uncooked meats or organs from either domestic or wild animals. Suspect meat should be well cooked first to kill the larval stages of the tapeworms. It is recommended that only meat from a registered abattoir (where meat hygiene is applied) must be fed to dogs. This meat is generally accepted to be free from the tapeworm cysts.

17.7.3. Unsuccessful control of worms

The factors which are conducive to worm re-infestation are crowding, restricted kennel space, wet conditions, constant supply of susceptible puppies, reactivation of dormant larvae in pregnant dams and very high egg shedding by late pregnant dams and especially the puppies, contaminating the kennel environment with very high worm egg burdens. Under these circumstances breeders often become despondent because their dogs are still infested with worms, despite regular treatment with expensive deworming remedies. These breeders will then often suspect that the worms have become resistant to the dewormers they use. This is rarely the case. Re-infestation is the most common cause of apparent failure to control worms. It is also important to realise that no deworming remedy can kill all the worms in the gut, especially in heavily infected dogs. Worm infections can never be totally eradicated by breeders, but at best be controlled. The aim is to control their numbers.

17.7.4. Strategic deworming versus routine deworming

Routine deworming implies deworming at regular intervals e.g. 2-4 times per year. Whilst this may work well for the breeder with a limited number of active breeding bitches, it may prove unsuccessful in the larger establishment. Strategic deworming implies doing regular checks on the faeces by performing egg flotations before and after deworming and amending the deworming regimen accordingly. This establishes whether there is a worm infestation in the first place, which dogs are affected, what type of worms are around, how severe the infestation is and whether the dewormer used is effective or not.

17.8. Heartworm (Dirofilaria immitis)

Heartworms are parasites which affect a number of mammals, including dogs, cats, and are widespread in numerous parts of the world. It is transmitted by mosquitoes which have fed on infected dogs or cats. Infected dogs may show signs of exercise intolerance, weight loss and respiratory problems. Treatment for infected dogs differs from therapy advised for prevention. In areas where heartworm infection is endemic, ongoing preventative treatment is indicated using one of many efficacious drugs.

17.9. Spirocerca lupi

Spirocerca lupi is a nematode (roundworm) which is found primarily in dogs (but also wild carnivores) and occurs throughout the world in warmer to temperate climates. It is not a new parasite but seems to be more prevalent in recent years in some parts of the world. The adult worm lives in the oesophagus of dogs where it embeds itself in the oesophageal wall and forms large nodules which may later become cancerous. Infected dogs will usually have 2-4 nodules but many more are also possible. Whilst in the oesophageal nodules, the adult worm produces eggs which are shed in the dog's stool. The eggs are then ingested by dung beetles which act as the intermediate host. The dog can be infected by directly eating the dung beetle or eating the lizard or bird which has ingested an infected beetle. The dung beetle implicated is the small Scarab beetle (few mm in length) and not the traditional bigger ones which are several centimetres. Once in the dog's stomach, the worm larvae enter intestinal blood vessels and travel to the aorta where they may mature (this may take up to 4-6 months). Following this migration they pass through the wall of the arteries into the wall of the oesophagus. En-route they cause damage to the blood vessels which may cause aneurisms. Aneurisms are weakened areas in the walls of arteries which in time may bulge (balloon). Dogs with aneurisms may not show symptoms and appear perfectly normal. Aneurisms require specialised equipment to diagnose and small ones may be missed. When the aneurism bursts however, the dog will die within seconds from massive internal haemorrhage. *Spirocerca lupi* is therefore a common cause of sudden unexplained death in areas where the worm occurs. Most frequently however, they just cause lumps in the oesophagus which slowly grow bigger. Initially when the lumps are about pea size they do not cause any problems and the dog shows no visible signs of infection. As the lumps grow bigger the dog may show a poor appetite, lose weight, start regurgitating food after meals, gagging, show a low grade fever and appear listless. Anaemia and presence of dark to black stool due to the presence of half-digested blood in stool (melaena) may also be noted in advanced cases. Although most worms will migrate to the oesophagus as final destination, in rare cases the worm migrates to other sites (called aberrant migration) and may end up in brain, eye, spinal cord, skin or any other tissues causing a variety of symptoms depending on location. In long standing cases, the lump in the oesophagus may become neoplastic (cancerous).

Although dogs of all sizes may be infected, dogs of large breeds are more commonly affected than smaller breeds. All ages may be affected with a peak incidence between 1-4 years. The habit that some dogs have to eat their or other dog's stools or even stools of other species (all called coprophagia), clearly increases risk of ingestion of dung beetles and thus infection. Agile athletic dogs which frequently catch birds, lizards or small mammals are also at increased risk. The risk increases if the dogs actually consume the meat of their catch. Dogs belonging to multiple dog households are more likely to be infected as are dogs residing on large properties. Co-habitation with other farm animals also increases risk of infection. The biggest risk factor of all appears to be the presence of at least one infected dog in the colony. This dog may act as source of infection to dung beetles and indirectly to other in-contact dogs. The practical significance is that if one dog in the colony is diagnosed with *Spirocerca lupi*, not only are the other dogs at risk for infection, but the chances are great that at least some of the dogs are already infected as well.

Even though the clinical signs may lead to the suspicion of *Spirocerca lupi* infection, special tests are required to confirm this. Radiographs of the chest and stool examination for worm eggs may be helpful in this regard but are not sensitive as many cases can be missed using these diagnostic modalities. Oesophagoscopy (looking down the oesophagus with a flexible endoscopic camera) is the most accurate means of diagnosis. Only the smallest nodules, as are found at the start of the infection, will escape detection. This procedure requires full anaesthetic. It is important that early diagnoses of infection are made whilst the nodules are still small as this favours outcome of treatment. Advanced cases with large granulomas respond poorly to treatment and if the lump has progressed to cancerous transformation, treatment is not possible. Advanced cases may therefore have to be euthanized. Surgical excision of the nodules has been attempted but is associated with high mortality rates and no longer recommended.

Treatment of infected dogs is the only option in dogs not euthanized as all untreated dogs usually die from complications. Earlier cases may respond to some avermectin containing formulations. Treatment may stretch over a period of 6 months or longer. Generally, the earlier the treatment commences, the higher the success rate.

Preventative measures include the regular removal of dog faeces to prevent colonization by dung beetles (which usually happens within minutes). The faeces should be disposed of in a manner that ensures it is not accessible to dung beetles, birds, small mammals and reptiles, which may all spread the larvae of this parasite. Dead birds either caught by the dogs or dragged into the garden by cats should be removed immediately to prevent ingestion by the dogs. In one study the administration of avermectins at regular intervals (4-6 weeks) did reduce the incidence of the worm infestation and reduced fatalities significantly. Breeders residing in areas where the risk of *Spirocerca lupi* infection is high, should strongly consider on-going preventative treatment using an avermectin containing product. Many breeders have been doing this for years in any event because it has some efficacy against other worms and very good efficacy against ear and skin mites. Numerous registered and unregistered avermectin containing products exist on the market in most countries which may both treat and prevent *Spirocerca lupi* infections. It is very important that breeders be aware that some breeds are genetically susceptible to adverse reactions to some drugs in the avermectin group. A single administration of these drugs to susceptible dogs may prove fatal. The known susceptible breeds are Border collie and other collie-types. Individual dogs of other breeds may also carry the gene determining susceptibility to these drugs, albeit very rare. Fortunately there is a genetic test available

Chapter 17 Internal Parasites (Endoparasites) of Dogs

to determine whether a dog carries the gene (MDR1) or not. Breeders whom have one dog which was diagnosed may opt to test all individual dogs for the presence of the gene prior to preventative treatment. Due to the cost of individual gene testing and very low risk in most breeds, some breeders opt to treat without prior gene testing. It is fair to speculate that the emergence of *Spirocerca lupi* and associated threat to dogs in some parts of the world, will lead to routine preventative treatment of all dogs in that area as is already the case with *Dirofilaria immitis* (heartworm). Affected breeders should consult their veterinary surgeons regarding treatment and preventative treatment options before randomly administering drugs to their dogs. Most anthelmintic (deworming) agents including heartworm remedies, used for routine deworming of dogs, are not effective in either treating or preventing *Spirocerca lupi* infections in dogs.

Chapter 18

External (Ectoparasites) of Dogs

Only the most common external parasites are discussed.

The most common ectoparasites are skin mites, fleas, lice and ticks. Breeders should, in consultation with their veterinary surgeon, devise a control program appropriate for their area. Because many ectoparasites require very close or direct contact for transmission it should be a breeder's first priority to make sure that they do not introduce these parasites into their kennels in the first place. This may not be that simple as many breeders show, train and socialise dogs, all practices which bring them into contact with other dogs and their parasites. It is therefore wise to pay particular attention to animals which have left the kennels and have had contact outside. It is a lot cheaper to treat these few animals preventatively against external parasites as opposed to trying to eradicate an introduced parasite which has established itself in the dog colony. Breeders should not be embarrassed at the discovery of any of the skin parasites on their dogs. These parasites are very successful and may very well visit any breeder, big or small. Having said this, no breeder can afford to let a puppy go with any of these parasites on the dog. New owners of puppies are not very understanding when it comes to finding all sorts of creepy crawlies on a newly acquired puppy. This discovery will lead to accusations of poor hygiene and substandard kennel management and be the cause for the label of bad or germ-infested breeder. Breeders may find themselves in a position where they are in the process of combating external parasites but may not have fully accomplished that goal. Under these circumstances, it is of vital importance that at least the puppy is properly treated and declared "parasite free" at the time of sale. It is important for breeders to realise that other animals they may own or their dogs have contact with, may also harbour parasites which may act as a source of infection for their dogs. This should be communicated with their veterinary surgeons and either treatment of or isolation from these animals may be indicated.

18.1.1. Ticks

Depending on area, ticks may be a huge problem in dog kennels. The lifestyle of the dog and areas they visit plays an obvious role. Regular access to water also affects the residual action of numerous ectoparasiticides. The main problem associated with ticks is the many tick borne diseases (Babesiosis, Ricketsiosis, Borreliosis and others) some of which are fatal. Breeders should understand that no product may claim to be a 100% efficacious in all cases. Breeders often think that if dogs are kept on cement surfaces they will have no ticks. Ticks do not necessarily need grass to thrive. All they need is a host to feed from. Also, many ticks may have as part of their life cycle a

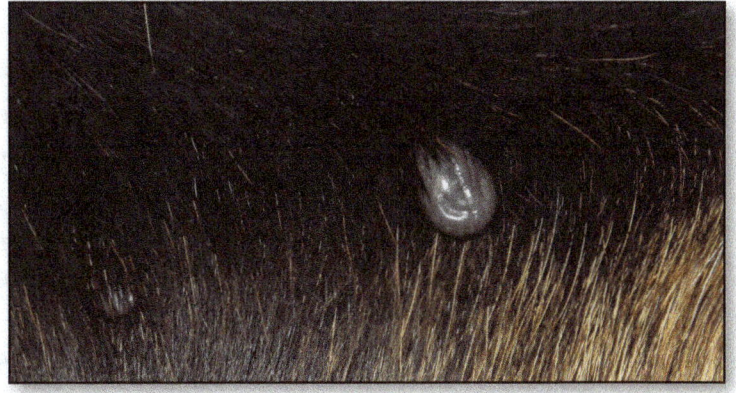

Ticks visible on dog's coat. Ticks are carriers of many diseases and require strict control.

Chapter 18 External (Ectoparasites) of Dogs

stage where they live on other hosts including rodents which are ever present wherever there is food (dog food scraps, garbage).

18.1.2. Skin mites and ear mites

Mites are parasites which are not potentially lethal to the dog but rather a stubborn menace. In a normal household situation with 2-3 pets, these parasites are easy to control. In stark contrast to this, in a breeding kennel this is not so easily achieved. It may take up to one season to effectively eradicate the mites and require regular routine control to prevent reintroduction into the dog colony. Some skin mites are very infectious and can spread like fire in a kennel. Sarcoptic mange (scabies) is a disease caused by the mite *Sarcops scabei*. Once introduced in a dog colony this mite will spread rapidly and most but not all dogs will show symptoms. These mites cause very severe itching and scratching. Dogs suffering from scabies will also have little crusts and hair loss. It may be difficult to find the mites on examination of skin scrapings. When suspected or confirmed, all dogs on the premises should be treated. This parasite can also infect humans and they will require treatment to rid them of this itchy bug.

Cheyletiellosis is a disease caused by Cheyletiella mites which live on hair and fur of dogs and cats and rabbits. In dogs this disease may also itch but scaling (dandruff) is a more prominent clinical sign. As with scabies, this mite is also a zoonosis and hence owners may show a rash as well particularly around their waist, arms and neck. Breeders will not rid themselves of mites overnight. Although adult mites are obligatory parasites and need a host to survive, they do lay eggs which may survive in the environment for some time, only to infect another dog at a later stage. Treatment for an entire season may be required followed by monthly treatments on an ongoing basis to prevent either reintroduction or re-establishment of the parasites.

The ear mite (*Otodectes cynotis*) is a parasite of mainly the ear canal but may also infect skin and is another example of a very stubborn menace. Ear mites cause an accumulation of brown/black waxy or crusty discharge in the ear canals. Itchiness of the ears and head shaking is also a standard feature of ear mite infestation. Local treatment of the ear mite in the ear canal using ear drops may not be enough to control this parasite. This may be because the mite is also found on the skin. Treatment which involves the use of appropriate drugs in ear and skin may be indicated. Ear mites have a tendency to re-emerge from apparently nowhere and long term treatment of the entire colony is indicated. The household cat may also be affected and should also be treated. The roaming nature of cats may bring them into contact with other infected cats leading to reintroduction of the mites into the household and ultimately the dog population.

18.1.3. Demodectic mange (Demodex canis associated mange)

This mite requires special mention because it is a problem in some breeds as well as in some lines of dogs. It is dealt with separately from other mites because it presents differently and requires different control. Unlike other mites, demodex does not have a highly infectious nature. It has to be assumed that most if not all dogs will have some demodex mites in their skin and the parasite should be considered cosmopolitan and a normal inhabitant of normal healthy dog skin albeit in very low numbers. All puppies acquire the skin mite during the first couple of days following birth from the dam. The mite is found in the hair follicles. In most dogs however, the infection will be very low grade and asymptomatic. The symptoms of demodex infection may be local or generalised. In the former the dog will have one to several small circumscribed areas of alopecia (hair loss), usually on the face or forelegs. The latter refers to large areas of hair loss over vast areas of the body or the entire body. In most cases the demodectic mange is not itchy but some cases may have skin infections on top of the demodectic mange skin lesion and become itchy.

It is not well understood what factors dictate whether the dog will remain an asymptomatic carrier or show clinically visible lesions. This problem seems to be poorly infectious as Demodex is never seen in an outbreak situation in even large dog populations. It is also almost impossible to infect a non-susceptible individual. A hereditary predisposition is strongly suspected and this explains why Demodex is over-represented in some breeds. Some dog breed lines also appear to be more susceptible. Given this, it is sometimes advised that strict selection against this is applied. In the past even culling of severely affected animals and parents was practised. This probably stemmed from the inability to treat some of the stubborn cases. This is no longer necessary as nowadays there are modern and safe drugs which are effective in treating the most stubborn of cases.

Topical treatment with insecticides often proves ineffective and should be combined with systemic drugs prescribed by a veterinary surgeon.

18.1.4. Fleas

Fleas are usually easily controlled in a kennel environment where the dogs do not frequent the homes of the breeders. This is because fleas cannot reproduce or complete their lifecycle when the ambient temperatures drop below 12°C. It thus follows that they are able to extend the flea season in heated homes and that cold to temperate areas have a distinct flea season whereas warm to tropical areas may be plagued by fleas throughout the year. As mentioned before, it is very important to treat dogs when they have contact with outside dogs. It is a lot cheaper to treat individual dogs than to treat entire kennels following introduction of fleas into the kennel.

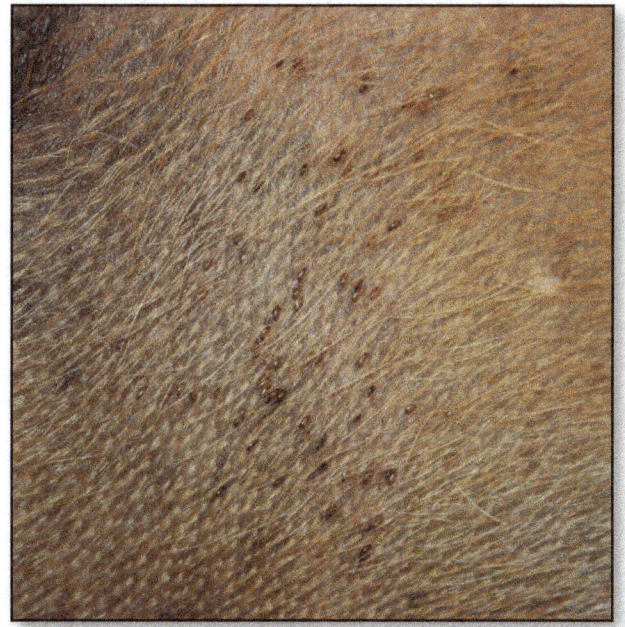

Fleas on dogs may cause allergies, carry disease and act as intermediate host for worms

Although fleas are not a direct threat to a pet's life, they may lead to flea allergies. Flea infestations carry with them the stigma of a poorly managed breeding kennel and if discovered by the new puppy owners after purchase, is the cause of disgruntled clients.

18.1.5. Flies and maggots

Biting flies cause mechanical injury, bleeding and crusting. They favour the ear tip in breeds with erect ears or the bend in the ear in breeds with hanging ears. Blowflies attack dogs which are wet, soiled and have weeping wounds. They also favour faecal and urine soiled sites and long haired breeds may fall victim to maggots in their perineal areas. Maggot infection (myiasis) can cause large lesions by liquefying the skin they feed on.

Chapter 19

Matters and Conditions Relating to Dogs Kept in Breeding Kennels

In a quest to make this book as comprehensive yet tidy and relevant as possible, many topics which do not strictly belong under previous headings have emerged. These are all included in this chapter.

19.1. Kennel management

Appetite and health checks should be executed at least twice a day to ensure early detection of problems with any dog in a kennel.

19.1.1. Hygiene and sanitation

By definition some extent of crowding is practised in all dog kennels. Spread of disease under these conditions is a considerable risk. Bacteria and viruses can spread directly from dog to dog or indirectly via food pans and also footwear of visitors and workers. Some infectious agents are airborne and others water-borne. Some are hardy whilst others are easily destroyed by disinfectants. The dogs may vary in their susceptibility to disease depending on their age, the presence of stress factors and general hygiene observed in the kennel. A clean kennel is one which is dirt free, free of disease causing viruses and bacteria, free of odours and harmful chemicals. Besides faecal and urine waste, dogs also produce significant amounts of fur which is shed daily. The ability to easily clean the kennel effectively depends on the kennel's construction. The type of floor surfaces used in kennels influence your ability to clean them. Grass and ground surfaces are impossible to disinfect and will be particularly worrisome during the rainy season when hollows are filled with water, creating mud pools. Grass camps are helpful as running and exercise camps and should be rotated and occasionally kept empty to allow for cleaning and drying.

Concrete is the most popular kennel surface because it is durable. Floors should be sloped away from the sleeping quarters to allow water and effluent to drain away towards a sanitation channel leading to some drainage system. The direction of wind and sunlight should be considered when building the kennel structures. At least part of the kennel should provide shelter from direct wind and rain and should preferably be raised to prevent water flowing into the sleeping quarters.

The choice of disinfectant should be dictated by its ability to kill the most important viruses and bacteria but must be safe for dogs. Besides disinfection it might be necessary to use a cleansing agent to degrease dirty surfaces from time to time in order to remove organic material from the kennel surfaces. The presence of organic material decreases the efficacy of disinfectants. Pressurised hoses are very helpful in removing stubborn dirt and organic material. Kennel floors and walls should be constructed from a concrete mix which can withstand the very abrasive effect of pressurised water hose systems. Natural sunlight has a sterilising effect through ultraviolet light and desiccation. Kennel designs should make maximum use of this free commodity.

Breeders in very cold countries often construct kennels indoors. Although it is easier to protect animals from the elements in these kennels, the effect of natural sunlight is negated as is ventilation

Chapter 19 Matters and Conditions Relating to Dogs Kept in Breeding Kennels

by wind. Ventilation is of no practical importance in open-air kennels. In high-density closed kennel situations, a well-designed ventilation system is crucial to help control aerosolised pathogens from spreading. Ten to fifteen air changes per hour is an ideal number for most kennels. Relative humidity should be kept between 50 and 65%, and ambient air temperature should be maintained between 20°C and 24°C. The later temperature ranges given is relevant only in breeding kennels and not for the kennelling of adult dogs.

Indoor kennels that house a large number of dogs should therefore be fitted with special ventilation vents to ensure that the air volume is replaced frequently and so avoid ammonia build up in the air. Good sanitation efforts and hygiene principles include regular stool removal and washing and disinfection of the kennels. Good maintenance of the kennel structure to prevent escapes and injury is necessary.

It is wise for breeders to consider the construction of a quarantine facility or sick bay area. This may be a small number of kennels which are geographically removed or temporary house pets which recently came from the veterinary hospital or require special attendance and or treatment in a "higher care unit".

19.1.2. Keeping breeding dogs and other animals on the same premises

It is true that dog lovers are generally lovers of other animals too. Premises permitting, dog breeders may keep other animals as well. These may include cats, rabbits, birds, horses and many others. This may require special socialization of the dogs with these animals to prevent injury and fatality to both dogs and the other animals they live with. Most diseases in animals and humans are species specific. That means that the pathogens have adapted and specialised to infect one specific species (host) and are unlikely to infect others. There are however some exceptions. As a general rule other animals kept in tandem with large dog populations may somewhat complicate the kennel management. This is so because it may be more difficult to maintain hygiene, control vermin, flies and ectoparasites, all of which can affect the dogs as well. Most of the breeders will however contend that this is a small price to pay for the joy their animals bring them.

19.1.3. Health and safety issues regarding kennel staff

Breeders may employ staff to help with kennel related chores. These kennel owners need to acquaint themselves with the liability issues regarding their members of staff. Working with animals expose the staff members to some risks. In most countries, employers have considerable obligations to their employees which are legally enforced. It is advised that kennel operators have in place health and safety manuals to protect their staff and ultimately themselves against legal actions and claims. There are a number of zoonoses (infectious diseases which are transmitted between species). Those will be discussed in another section. Breeders may also consider vaccinating themselves, their family and staff against tetanus and rabies if those are a risk in the individual kennel and if advised by their physician. All bite wounds should be attended to by a physician. Kennel owners should not underestimate the very severe infections and potentially fatal complications of infected dog bite wounds. High incidence of human immunodeficiency virus (HIV) infection and aids is a statistical fact in many parts of the world. Affected individuals are more likely to suffer from complications from even small or superficial bites. Improper training of dog handlers is the most common reason for dog bites to the handlers. Also, breeders should abandon the naïve notion that "my dog will never bite". There are individual animals of many breeds which may be dangerous and unpredictable. Increased vigilance is required for those individual dogs of big and powerful breeds.

19.1.4. Positive identification of dogs

There are many reasons why positive identification in dogs is required. Certification of dogs for whatever reason is pointless without being able to categorically link the certificate to the dog. Another is to establish a database with the positive identification of the dog linked to an owner's contact details. These databases are invaluable in reuniting lost pets with their owners and aid in vastly reducing the alarming numbers of lost pets destroyed annually.

Dogs may be identified using tattoos, transponders (so called microchips) and more recently via DNA profiles. Although tattoos are perhaps a cheaper way of identification, it has the major disadvantage that

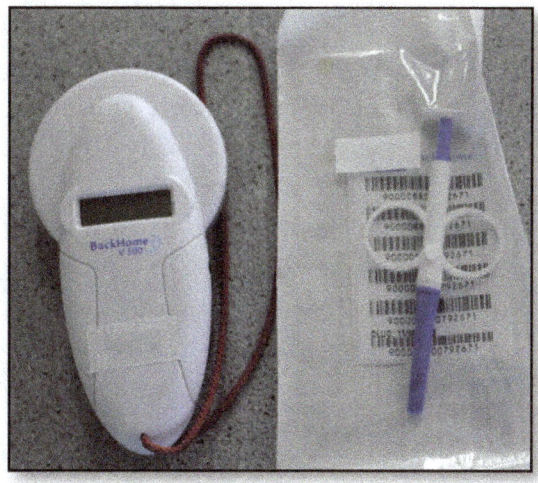

Transponder reader left and and transponder applicator on right

it is not unique like a transponder number and may not always be readable and may deteriorate with time. Some oppose the use of tattoos due to the pain inflicted when tattooing. The ear is most common place of placing the tattoo. Currently, use of microchips is the most popular means of identification in dogs. Although generally very reliable, microchips have been known to fail. Microchips require expensive apparatus (readers) to detect the number. The main reason for DNA profiling to date has been to confirm parentage. Some dog registering bodies are now insisting on DNA as means of identifying puppies for identification and registration purposes. This has the main advantage that it is relatively tamper proof and not dependent on individual integrity. Another advantage is that reliable genetic studies can be conducted once large numbers of animals are represented on such databases.

19.2. Self-treatment by breeders

Considering the large number of dogs which breeders have, it is inevitable that they will in many instances elect to self-treat. Experienced breeders have a reasonable understanding of the most common illnesses and ailments afflicting dogs. They therefore often insist that they should have access to basic treatment protocols and have available to them medicines to deal with minor cases in their kennel. However, it is always recommended that breeders only treat dogs in close consultation or under direct instruction from their veterinary surgeon. Breeders must understand that veterinary surgeons are prohibited by veterinary legislation to dispense scheduled medicines without having seen the patients for the condition the drugs are being dispensed.

19.3. Alternative healing methods

Most conventional veterinary surgeons are not trained in alternative medicines and will practice veterinary science with medicaments which are mostly proven, registered with proven claims and use methods and medication which are peer reviewed. This does not imply that alternative medicines and healing methods are harmful or do not work but merely that most conventionally trained veterinary surgeons have no experience of these methods. Alternative medicines can take many forms, like homeopathy, herbalism, tissue salts, T-touch, acupuncture, magnetism and many more. As many of these alternative healing methods are becoming more and more accepted, there is a trend towards combining the alternative method with the conventional.

19.4. Performance enhancing drugs

When an ergogenic aid is a substance, it may also be known as a performance enhancing substance. Administration of performance enhancing drugs, also known as "doping", refers to chemical or medicinal intervention, normally to enhance athletic performance in the show ring or working trials. It is the client's responsibility to familiarise themselves with the rules and regulations of the respective associations and dog clubs regarding the use of these products. It is however important to realise that the possession of scheduled drugs without prescription by a registered physician or veterinary surgeon is a criminal offence in many countries. Until spot checks or routine testing is performed, we will not know what the scale of the use of performance enhancing drugs in dogs is. Performance enhancing drugs typically include anabolic steroids and testosterone. Some other drugs including corticosteroids, non-steroidal anti-inflammatory agents and sedatives are not typical performance enhancing drugs but they may be used to mask pain or hide behavioural problems and so "enhance" the dog's performance on the day.

19.4.1 Corticosteroids
Used to hide lameness and increase dog's activity on the day.

19.4.2 Non-steroidal anti-inflammatory agents
Anti-inflammatory drugs are used topically and systemically to mask the symptoms of pain which result in lameness or poor posture. Non-steroidal anti-inflammatory agents are used daily by veterinary surgeons and have many therapeutic indications. These substances cannot increase performance in any way but may however be used to mask the symptoms of pain which result in lameness or poor posture in the show ring or working arena. They are also sometimes used to hide lameness from prospective buyers.

19.4.3 Behavioural modification using drugs
There is alleged use or "abuse" of behavioural modifying medication in dogs to control aggressive behaviour, fear and excessive excitement in the show ring. Sedatives, tranquilisers and mood altering drugs are therefore sometimes used to mask undesirable temperament and or nervousness. In these instances the evaluation of true temperament cannot be evaluated and this practice is regarded as unethical in most circles. The drugs used for this purpose vary from over the counter medication to highly scheduled drugs only available from veterinary surgeons.

19.4.4 Anabolic steroid abuse in dogs
Anabolism refers to the synthesis of cells and tissues and from this was derived the word anabolic steroids which refers to steroids (type of endocrine substance or hormone) which increases the rate of protein synthesis, most noticeable in muscles. Anabolic steroids also have androgenic and virilising (male) effects. Anabolic steroids are available in injectable form and oral tablets and pastes. Anabolic steroids in animals have perfectly legal therapeutic uses in veterinary science but many veterinary surgeons refrain from using them because their use seems to have become stigmatised. Perhaps there is fear of allegations of abuse or misuse in their clinics? They are useful in the treatment of convalescence, anaemia and for treating catabolic side effects of chronic corticosteroid use or chronic renal failure. Increasing muscle mass may be required in orthopaedic and other conditions. Increased appetite with their use may also be helpful in some conditions. The single use or limited course of anabolic steroids consisting of 2-3 administrations with a week or more intervals is unlikely to cause harmful side effects in adult animals. Repetitive or chronic use is not recommended. In breeding animals

it is not advised at all. Risk associated with anabolic steroid abuse is increased cholesterol, hypertension, liver damage and pathological thickening of the heart muscle walls. Use before puberty may cause premature closure of the growth plates and short stature. Because anabolic steroids have some androgenic action similar to that of testosterone, it may have numerous reproductive and endocrine harmful effects. In bitches they include anoestrus (cessation of heat cycles), male behaviour, and excessive clitoral enlargement. In male dogs it may cause prostatic hyperplasia, suppression of endogenous testosterone in studs ultimately leading to decreased sperm production, decreased libido and ultimately testicular atrophy.

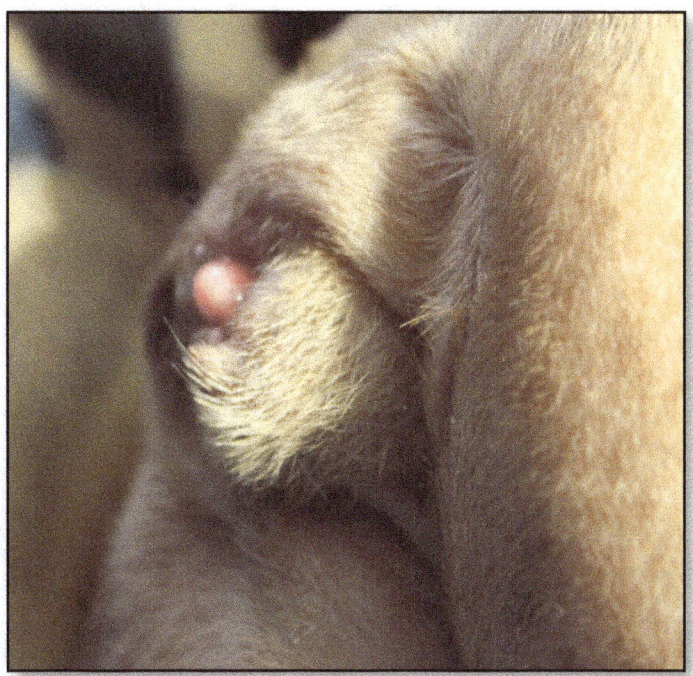

Clitoral enlargment may be seen with anabolic steroid abuse or endocrine related disorders

The use of testosterone has similar but more pronounced effects on reproduction.

19.5. Behavioural aspects in dogs

19.5.1. Socialization, critical factors for socialising of companion dogs

During the first 4 months of a dog's life its behavioural development can be influenced by stimulus in its environment. Adult behaviour is dependent on events during this early period of behavioural development. Repeated exposure to a stimulus during this period allows the dog to "imprint" on this stimulus and hence regard this stimulus as being a normal part of its environment, with effects often persisting into adulthood. This is known as socialisation to a particular stimulus or group of stimuli. Socialisation in the dog is not restricted to inanimate objects. Dogs can be socialised to various species

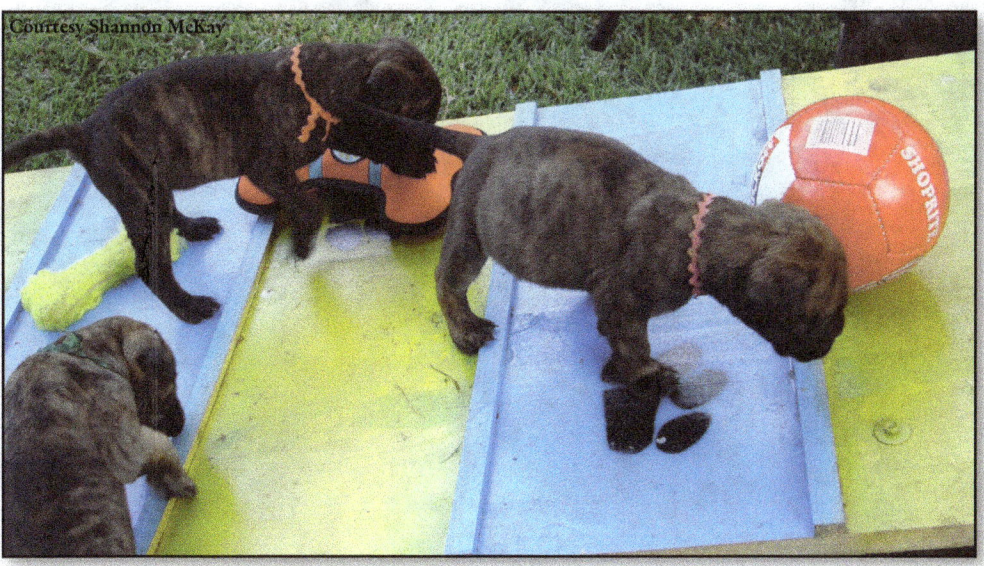

Chapter 19 Matters and Conditions Relating to Dogs Kept in Breeding Kennels

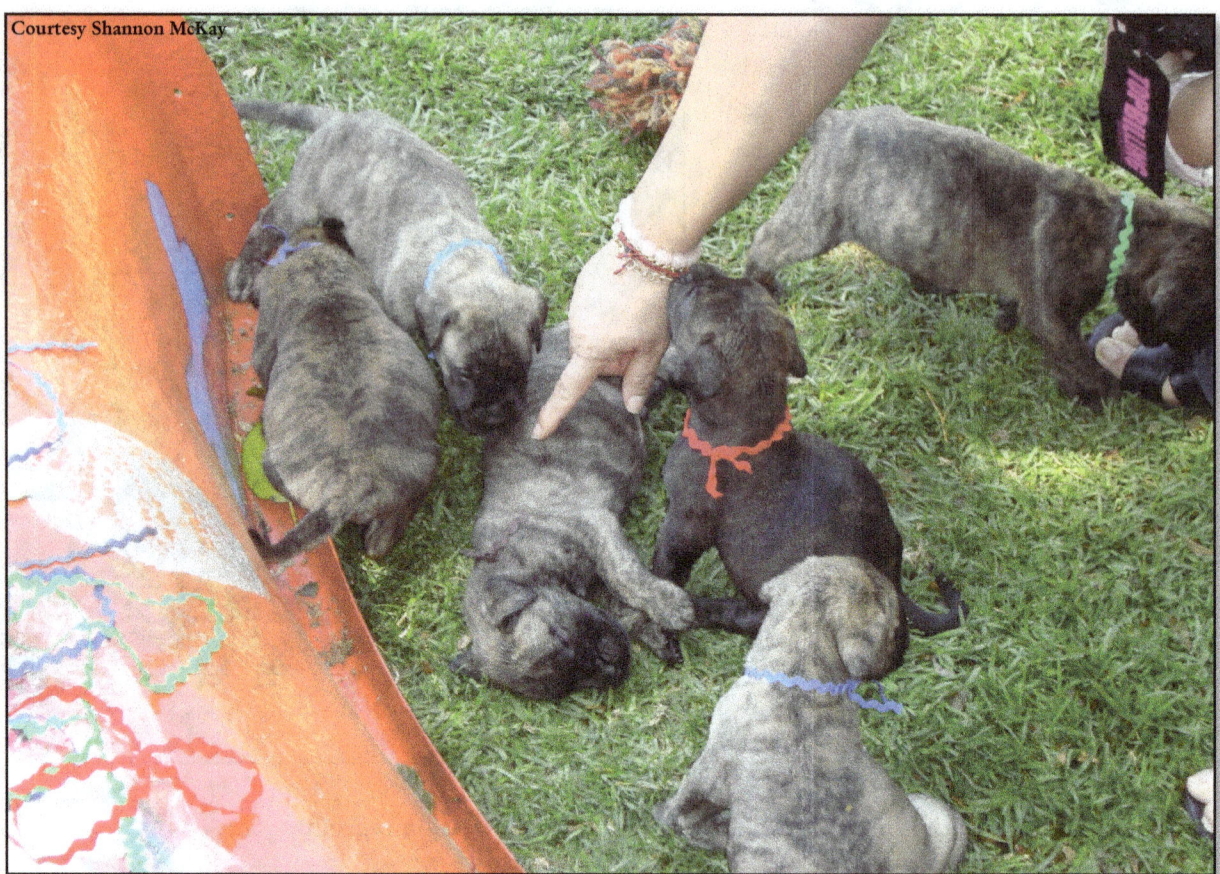

Socializing dogs with each other

during the critical period of socialisation and hence develop longstanding social bonds both within and across species. It is this plasticity of the dog's behavioural development which allows for dogs to be companions to humans and peacefully interact with non-human species as well. If a dog were not to receive socialisation with humans during the socialisation period, the dog would be averse to humans as an adult.

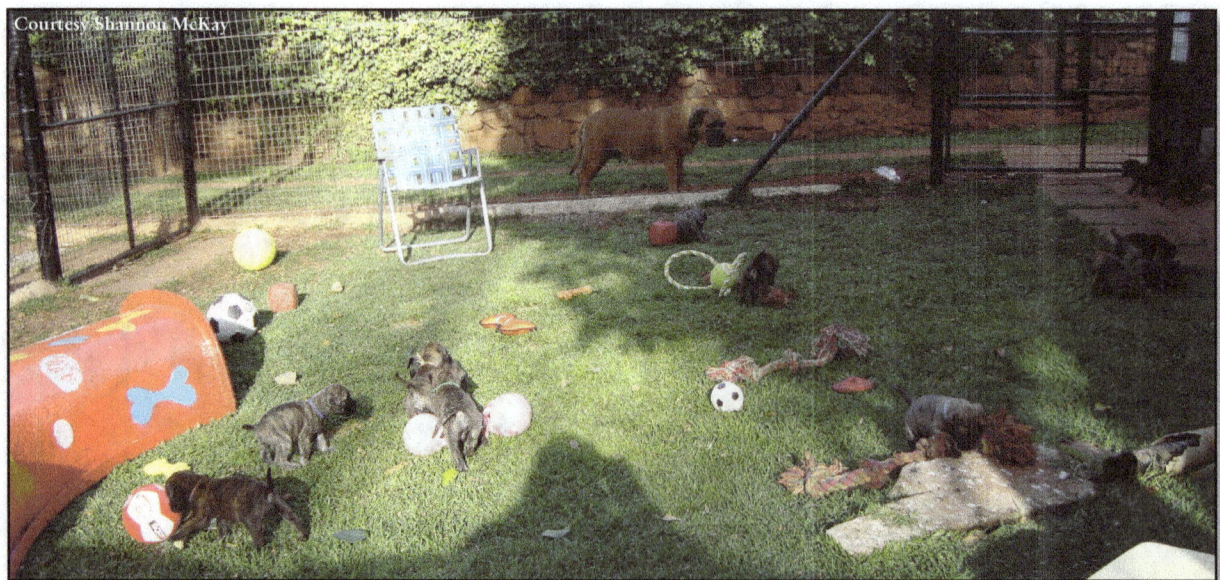

Stimuli exposure at training school

Chapter 19 Matters and Conditions Relating to Dogs Kept in Breeding Kennels

A typical example of dog to non-human socialisation is livestock guarding dogs. These dogs are raised from the age of approximately 8 weeks with a flock of production animals (normally sheep or goats). The puppy receives constant socialisation with the flock and accordingly develops social bonds with the flock, resulting in the dog remaining in close proximity with the flock and protecting the flock from predators as an adult.

Puppies require exposure to the species which they are intended to co-exist with as adults. If this experience is lacking the dog could behave with aversion or aggression to the other species, which is detrimental both to the dog and potentially the other species. It is thus crucial to ensure that puppies are well socialised.

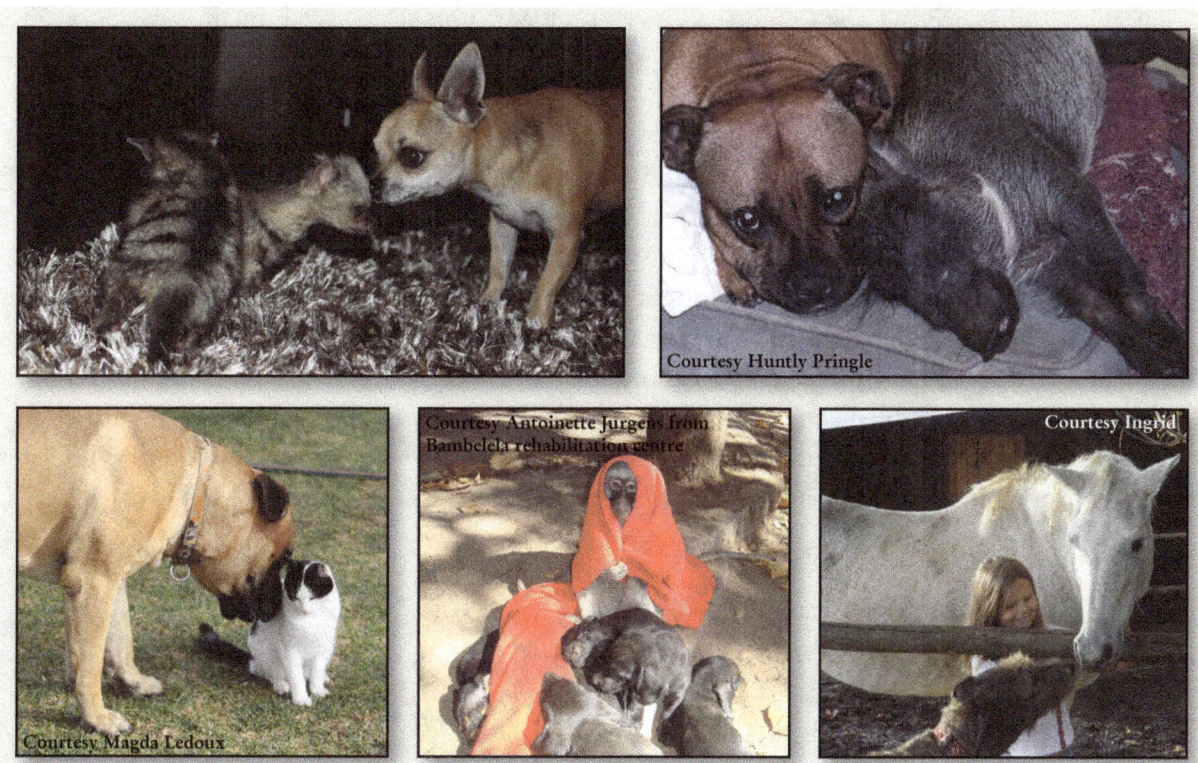

Socialising a puppy to another species requires the following:
- Repeated exposure to the stimuli in question
- Socialisation incidences either to be neutral or with a beneficial outcome for the puppy e.g. such as a child calmly petting a young puppy as opposed to the child hurting or scaring the puppy
- Variety in the relevant stimuli i.e., a puppy will require socialisation to a broad spectrum of individuals within a species before it could be said that the puppy is socialised to that species
- Short, frequent socialisation sessions during the critical period of socialisation are more beneficial to socialisation outcomes than long, infrequent sessions
- Should the puppy display any aversion to a stimulus it is critically important not to force the puppy to approach the stimulus. The puppy should be allowed to explore the stimulus in its own time. Forcing a puppy to interact with a perceived threat during the socialisation period can instil a lifelong aversion towards that stimulus
- The capacity to become socialised to various stimuli varies within breeds and individuals, therefore suggesting a genetic predisposition to socialisation ability and capacity

- Dogs can become "de-socialised" and therefore on-going socialisation is recommended after the most critical period of socialisation of 4 months of age
- Health concerns exist around puppies with an incomplete vaccination schedule being socialised with other dogs. This is a valid concern and therefore all attempts must be made to ensure that socialisation instances occur in a safe and controlled environment, such as professional puppy socialising classes, and not in unregulated dog areas such as dog parks, where the health status of all dogs is unknown

The socialisation period is a powerful period for altering the behavioural development of dogs. Completing a comprehensive and sensible socialisation programme during this period (and maintaining intermittent exposure to stimuli after this period) could maximise a dog's ability for socialisation and hence the dog's ability to be a confident, non-aggressive human companion in a demanding social environment.

19.5.2. Puppy temperament assessments

Dogs are utilised in many working applications across the globe (police dogs, guide dogs, detection dogs, service dogs) as well as in sporting activities, such as field trials and competitive obedience.

The training of these animals requires resources both in terms of time and money. Not all candidates enrolled in these training programmes succeed at the eventual task. The question has therefore been asked whether there are any predictive behavioural factors in candidate dogs which can be identified prior to training being implemented. If this is so, unsuitable candidates could be excluded from entry into such training programmes and therefore allow for more resources to be allocated to candidates which are expected to have a greater chance of success in the eventual task.

This question has been explored in the past and "puppy temperament testing" more scientifically referred to as puppy temperament assessment (PTA) has been devised as a tool to attempt to identify traits in the young puppy which are predictive of adult behaviour. PTA elements are varied between testers, but most include social drive, play drive, prey drive and response to novel stimulus as a basis for establishing predictive adult temperament in the puppy. Tests are typically conducted at an age of 49 days, when the puppy is assumed to have adult motor skills, but a "clean state" from a behavioural perspective.

Whether PTA does provide a reliable tool for predicting adult behaviour in dogs is debatable. A scientific review of the topic suggested that tests of young puppies are not valid predictors of their future behaviour. Given that puppy tests are widely used but their validity is rarely examined, this finding has huge implications for work in applied and research contexts. Future research is urgently needed to examine this possibility directly. Despite scepticism by scientific scrutinizers, many breeders are

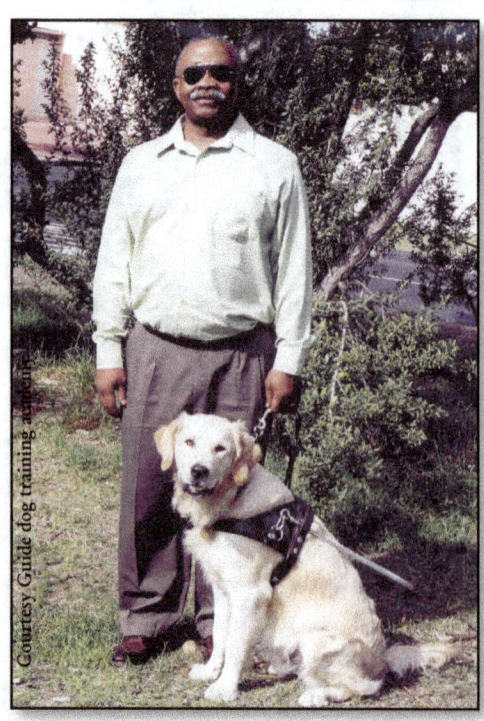

Guide dogs must have special temperaments and puppy aptitude tests and others may help in selecting the best puppies for the task intended

strong believers of PTA as a reliable and effective predictor of adult behaviour, but it is possible that a report from a tester alters the way in which the puppy is treated and the report's conclusion becomes a self-fulfilling prophecy! Nonetheless PTA could be useful to identify extremes in behaviour, which is useful to the breeder when selecting the most appropriate type of home for a puppy e.g. if a puppy shows excessive prey drive during PTA then this puppy would more than likely be unsuitable for a family home with small children.

Not everyone believes that PTA (as it currently exists) is able to detect small variances in behaviour between puppies which will be predictive of adult behaviour. This is because the test is a mere "snapshot" in time and can be influenced by multiple uncontrollable factors. Also the responses shown by puppies in these tests are subjectively interpreted by the tester. Validity of some of these tests is questioned because of lack of precision. Some argue that improved testing methods and increased objectivity and standardisation by testers are much needed in order to fulfil the expectations by breeders of PTA.

Despite controversy surrounding PTA, it may be concluded that PTA, despite its shortcomings, is beneficial as it can highlight extremes in behaviour. Even sceptics of PTA would have to admit that at the very least, it is a valuable socialisation experience for the puppies during a critical period in their behavioural development.

It is important that PTA is to be done by a stranger in a novel environment.

19.5.3. Stress and associated conditions

a) What is stress

Stress refers to the combined effect on any living being by any factor (stressor) that may adversely affect that biological system and immune system by making them more vulnerable to disease. Common stressors are pain, anxiety (especially separation anxiety), discomfort, fear, hierarchical conflict, noise, social isolation, boredom, malnutrition, lack of protection from the elements and spatial restriction. Dogs which have been appropriately socialised with other people, dogs and surroundings are less likely to stress. The mechanism by which stress will affect the pet's immune system is not fully understood but is in part mediated by the release of endogenous cortisol and other hormones. Stress is sometimes objectively gauged by measuring cortisol levels, blood pressure and heart rates. It is scientifically proven that even small changes in a pet's life can have significant impact and act as an immense stressor. Typical stressors are, change in diet, transport, change of environment, introduction to new handlers, caretakers, and introduction to new animals.

b) Methods to reduce stress

Noise levels in dog kennels deserve discussion. Noise produced by large numbers of dogs howling, barking and yapping may be very disturbing to humans (neighbours) and physically stress dogs and lead to behavioural, physiological and anatomical responses. A common trigger for dogs to start vocalising is when they see other dogs, especially when they see other dogs receiving attention outside of their confinement. This stems from the dog's desire to be with the other dogs they see or engage in the same activity or want the same attention. Kennel design with partitioning walls may prevent dogs seeing each other and thus reducing noise levels and stress. Some kennels have employed the use of a stereo sound system to play soft soothing music and claim that it has a harmonious effect, settles the dogs down and tends to reduce barking. Could it be that music introduces some familiarity in the kennel environment?

Chapter 19 Matters and Conditions Relating to Dogs Kept in Breeding Kennels

Cohabitation (sharing of kennel space) may also reduce stress levels. Dogs housed in social groups vocalise less, sleep more and show fewer abnormal behaviours. Few dogs can however be trusted together. There is a real risk that dogs housed together may fight and cause serious trauma and even death. The ever-friendly pooch may very well prove to be a killer in the kennel. This may also be true for dogs which were brought up together and were always in harmony according to the breeders.

Stimulation through human contact and regular exercise also reduces stress as may the provision of chews to keep dogs occupied and distracted.

Behavioural modification may be required to control obsessive compulsive disorders, aggression, separation anxiety, excessive fear, elimination disorders, travel anxiety and sickness and many more. A qualified animal behaviourist should be consulted in these instances as they can make a huge difference with simple training. In addition, medication may be required to control or ameliorate the condition. The veterinary surgeon may also prescribe an anti-depressant drug registered for use in dogs which may help some of these cases. Behavioural modification may also be achieved by the use of appeasing pheromones to settle dogs down. Pheromones are chemicals constituted mainly of fatty acids. Plants, insects and mammals use pheromones. The vomero-nasal organ which exists in the mouth detects pheromones. In dogs the pheromones have mainly relaxing effects.

These appeasing pheromones are commercially available in sprays and collars. Some pet owners prefer to explore "natural" alternatives. For those owners, L-tryptophan, an essential amino acid, may be considered. It is metabolized and converted to 5 - hydroxytryptophan and finally serotonin, which is a well-known "mood lifter". Another popular natural aid is flower essence such as "Rescue Remedy". It is an extract of flowers and is claimed to have a calming effect. There are many more. Consensus on the efficacy of these vary but some insists that it works. Irrespective it cannot harm.

c) Kennel vices

Stereotyped behaviour or repetitive behaviour is also called obsessive-compulsive disorder (OCD) and is frequently associated with boredom related stress. An obsessive compulsive disorder is a disorder which the dog intentionally, stubbornly and repetitively acts out. Some breeds are more prone to develop OCD than others.

Boredom is defined as restriction from range of sensory experiences or behavioural opportunities. Examples of kennel vices are; pacing, digging, kennel scratching, head bobbing, weaving, circling, tail chasing, incessant barking, trembling, fence fighting, wire biting, kennel licking, swallowing foreign objects, pica, excessive grooming including obsessive licking resulting in lick granulomas, self-mutilation, paw lifting, coprophagia, pica and destructive behaviour. Although these are frequent stereotyped behaviours encountered in kennel confined dogs, this is not unique to kennelled dogs. Ordinary household pets may also be plagued by OCD. Kennel design and management can reduce the incidence of these vices. Medication for separation anxiety disorders in dogs may also be helpful in treating OCD related problems in dogs.

d) Kennel associated ill thrift

Ill thrift is a layman's term often used to describe dogs which appear in poor condition. Ill thrift may obviously be the result of very many other conditions and any dog suffering from poor body condition should be subject to a thorough veterinary examination. A comprehensive diagnostic workup to establish what the underlying cause may be. There are dogs that adapt poorly to the stress associated with kennel confinement and may suffer from "kennel associated ill thrift". In these dogs veterinary examinations fail to reveal a medical explanation for their condition. These dogs may be seen to suffer from a "psychosomatic" disorder. Most of these dogs suffer from a poor appetite. Although this condition may occur in any breed, some breeds appear to be over represented.

19.5.4. Aggression in dogs

Breeders collectively often have a tendency to romanticise their own breed and hence have a problem to objectively evaluate negative traits within the breed. One such trait is aggression. The immense strength of a dog's jaws and neck muscles should not be underestimated. The males of many breeds are often intolerant of other males and poorly sociable with other pets in general. These traits are highly prized in some breeds for their immense presence and formidable stature and hence guarding properties. Clearly, with the breeding and owning of such breeds comes a huge responsibility. Although some of the medium and larger breeds could be singled out, it should however be recognised that there are individuals within any breed which may possess uncontrolled or unstable characteristics. With aggressive traits, size surely matters. For instance, if a nasty little Fox Terrier bites a kid, this is unlikely to make the local headlines. However, if a huge mastiff does, devastating injuries are more likely to result which could even make national headlines. Not to mention legal implications and guilt.

Fighting dogs may lead to very severe injury and death. This should be a warning against sharing kennels. Breeders should also beware of the fact that even small breeds which appear pretty docile and reputed to be "loving little darlings" may indeed turn out to be killers when confined in groups in kennels. It is fact that in huge groups, the pack may turn on a kennel mate for a multitude of reasons. It is also important to note that even apparent innocent bite wounds may turn septic and result in serious complications which may include death. The general rule is that if a dog has bitten another once, history is likely to repeat itself.

In conclusion, there should be active selection against aggressive traits in any breed. Specialists should be consulted regarding puppy aptitude testing (previously referred to as puppy temperament assessment) and early selection for and against behavioural traits.

19.6. Common conditions in dog breeding kennels

19.6.1. Respiratory infections (kennel cough)

Canine infectious tracheobronchitis also commonly called kennel cough, is a highly contagious respiratory disease of dogs. Kennel cough is not a single specific disease but rather a collective name for the symptoms caused by a tracheobronchitis. The latter can be caused by any one or any combination of a multitude of respiratory tract pathogens (organisms that cause harm). The primary causes of infectious tracheobronchitis are *Bordetella bronchiseptica*, Canine Parainfluenzavirus, Canine adenovirus type 2 and Canine distemper virus (CDV). Once the virus has caused its initial primary damage then secondary bacterial infections ensue. Infectious tracheobronchitis is rarely life threatening, but it certainly threatens the public image of boarding facilities. Breeders whom regularly board dogs from other breeders or for the public for extra income should take extra care because they are at increased risk. Pets which are entrusted to the care of boarding facilities are frequently returned coughing and gagging to their disgruntled owners. The owners of these pets are even more upset when

Chapter 19 Matters and Conditions Relating to Dogs Kept in Breeding Kennels

they discover that kennel cough is an infectious condition and infects their other dogs. Kennel cough is mostly known as a nuisance disease which is self-limiting. It is typically characterised by chronic coughing and bringing up of phlegm. Exercise or excitement frequently exacerbates the coughing. Some dogs may have a nasal discharge ranging from watery to pussy. In complicated cases, there may be a severe cough for up to 3 weeks associated with weight loss and listlessness. In exceptional cases, some dogs may even develop pneumonia. There is a possibility that bitches which contract kennel cough in early pregnancy may lose the pregnancy. Mild cases of kennel cough may not require treatment whereas in complicated cases, antibiotic therapy is indicated. Cough suppressants may be indicated to alleviate symptoms. Kennel cough vaccines are strongly recommended when dogs are to frequent areas where there are many dogs.

19.6.2. Musculoskeletal disorders

a) Hip dysplasia (HD)

Hip dysplasia is a developmental condition of the coxofemoral (hip) joints. The word developmental in this case means that affected puppies are born with normal hips but develop HD as they grow.

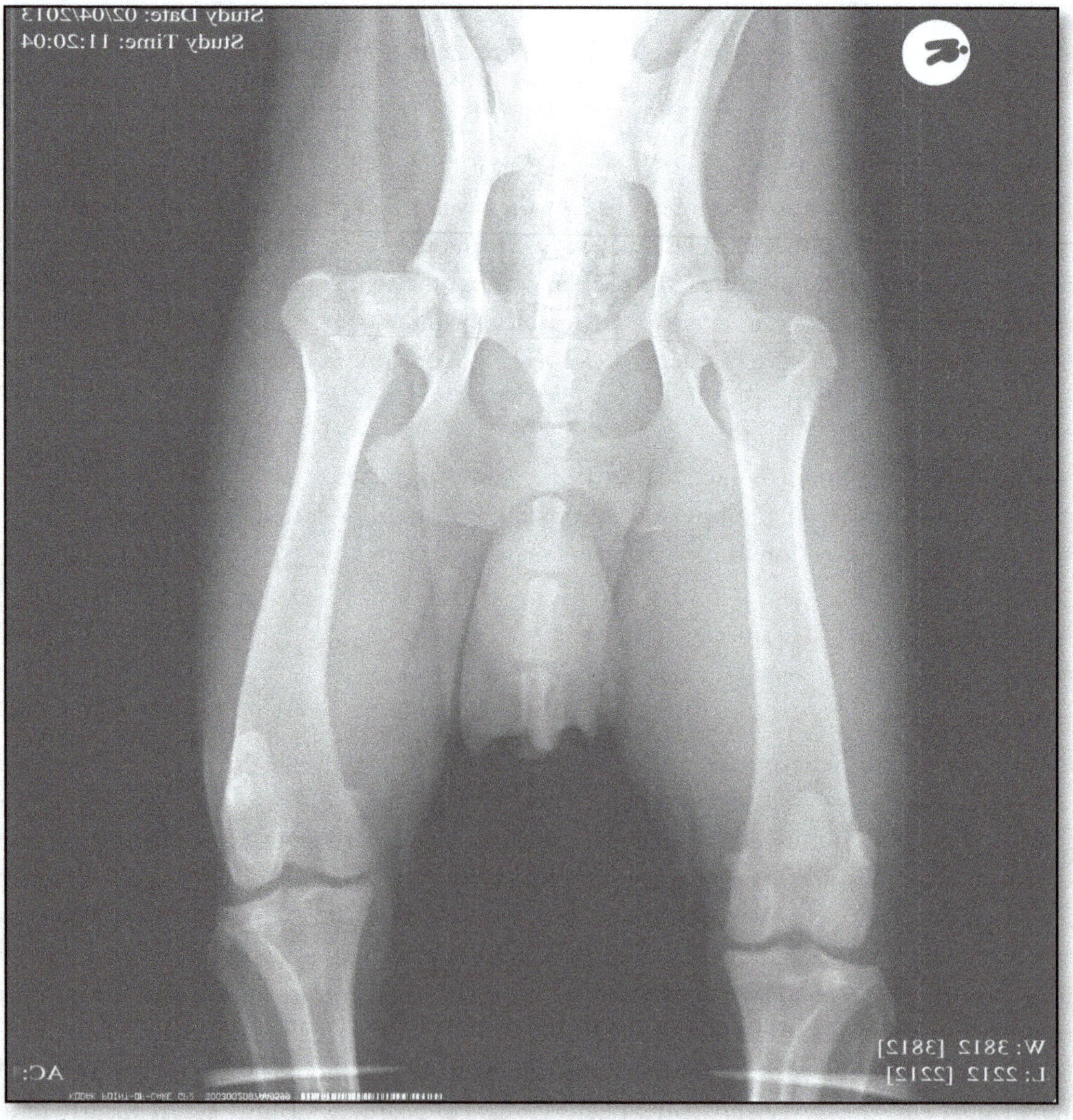

Hip dysplasia in left hip and near normal right hip

The basic problem in HD involves failure of the head of the femur (ball) to fit properly into the acetabulum (socket of the hipbone). If the fit is not satisfactory, the femoral head may be loose (hip laxity). This results in excessive rubbing, dislocation and eventually osteoarthritis of the joints. The defect may occur in any breed, but the larger breeds are the most affected. Larger breeds are also much more likely to exhibit clinical signs. There may be a poor correlation between radiological signs of hip dysplasia and clinical signs shown in dogs with hip dysplasia. Some breeds may have pronounced radiographic signs of HD, but show few clinical signs and sometimes none at all. This may partially be attributed to their high muscle mass in the pelvic area (Bulldog, Staffordshire Terriers and others). In these breeds a much more severe grade of HD is generally required to result in clinical signs.

The clinical signs of HD, as well as age which they will first display these signs may vary widely depending on severity of HD, breed, size and lifestyle of the dog. Dogs showing HD associated clinical signs at an early age (4–10 months of age) are generally (but not always), amongst the larger breeds with a fast growth rate. These dogs show clinical signs consistent with joint laxity as they may not yet have developed arthritis in the hips. They have poor hind limb muscle development, lameness, difficulty in getting up from the sitting position and may "bunny-hop" when running. In older dogs, the clinical signs are more consistent with the development of osteoarthritis. These dogs will show stiffness when getting up and be reluctant to exercise. When they have warmed up somewhat they may improve only to show increased stiffness following a rest after exercise. These dogs may show lameness and muscle wasting in their hind quarters as well.

Causes of hip dysplasia in the dog have been the subject of considerable research. Early reports concluded that the underlying problem in HD is primarily a genetic predisposition and that HD is inherited as a polygenic dominant trait with incomplete penetrance. Today, more emphasis is placed on the multifactorial aetiology of HD. The involvement of many genes are recognized but they may be of smaller consequence than previously assumed. There is some evidence of major-gene involvement in HD in some dog populations.

A complex interaction of factors other than genetic factors is involved in the ultimate development of hip dysplasia. This requires explanation. It is thus clear that the underlying problem is at least partly genetic but that environmental factors are needed to affect the severity of the problem. It does not imply that if all the environmental factors are ideal, one will have a 100% success rate in preventing manifestation of radiographic HD. Getting all of the environmental factors "right", increases the breeder's chances of both reducing incidence and severity of radiographic HD. If the dog does not have any genetic predisposition for HD at all, it does mean that it would not be possible to induce HD with any set of environmental factors. Very few, if any such breeds however exist. The debate of exactly how much does genetics and environment contribute to HD is futile. The bottom line is that breeders should try their utmost to eradicate the genetic component of HD in their breed and in tandem with this, advocate the rearing of puppies to minimise the incidence.

The environmental factors are diet, growth rate and exercise in the developmental stages. With regards to diet it is vital that the diet is appropriate for the breed. With regards to growth rate it is important not to overfeed the puppies thereby inadvertently exacerbating the problem. Overeating can lead to too rapid skeletal growth and obesity. Breeders must realise that new owners of large and giant breeds will frequently deliberately overfeed their puppies in order to get as a result the biggest possible dog. In other cases, work commitments may prevent owners from supervising the

Chapter 19 Matters and Conditions Relating to Dogs Kept in Breeding Kennels

food intake and exercise regime. Puppies with excessive growth rates are at greater risk of developing HD and at greater risk of more severe hip dysplasia. The critical ages are between 9-16 weeks of age. Keeping growing puppies of HD prone breeds lean during this stage can aid in reducing its incidence. Regular moderate exercise helps with joint, tendon and muscle development in growing puppies and prevents joint laxity indirectly reducing HD in that way. It also aids in keeping their weight under control. In conclusion, puppies which are kept lean and well exercised show less HD than those in which this was not done.

Breeders often ask whether an injury could have caused the hip dysplasia. This is more frequently of concern when the hip dysplasia appears to be unilateral. Theoretically, it is true that an injury could indeed lead to HD. An injury may cause inflammation and secondary arthrosis which may later be regarded as HD. This may lead to a reduction in weight bearing. This causes the affected hip to become shallower in time with weak muscular and ligamentous appendages leading to laxity and HD. Although the injury theory is possible, it is almost impossible to prove and it is not known how frequently this occurs. In conclusion, further research is required to conclusively prove or disprove whether unilateral hip dysplasia has a genetic origin or not. The implication is this, if it is proven correct, then we are correct in discriminating against unilateral cases of radiographic HD. If not, the rule would have to be changed. Until then unilateral HD will be assumed to be of genetic origin in all cases by most breeding authorities as otherwise they would be overwhelmed with "unproven claims" of injury and the eradication system would not work.

Hip dysplasia is diagnosed by radiography of the hip joints. The positioning of the dog may erroneously make a hip look slightly better or worse. Breeders need not be concerned about this technical error as expert radiologists will usually not issue certificates in case of poor radiographic technique. Numerous classification systems exist to grade the hips. They all amount to the same, namely grading hips (hip score) from normal, mild, moderate to severe hip dysplasia using different nomenclature. In the breeds that recognise HD as a defect requiring control, breeding recommendations are made. They usually advise breeding up to a grade that is considered acceptable as well as making recommendations as to what grades are permitted to breed with another. For instance they may permit breeding of a moderate hip dysplasia provided it is with a grade better than itself.

The outcome of all these hip dysplasia eradication schemes in many breeds is that they are effective in reducing the incidence quite dramatically in the first 10 years of the scheme and thereafter they are unable to make much more progress. The initial progress made may be brought about by a combination of factors. Part may be because of true genetic progress and part nutritional influence. Unfortunately, a more sinister reason is the practice of pre-screening the hips of young dogs. The latter dogs are excluded from official records because they will not be submitted once the breeder has discovered they are showing radiographic signs of HD. This they do to protect the reputation of themselves and their dogs. In many large dog breeds the incidence of HD remains at 20-40%. This should not be surprising as the trait is inherited as a polygenetic trait and selection against a number of genes has less chance of success and progress when compared to cases where few or only one gene is involved. The biggest problem that some critics of HD eradication schemes have, is that the radiographic hip scores (ratings) might not reflect a dog's genotype accurately. They further contend that relying only on phenotypic trends rather than genetic trends is a serious impediment to progress. Also, in their opinion, implementation of estimated breeding values should be a priority to substantially increase the effectiveness of selection against HD.

Even though there may be truth in this, eradication schemes are the best a breeder has currently. Work is in progress regarding gene testing and genomics and these technologies promise more accurate identification of genotype. It is regrettable that there are still many breeders in many countries who oppose hip eradication schemes.

Early radiographic screening for hip dysplasia is possible. Hips do normally not get better with age but usually deteriorate. Depending on breed, the age at which hips may be officially certified varies from 12-24 months. This is a long time for breeders to wait. During this time there is a substantial monetary as well as emotional investment. For this reason, methods to screen hips early have been developed. Early screening of hips (4-6) months may be a money saving event but should be done professionally and preferably be part of a hip screening eradication scheme with a formal veterinary radiologist. The reliability of early radiographic evaluations for canine hip dysplasia obtained from the standard ventrodorsal (on back) radiographs is generally reliable and is particularly accurate in identifying the bad grades of hip dysplasia. Early screening methods which involve measuring distraction indexes (PennHip method) as well, may improve accuracy. It can never however be as accurate as radiographic hip evaluation at the age of certification. There may be an estimated error of around 15% in dogs which scored well at 4-6 months because their hips may have deteriorated in time. In contrast, the error of falsely identifying bad hips at 4-6 months is either very rare or non-existent. Early screening of hips for hip dysplasia makes a lot of sense. It offers the breeder the opportunity to rid themselves of the affected stock long before they invest too much in the affected individuals. This investment is both monetary and emotional. Early screening methods also have some potential dangers. If screening is performed by inexperienced operators, erroneous evaluations may be made. If at all possible, the early screening should also be left in the hands of board certified specialist radiologists. Another problem is that breeders may use the early screening to identify problem animals and sell them to other non-suspecting individuals. Dogs identified early may also not enter the official eradication scheme as they are either euthanized or sold to pet homes. The official scheme is then left with a population of already selected stock rather than a random sample of the population. This may erroneously identify parent stock as being producers of above average hip score offspring.

There are different surgical options available to owners of dogs which have been diagnosed with HD. These are only mentioned to make the breeder aware of them and to help them make informed decisions. For further details it is advised that breeders consult a specialist surgeon. In very young dogs, juvenile pubic symphysiodesis can be performed. This procedure is ideally performed in puppies 10-14 weeks of age but before 16 weeks. The practical problem with this method however lies in the accurate identification of suitable surgical candidates at this young age. There is no reliable method at this age and therefore the risk exists that many dogs will undergo an unnecessary procedure. Some hold the opinion that this is an invalid procedure for this and other reasons. In dogs slightly older, a triple pelvic osteotomy may be performed to help prevent severe arthritis developing in time. Contrary to some years ago, this procedure is less commonly advised nowadays. In adult dogs where there is already in existence advanced stages of arthritic changes, a total hip replacement is the ideal option but is not always affordable or available. Femur head excision osteotomy (removal of femur head = ball in the socket) is a procedure which may be considered when medical therapy has failed. This operation gives a reasonable degree of functionality and good pain relief in most cases. It was previously believed that this procedure is to be reserved for small dogs of 20 kg and less but increasing numbers of veterinary surgeons are recommending the procedure for larger and even giant breeds. The latter may have extended recovery times. There are medicinal options for dogs already affected by HD. These products may help repair the cartilage which is chronically being insulted in the affected hip joint. It cannot however help in the prevention of HD but only help to control the symptoms. Because they lack efficacy in pain control, they are usually only used as an adjunct to other treatment options. Many non-steroidal anti-inflammatory agents are in use for hip dysplasia associated pain and discomfort. They are not curative but only control the symptoms. It is very important that breeders choose a drug which is least likely to result in serious side effects when given to the dog for extended periods or even lifelong treatments. Only a few drugs are registered for long term use in dogs. Irrespective of choice of drug and albeit rare, they all have the potential for adverse effects such as gastro intestinal ulcers, bleeding tendency, nephrotoxicity (kidney damage) and hepatotoxicity (liver damage).

b) Elbow dysplasia

Elbow dysplasia ED is a defect of the growth processes of the elbow joint in the forelegs and usually occurs at about 4-6 months of age. Either one or both legs may be affected, with one usually worse than the other. There are five different pathologies of the elbow joint which are grouped under the same heading of ED. These are: fragmented medial coronoid process, osteochondritis of the medial condyle, osteochondrosis, elbow joint incongruency and ununited anconeal process. Dogs suffering from ED will have at least one or more of the mentioned pathologies. Elbow dysplasia is generally found in large breeds and often shows a very high rate of heritability. High growth rates as suggested in HD may also contribute to increased incidence of ED. Dogs with elbow dysplasia may either show no lameness or varying symptoms of front leg lameness. In some cases the joint may appear swollen, hot and painful to touch.

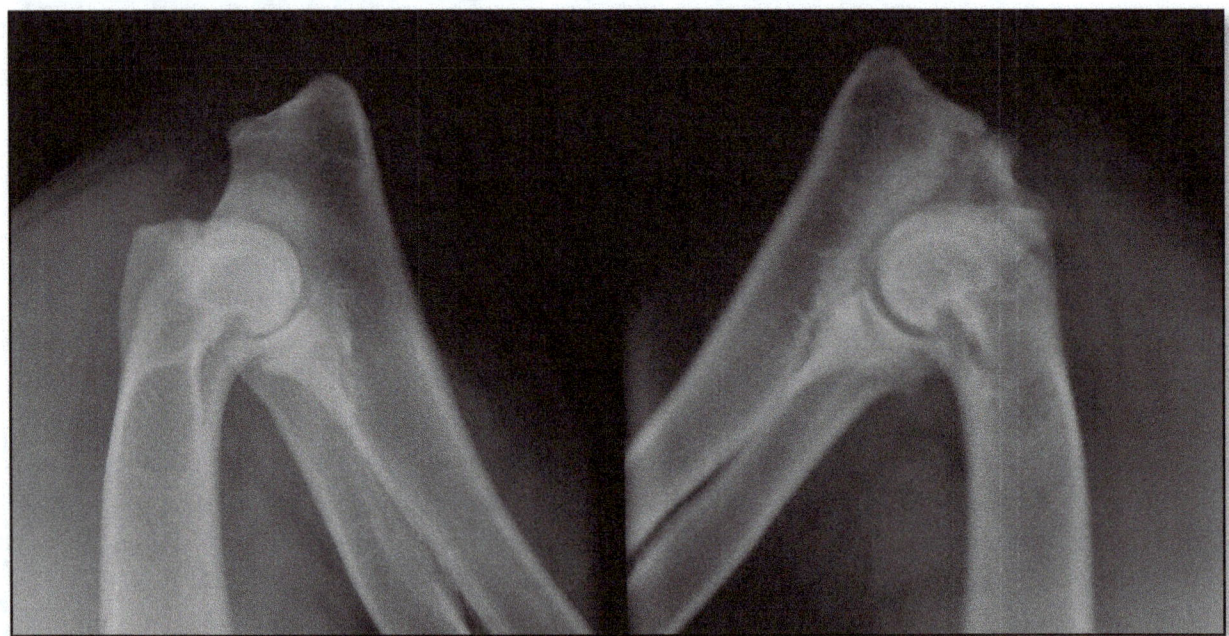

Normal elbow on left and severe dysplastic elbow on right

The diagnosis rests upon demonstration of any of the mentioned pathologies on radiographs. Again there may be a poor correlation found between severity of radiographic signs of ED and clinical signs. Dogs suffering from clinical ED will get down slowly without bearing too much weight on their front limbs. These dogs go down slowly and get up slowly.

It is very rare in small breeds but common in large breeds. Some breeding authorities insist on elbow dysplasia screening, whilst most others strongly encourage it. The incidence of this defect may be so rare in a breed which does probably not warrant routine screening and certification as is the case in Hip Dysplasia. It is advised however that new acquisitions be screened prior to breeding. The diagnosis should be made at around 6 months of age but before 9 months of age in order to render optimum surgical results. Specialist certification can only be performed at 12 months or older.

Surgical correction is possible with varying results. The genetic basis to the defect is that of a polygenic threshold character. The earlier the diagnosis is made and surgery is performed, the better. It seems that the expression of this gene is also dependant on nutrition and caution is advised when feeding high caloric diets.

c) Panosteitis (enostosis, also known as "growing pains")

Panosteitis is a relatively common condition in many large breeds. It causes pain and lameness in mainly young (6-18 months) and occasionally somewhat older, medium to large breed dogs. It is characterised by inflammation in the long bones of the front and hind legs. The cause of this condition is unknown.

The main symptoms are the appearance of a sudden lameness. It does happen that the lameness may disappear and show up in another leg, hence this condition is sometimes said to cause a "shifting" lameness. The inflammation in the legs may cause partial anorexia, fever and lethargy. The diagnosis is by radiography but some may show very little or subtle radiographic evidence of the condition.

Many cases will resolve spontaneously but some may require anti-inflammatory agents combined with restricted exercise.

d) Patella luxation

Patella (kneecap) luxation (slipping off) is a very common orthopaedic condition of the hind limb in many breeds of all sizes. It is a developmental condition and a heritable basis for the disease has been suggested. The cause of the dislocation is due either to a too shallow groove in the femur in which the kneecap slides or inadequate ridges on each side of the groove which help to retain the kneecap. Dogs with bow-legs may have a higher incidence. The luxation can occur at any age, but it is usually diagnosed in dogs aged about 4-6 months. The degree of luxation may vary from a partial dislocation to one in which the patella becomes fixated. Many dogs with luxating patellas may show no or little symptoms. As with many orthopaedic conditions, large dogs are much more likely to show clinical signs associated with patella luxation than small dogs. Most dogs below 3-4 Kg may not show symptoms of patella luxation despite their patella's having attached onto the structures on the inside of the knee, (patella fixation).

e) Cruciate ligament rupture

Cruciate ligament rupture is a very common cause of lameness in dogs of many breeds of all sizes and at all ages. Dogs with ruptured cruciate ligaments may show lameness of various degrees. The rupture of these ligaments is usually not traumatic in origin but due to inherent weakening of the ligaments with subsequent spontaneous rupture (age related degeneration). The high incidence in some breeds and almost a total absence in others, suggests a hereditary basis. Numerous surgical methods may be used to correct the defect and the prognosis for full recovery is good in most cases. It is important to first radiograph the hips prior to performing a cruciate operation. This is to exclude HD as a possible cause of the lameness and to help estimate the length and extent of recovery.

f) Soft pad

Soft pad is a condition where the pads of the dog are totally worn and very smooth. Soft pad is a condition which is frequently encountered in kennelled dogs. Due to the fact that it is not a scientifically documented condition, it is not well known amongst veterinary surgeons. The causes are believed to be the following: The epithelial turnover of pad tissue is enhanced when stimulated by exercise in the same fashion that a bricklayer would develop calluses on his hands. Suddenly exercising the animal on abrasive surfaces will erode the epithelium away and lead to soft tender pads. Affected dogs may appear lame in all fours and may look like they are 'walking on eggs'. Inspection of the pad surface will reveal absence of the normal epithelium pedicles or spiky spurs and the surface will be very smooth, soft, and tender to touch. Another cause is believed to be continuous wet conditions on the kennel surfaces. Some kennelled dogs are subject to wet kennel surfaces for days on end particularly during the wet season and this leads to the following: the epithelium gets soft and swells in the same way that the skin on our hands gets soft when we stay in the bath for too long. The epithelium can now easily be scratched off when the animal moves about on the rough kennel surface leading to soft pads. The condition is easily treated by eliminating the underlying cause and treating the pad itself with an agent that hardens the pad epithelium like formaldehyde containing products. Interdigital dermatitis, which is a rash between the toes, is often associated with soft pads particularly when wet conditions were the contributing factor to the soft pads.

19.6.3. Pressure point hygroma

a) Occipital hygroma

This is an accumulation of fluid underneath the skin at the base of the skull as a result of trauma at that particular point directly above the occipital protuberance, which is a bony point at the base of the skull. This occurs more often in young dogs than older ones. The typical cause is where the dog keeps on bumping their head against the table or entrance of its kennel. The prognosis for recovery is 100% but it may require surgery and instillation of a drain. Removal of the lump is associated with high risk of wound dehiscence and is not recommended.

b) Elbow/Hock hygromas

These are accumulations of fluid underneath the skin over pressure points on the dog's body e.g. elbows; hocks; lateral knee aspects; hipbone and carpal (wrist) areas. These areas may become swollen, thickened, blackened and filled with fluid. Later on, these areas may become badly infected. These infections may prove extremely stubborn to treat and surgical and medical treatment is often unrewarding and in extreme cases necessitate euthanasia. Prevention is to make these heavy dogs lie on soft padded surfaces. Surgical removal can be disastrous. It is best to insert drains and leave them in for up to 2 weeks.

19.6.4. Miscellaneous conditions.

a) Tail tip injuries

Tail tip injuries typically occur in dogs that have an "over-enthusiastic" tail and keep on knocking their tail against hard surfaces. Tail tip injuries may also result from smacking it against the walls of its enclosure. The tail tip becomes denuded, sensitive and may start bleeding. The dog is usually presented to the veterinary surgeon for bleeding of this tail tip. Haemostasis is applied and the tail is then usually bandaged. However, the dog only needs to smack his tail against a wall once and the tail starts bleeding all over again even through the bandage or the dog pulls the bandage off. Care should be taken to protect the tail tip against continued injury. Proper padding should be applied to the tail tip and the bandage properly secured. Doing this, the extent of tissue damage is minimised when the dog inadvertently hits its tail against a hard surface again. Failing to achieve this, there is a real likelihood that frustration may prompt owner and veterinary surgeon to amputate the tail. When amputation becomes necessary, the tail should be amputated as high up as possible. This is because otherwise the episode of tail injury and further amputation is going to repeat itself (so called salami slicing amputation technique).

b) Cherry eye (prolapsed gland of third eyelid)

Hypertrophy and prolapse of the gland of the nictitating membrane (cherry eye) is common in young dogs. In the acute stage, the red mass swells and protrudes over the leading margin of the nictitans, and there is a mucopurulent discharge. Although the swelling may recede for short periods, it eventually often remains prolapsed. Because it contributes to tear production, it should be preserved. The gland should be replaced and anchored with sutures. Complete excision may predispose to keratoconjunctivitis sicca (dry eye).

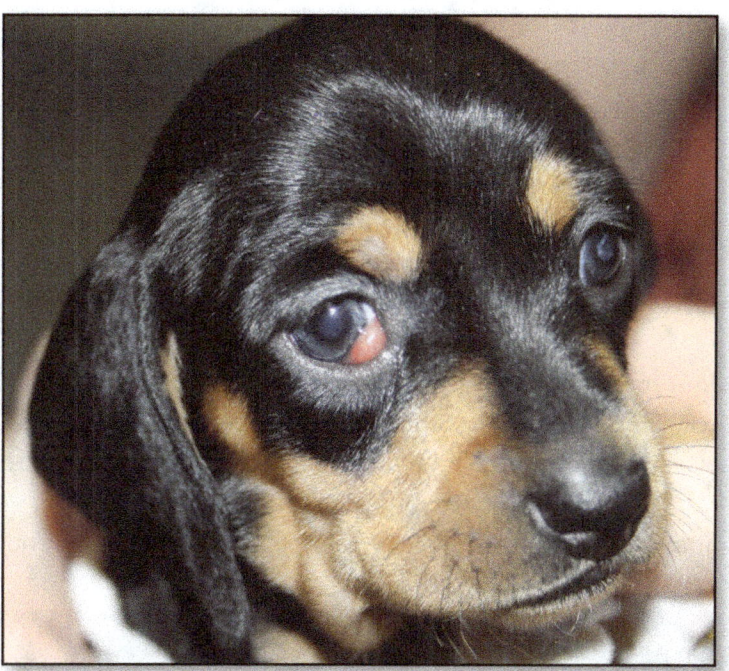
Prolapsed gland of third eyelid "cherry eye"

c) Retained deciduous teeth

Normally the deciduous tooth's root is resorbed, making room for an adult tooth. Should this fail, the adult tooth may deviate from its normal position, producing malocclusion. The resulting double set of teeth overcrowds the dental arch, causing food to become trapped between the teeth, leading to early periodontal disease. A retained deciduous tooth should be extracted as soon as an adult tooth is noted in the same area as the baby tooth. If extraction is performed early, the abnormally positioned adult tooth usually moves to its normal location. Many toy breeds are affected but Yorkshire terriers are over-represented.

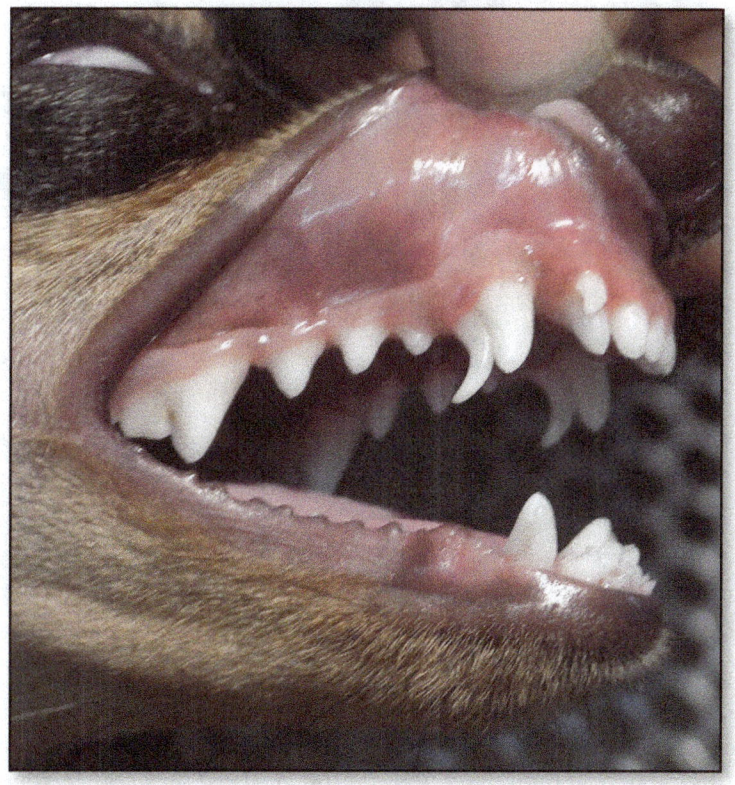
Retained deciduous teeth

d) Megaoesophagus

Megaoesophagus is a condition where there is dilation of the oesophagus due to a loss of normal peristaltic (contractility in circular fashion) movements in the oesophagus. Part of the oesophagus or the entire oesophagus may be affected.

Dogs suffering from megaoesophagus will appear to vomit the food soon after ingestion. This "bringing up" of food is not truly vomiting but rather regurgitation. The difference is that when vomiting, the food has already reached the stomach and there is a strong abdominal contraction component seen when dogs vomit. In contrast, whilst regurgitating food, there is no abdominal contraction and the food passively leaves the mouth usually in a sausage shape of undigested food.

Megaoesophagus may be congenital or acquired. Puppies born with the condition may only show symptoms at the time of weaning when they start consuming solids. These puppies may also fail to thrive and make unusual respiratory noises.

In some acquired forms of megaoesophagus there are some treatment options. In most others and the congenital form the problem cannot be treated but only managed. Feeding small quantities from an elevation to help the food down may help reduce the regurgitation.

Some dogs will do well whereas others don't and may require euthanasia.

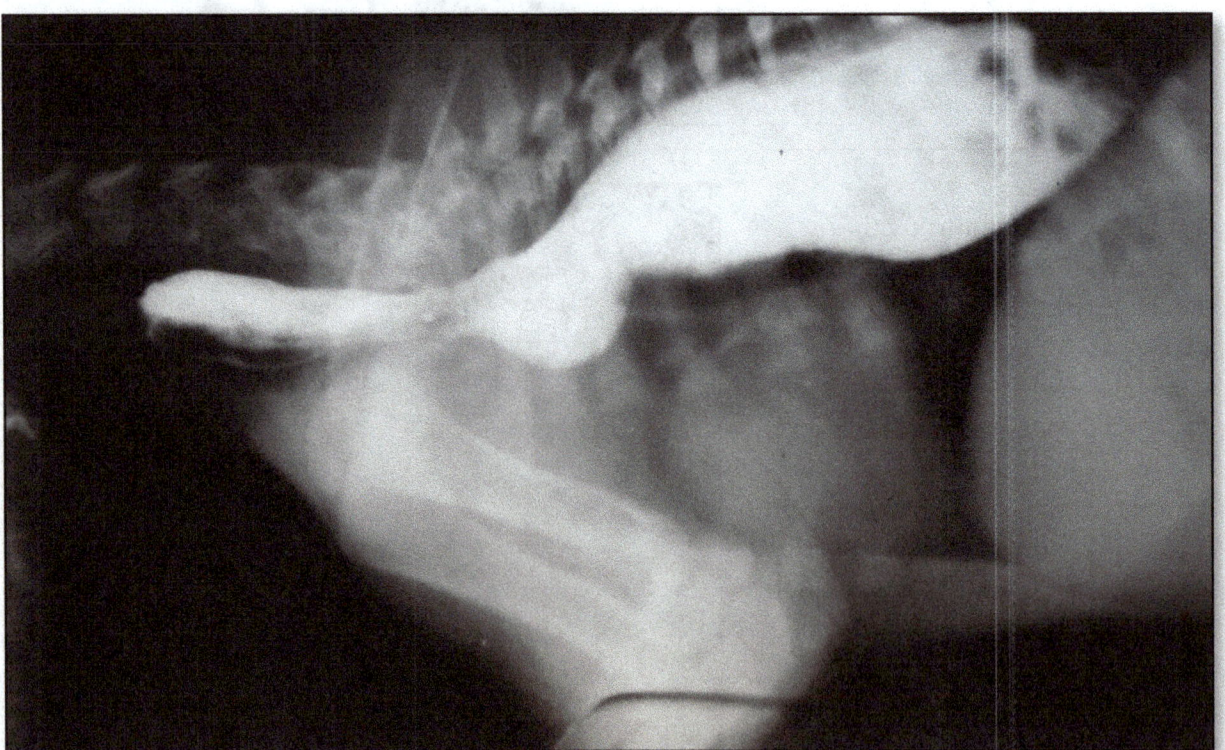

Megaoesophagus, note white barium clearly visible on radiograph indicating inability of food to pass into stomach

e) Lick granuloma

Lick granulomas are also known as acral pruritic nodules and acral lick dermatitis. This is a complex disorder in which dogs lick continuously at an area on their leg, which becomes raw, weeping, and ulcerated. The cause is unknown but inheritance may play a role, since certain breeds are affected more commonly. Other possibilities include a disorder of the sensory nerves, or an obsessive-compulsive disorder. Boredom and frustration are thought to play a role in this condition, which is often seen in highly strung dogs. The most common place is the carpus of the dog but any other spot on the legs is possible. Lick granulomas can be difficult for veterinary surgeons to treat, and frustrating for the owner. Because boredom and frustration are thought to play a role in this condition, your veterinary surgeon will likely discuss environmental enrichment and behaviour modification for your dog. Local treatment, treating secondary bacterial infections at the site and prevention of further injury through bandages and collars should all be explored.

f) Allergic dermatitis

Most allergies in dogs result from allergic components in the air. It is therefore sometimes referred to as inhalant dermatitis or atopic dermatitis. It can be considered the canine equivalent of hay fever in humans. It is a common ailment in dogs. Allergic skin disease in dogs is frequently complicated by secondary bacterial skin infections (pyoderma) often yeast (Malassezia) infections as well. Dogs suffering from atopy are genetically programmed to become sensitised to allergens in the environment. Allergens are "things" that dogs may be allergic to. These allergens may be inhaled, cause irritation by direct contact to the skin or ingested. The main allergens for dogs are dust mites, fungal spores and pollens from any variety of plants. Unlike humans where the primary target organ for allergies is the airways, the skin is the primary target organ in dogs. Once exposed to the allergens, the dog reacts via an inflammatory response in the skin.

The age of onset is generally between 6 months and 7 years, but most animals have clinical signs by 3 years of age. The condition usually occurs on a seasonal basis initially, but most of affected animals become pruritic (itchy) year round with time. The paws, face, ears, axillae (armpits) and abdomen are the most frequently affected areas but severely affected animals may start scratching everywhere. Lesions develop secondary to self-trauma by scratching and include alopecia (hair loss), erythema (reddening), scaling and later hyperpigmentation (skin becomes blackened and often thickened with deep wrinkles resembling elephant skin). Secondary to self-trauma; a deep skin infection (pyoderma) may develop. An otitis externa (outer ear infection) is a common secondary complication. The exact mode of inheritance is unknown. Where both parents are allergic, there is a very strong likelihood the offspring will be as well. There is a strong breed predilection for this condition, and marked familial involvement.

There are many skin diseases which cause itching, and they can all look rather similar on physical examination. Your veterinary surgeon will ask questions about your dog's diet, environment, any kind of skin care already provided, whether any other pets or people in the house are itchy, where and how quickly did the skin lesions start, and is there any seasonal pattern to the itching. The answers, as well as the age and breed of your dog, will provide diagnostic clues. There is no definitive diagnostic test for this condition and diagnosis is made by symptoms and exclusion of other causes. Immunotherapy based on serum allergy test results may help some cases and is advised for those very stubborn cases. Food allergies are a particular problem as they are very difficult to confirm. Avoidance of the suspected food followed by improvement increases the suspicion index. Dogs are allergic to a particular ingredient (usually a protein) in the food and not to a particular food brand or label. Dogs which suffer from a true food allergy may benefit from a special "allergy diet".

Some breeders will claim that a particular shampoo may have a particular effect or induce allergy. This is however very rare. Most dogs with an itchy skin will scratch more after having been bathed with

Chapter 19 Matters and Conditions Relating to Dogs Kept in Breeding Kennels

whatever due to the fact that their skin has become agitated by the handling and irritation from brushes. Hence, the common practice of blaming the parlour and shampoos following grooming of dogs. Grooming sometimes precipitates an underlying allergy which was bound to manifest soon anyway.

It is important to note that in most cases of allergy the cause cannot be found, cure is normally not a realistic expectation but relief is. Lifelong treatment and supplementation is normally required and corticosteroid therapy at intervals is frequently required through the affected dog's life.

The therapeutic options available for management of Atopy are: avoidance of the offending allergens (which is mostly impossible), corticosteroid therapy, use of skin moisturising agents, long term use of omega-3 and omega-6 containing oils (special diets) and immunotherapy. All these options should be discussed with the attending veterinary surgeon. Although difficult and frustrating, most cases can and will get relief following an extensive work up and trial and error attempts of the various treatment options and compliance to treatment protocols.

19.7. Sudden death

Sudden death of a dog in a kennel which was previously in apparent perfect good health hours before can be very distressing but is a reality. A post mortem will usually reveal the cause of the death. Some common causes of sudden death are discussed in this section.

19.7.1. Gastric dilatation and volvulus (stomach torsion)

Gastric dilatation and volvulus (GDV), also known as gastric torsion is almost unknown in small and medium breeds but common in large and giant breeds. GDV tends to primarily affect large, deep-chested dogs. There is no apparent sex or age predisposition, but the incidence increases with age, being most common in 7-10 year old dogs. A familial tendency is suspected. Dilatation occurs secondary to the accumulation of gas or fluid (or both) within the stomach when the outflow of gas and fluids is obstructed. This obstruction occurs when the stomach twists along its longitudinal axis and kinks the oesophagus and duodenum. The early symptoms include an acute onset of restlessness, apparent discomfort, abdominal pain, repeated unproductive retching, excessive salivation and abdominal distension. GDV is a life-threatening emergency. Successful management depends on prompt diagnosis and appropriate medical and surgical treatment within literally hours of the torsion having occurred.

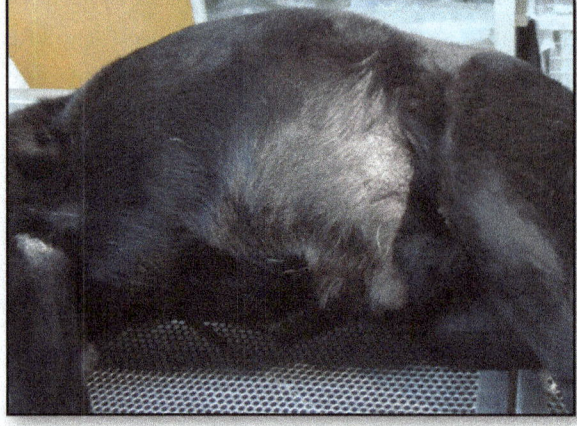

Gastric dilatation and volvulus in a dog

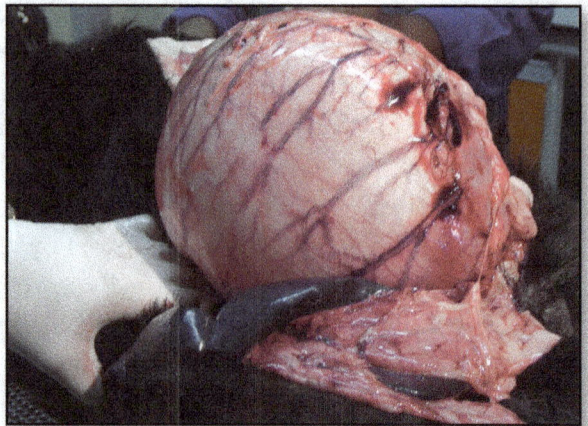

Postmortem of GDV dog showing massively distended stomach

During the surgery it is advised that a gastropexy is performed. That involves surgically suturing the stomach wall to the abdominal wall to prevent a GDV from repeating. The principal goals of initial treatment are to stabilize the animal and decompress the stomach surgically immediately. Dogs with a tendency to develop dilatation and volvulus should be fed smaller meals more frequently over the course of the day. Excessive exercise should be avoided to decrease the likelihood of twisting, and consumption of large volumes of water after exercise should be avoided to limit gastric distension. The vast majority of GDV cases veterinary surgeons get presented with during late evening or day hours will survive whilst those presented in early hours of the morning have a worse prognosis. This is probably due to the interval from start of the GDV and first detection of the problem. In day or early evening, the owners are more likely to spot a problem. If one thus has a regimen that the last feed is at say 1 pm and the last kennel inspection is at say 6 pm there is less likelihood that an early case of GDV be missed. As GDV mostly occurs within a couple of hours of a meal, some breeders do not feed their dogs after early afternoon. This increases their likelihood of detecting the GDV before their last kennel check. A preventative gastropexy can also be performed and this is sometimes done at the time of sterilisation in pet dogs at risk. This procedure is sure to gain more attention and breeders of at risk dogs are now advising this and having it performed on their breeding dogs.

19.7.2. Heart conditions

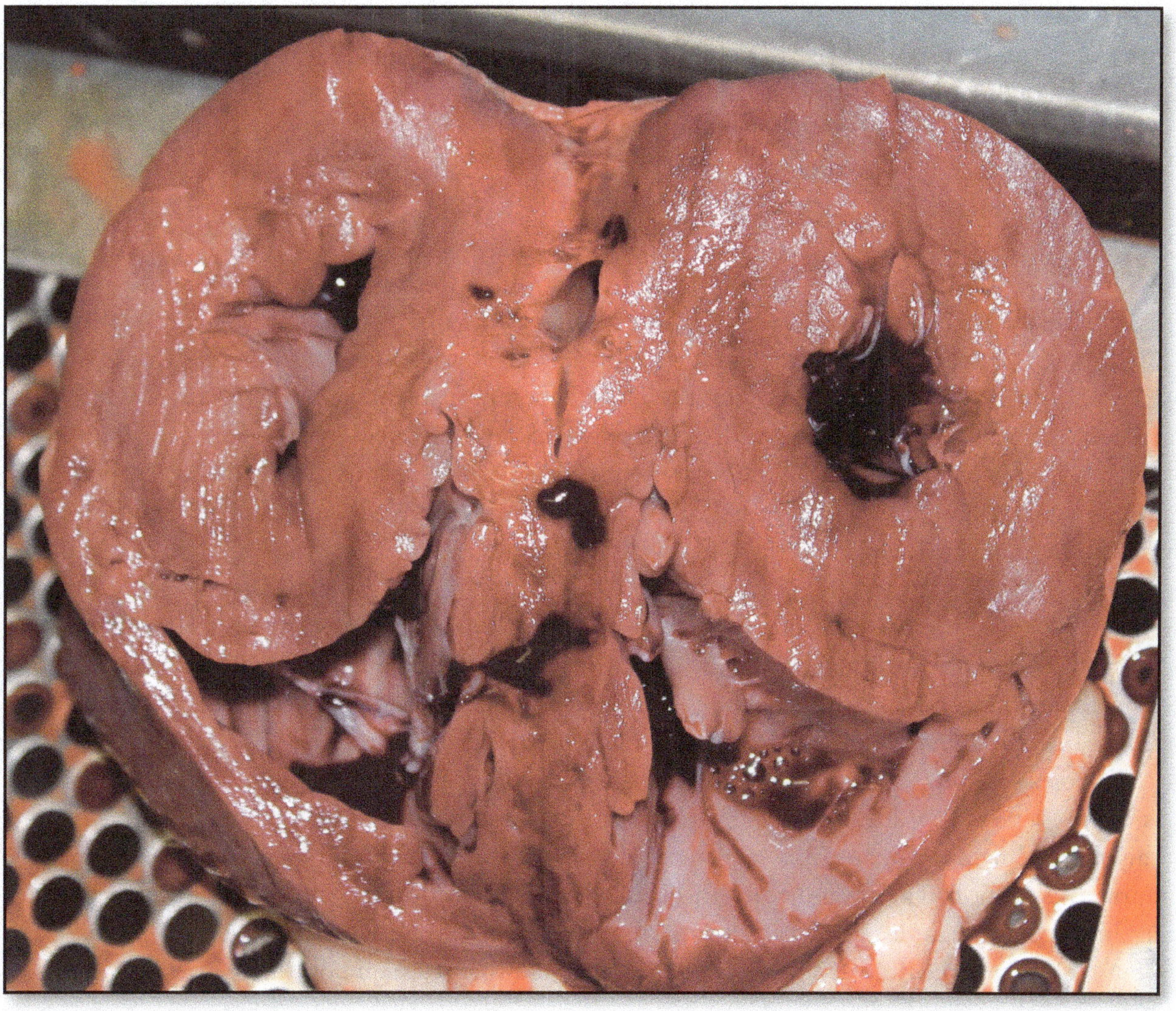

Hypertrophic cardiomyopathy is one of numerous causes that may lead to sudden unexpected death in dogs

Chapter 19 Matters and Conditions Relating to Dogs Kept in Breeding Kennels

There are numerous heart problems in dogs which may go entirely undetected by the breeder or veterinary surgeon and may only be evident on specialist echocardiography (heart examinations). Dogs which suffer from serious heart problems may have been in apparent good health before their sudden death. In some cases, clinical signs such as shortness of breath, coughing, weight loss and exercise intolerance may be noticed beforehand.

The exact nature of the multitude of heart conditions will not be fully discussed. Vascular ring anomalies, heart valve disease, hypertrophic and dilated cardiomyopathies are but a few of the common heart problems which may lead to heart related sudden deaths.

19.7.3. Heat exhaustion (hyperthermia)

Heat stroke is also known as hyperthermia. This occurs when the dog is unable to keep its own body cool. Dogs have limited ability to rid themselves of excessive body heat. Unlike humans which sweat, dogs have no significant sweating capacity and are reliant on panting and evaporation over the tongue for thermoregulation. Exercise and excitement may lead to increased heat production whereas high ambient temperature, high humidity, poor ventilation (e.g. in car) and obesity contribute to reduced ability to rid the body of heat. In nature dogs will avoid heat stroke by seeking cool spots and avoiding activity during hot times of the day. Dogs with restricted airways (especially brachycephalic breeds) are more prone to heat exhaustion. Heat exhaustion is a medical emergency and needs to be addressed immediately by cooling the dog even before arrangements are made to transport the dog to the veterinary surgeon. The dog should be sprayed or dunked in cold water, placed in a very cool place or air conditioned vehicle. If cold water is not available, the dog can be wetted and placed in front of a fan. Veterinary treatment involves continued efforts to cool the affected dog down and administering intravenous fluids. Heat exhaustion is often fatal particularly if it continues for too long and treatment is delayed.

19.7.4. Restricted airway syndrome

Brachycephalic airway obstructive syndrome in dogs is discussed separately. Even though it may predispose the dog to heat exhaustion as explained, it may be a primary cause of death even before heat exhaustion sets in. As the name implies it is common in brachycephalic breeds and some related or descended breeds. The syndrome involves suffering from at one or more of the following defects: elongated soft palate, stenotic nares (narrowing of the nostrils), everted laryngeal saccules, hypoplastic trachea and everted tonsils. Affected breeds are in many cases more prone to snoring and open mouth breathing.

Affected dogs not only have poor tolerance to heat but also to exercise. Some are so severely affected that even at rest they have difficulty in delivering enough oxygen to their system. Obesity exacerbates the condition. Affected dogs which simultaneously suffer from a slight respiratory or throat infection (pharynx or larynx) will also show more severe respiratory distress. When affected dogs are exposed to the slightest bit of exercise, excitement and excessive barking, the condition is compounded. The dog will attempt to compensate by hyperventilating. This is turn may dry the mucous membranes and also expose the already restricted upper airways to negative pressures during inspiration. The combined effect of the latter leads to oedema (swelling) of the membranes in the upper airways, leading to an even more restricted airway. The outcome of such episode may be anoxia (insufficient oxygen delivery to the body) fainting and rapid death.

Surgery, although not totally curative, may greatly improve the dog's quality of life and reduce risk of fatality. Selection against this syndrome is clearly important and very much needed.

Although not strictly part of the brachycephalic obstructive airway syndrome, laryngeal paralysis also needs mention under this heading. In this disorder, there is some loss of function in the laryngeal muscles which normally open the larynx/vocal cords when an animal inhales. The result is also airway obstruction to varying degrees, causing loud and laboured respiration and coughing or gagging when eating. It is a confirmed genetic defect in some breeds and strongly suspected in others, therefore breeding of the parents (carriers of the disorder) and siblings (suspect carriers) should be avoided.

Although tricky, surgery is either curative or vastly improves the condition and also reduces the risk of related fatality.

19.7.5. Bee sting attack

Three distinct syndromes may be associated with bee sting. The first is some simple local swelling and pain where the bee has stung. Dogs get stung mostly on their face and more specifically the eyelids and lips. This is usually inconsequential and disappears within hours without special attention or treatment. The second and third bee sting associated syndromes are bee venom allergies and massive bee sting envenomation.

Unlike the European honeybee, the African honeybee is an aggressive bee which attacks easily with little provocation. The African honeybee's venom is no more poisonous but the problem lies with its aggression and tendency to attack in large numbers resulting in massive volume of poison injected into the individual victim. African honeybees truly deserve the name "killer bees" because of their deadly attacks on people and domestic animals. Once the first bees start stinging, a pheromone is released (smells a bit like citrus peel) which prompts other bees to sting as well. African bees are becoming an invader species in temperate to warm areas of the world where they have been introduced. In some of these areas, people unfamiliar with African honeybees may sometimes not show the necessary respect and fall victim to bee sting attack.

One needs to distinguish between the allergic individual which develops problems from a single bee sting versus massive bee sting envenomation as a result of large numbers of bees attacking the pets.

a) Bee venom allergy

A human which is allergic to bee sting, is at more risk than a dog which is allergic. This is because humans may develop an asthma attack in response to histamine whereas dogs develop a skin reaction. A normal non-allergic dog may show very little signs to a small number of bee stings other than some local swelling and sensitivity. An allergic dog will develop urticarial (wheals) over the face and trunk and legs. The dog's face, lips, eyelids and ears may swell considerably. These animals will seldom show respiratory signs. This type of reaction looks very alarming, but is easily treated and the symptoms may even disappear without any treatment. Although best attended to by a veterinary surgeon, it is not a dire emergency.

b) Massive bee sting envenomation

Massive bee sting envenomation may occur when an individual dog is stung by 20-30 bees or more and is a dire emergency. The severity of the envenomation depends on the sensitivity and mass of

Chapter 19 Matters and Conditions Relating to Dogs Kept in Breeding Kennels

the victim but most importantly, the number of bee stings acquired. Typically, bee sting attacks are characterised by victims which have been stung by bees in the order of several hundreds of stings. Many of these may have a lethal outcome despite treatment. Prognosis is poorer when treatment is delayed. When attacked by large numbers of bees, clinical signs of massive envenomation will commence in under an hour. These are vomiting, a very severe diarrhoea, rapid dehydration, red discoloured urine, trembling, shock, hyperventilation, incoordination and later total collapse. Severely affected dogs may also develop respiratory distress. These dogs will not show signs of facial swelling. The dogs will typically die within a few hours. Avoidance of bees in the first place is the best strategy against bee stings attacks. Bees will start a hive almost anywhere they can find shelter, trees, buildings, drainpipes and holes in the ground. It is therefore wise to make sure one discourages bees from colonizing your property by securing the entrance to potential hive sites. The sound of humming bees and increased bee activity should alert the breeder to take evasive action. When bees swarm, they are looking for a new home and are particularly aggressive. Loud machinery, vibration and barking dogs can all irritate bees. When there is bee activity, do not use the noisy apparatus close by, as this is known to trigger bee attack. The best is to lead the dogs away from the bees. There are no efficacious first aid measures one can take in dogs following massive bee sting envenomation. Prevention of more stings is the most important and practical as well as seeking veterinary attendance as soon as possible. Treatment involves administration of antihistamines, cortisone, adrenalin and intensive fluid therapy. The prognosis depends on the time interval from the bee sting attack to the start of treatment, sensitivity of the individual, size of individual as well as number of bee stings. The severely affected animals will die within hours. Some dogs may suffer from jaundice and anaemia and make a full recovery following a long stay in intensive care. Unfortunately, some dogs may show an apparent recovery and later die from renal failure or other complications.

19.7.6. Strokes

Not unlike people, dogs can also suffer from a stroke. In both humans and dogs, there are two types of stroke: A stroke may be a cerebrovascular incident whereby the blood vessel gets clogged up by a thrombosis (blood clot) or there is bleeding in the brain which results in anoxia (lack of oxygen) to the brain. Typically the dog will appear normal one moment and have symptoms of balance loss; head tilt and in some cases suffer from uncontrolled eyeball movements (nystagmus). Partial paralysis on one side may be noticed in some cases.

Although very rare, a cerebrovascular incident may lead to the dog's death quite unexpectedly and leave very little signs on the post mortem unless the brain is properly examined. A stroke is a medical emergency. Most dogs suffering from a stroke will make a full recovery within a few weeks following appropriate treatment.

The causes of stroke includes mainly age related problems and blood clotting disorders. Older dogs should be presented for their "senior" check-up to address any age related problems such as diminished organ function and blood pressure problems.

19.7.7 Snake bite

In many parts of the world snake bites to humans and pets are a real threat. It is quite possible that because of the inquisitive nature of dogs the incidence of snakebite is higher in them than in humans (who generally fear snakes). It is also fair to speculate that dogs are more likely to suffer from multiple snake bites than humans because of their investigative persistent nature.

The type of snakebite encountered varies according to the geographic location and distribution of the various snakes. Examination of the live caught or dead snake enables positive identification and will help the veterinary surgeon in treating the dog which fell victim to snake bite. The most common and logical approach to treating snakebite without knowing the species of snake concerned is to follow the syndromic management of snakebite. This entails identifying three syndromes: painful progressive swelling (PPS), progressive weakness and bleeding.

Complications of snakebite associated with PPS are bite-site infections, necrosis (tissue destruction and death), compartment syndrome (occlusion of blood vessels by surrounding swollen muscles), deep vein thrombosis (blood clots) and respiratory complications. Broad spectrum antibiotic therapy is indicated for snakebite victims with tissue necrosis. If the snake is positively identified, specific treatment using antivenom (snake venom antiserum)

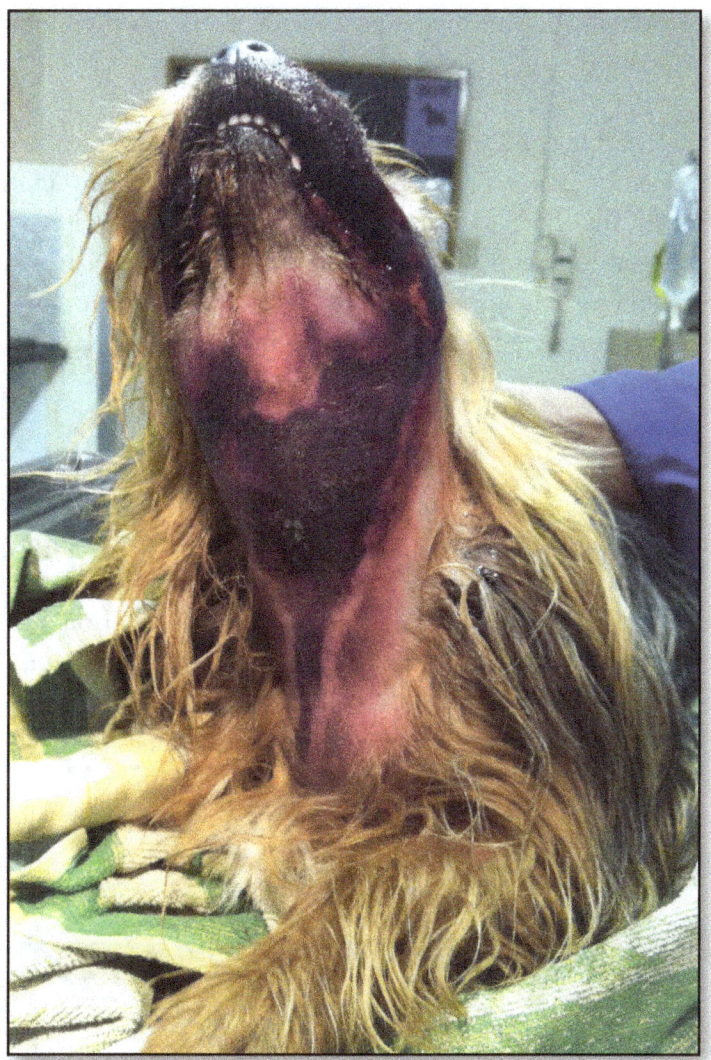

Lesions on dog's neck caused by snake bite

may be indicated. Partial consumption of the snake is often noticed when dogs are bitten by snakes. Authentic signs of snake envenomation after eating a raw whole snake have been reported in man and from this it must be deduced that this mode of envenomation is also possible in dogs.

Since antivenom related allergic reactions in humans are frequent and may be fatal, veterinary surgeons are also reluctant to administer them. The literature however suggests that the incidence of such reactions in dogs is rare. An effective vaccine against rattle snake poison is available and this suggests that this mode of protection is potentially possible for other snake venoms as well. First aid methods known to be effective for humans against snake bite may be helpful in dogs as well but seeking immediate veterinary attendance is recommended with all snake bites in dogs.

19.7.8. Canine red gut (clostridial enterotoxaemia) (mainly of interest to veterinary surgeons)

Red gut is a name arbitrarily assigned to a fatal condition of dogs based on its appearance on post mortem. This condition is suspected to be an exclusive condition of German Shepherd dogs. This book, with the odd exception, deliberately avoids singling out breeds with regards to incidence of specific conditions. This is because the book focuses on breeding dogs in general and its nature was

Chapter 19 Matters and Conditions Relating to Dogs Kept in Breeding Kennels

not intended to be breed specific. The author however has specific interest in this condition because it is poorly understood, mostly unknown and because the inclusion of this condition in this book may very well spark some interest from the scientific community regarding this very interesting yet devastating condition. The complex nature of this discussion may be of more interest to veterinary surgeons than breeders but it is nevertheless the opinion of the author that it has great value in advancing the health of the very many German Shepherd Dogs owned by breeders and pet owners. Red gut is a per acute necrotizing haemorrhagic gastro-enteritis syndrome suspected to be mediated by enterotoxins produced by the disturbed enteric flora of affected dogs. In the experience of the author it only occurs in German Shepherd Dogs but some veterinary surgeons and pathologist may dispute this and the possibility that it exists in other breeds should therefore not be excluded.

It is a dramatic disease with a very rapid onset characterised by initially mild and later severe depression, bloated abdomen, rapid breathing, increased pulse rate, lethargy, very pale mucous membranes (gums) which may later become cyanotic (purple) as the condition progresses, abdominal pain and ultimately death. Some dogs present with acute haemorrhagic diarrhoea with frank blood in the stool mixed with liquid faeces. Without exception, this condition is always fatal despite aggressive treatment attempts and death usually occurs in less than 12 hours of having diagnosed the condition.

The vast majority of cases at home or in kennels die acutely with very few symptoms.

The ante mortem (live dog) diagnosis is based on the suggestive clinical signs and some basic laboratory tests. Dogs suffering from red gut have the paradoxical observation that they have a very

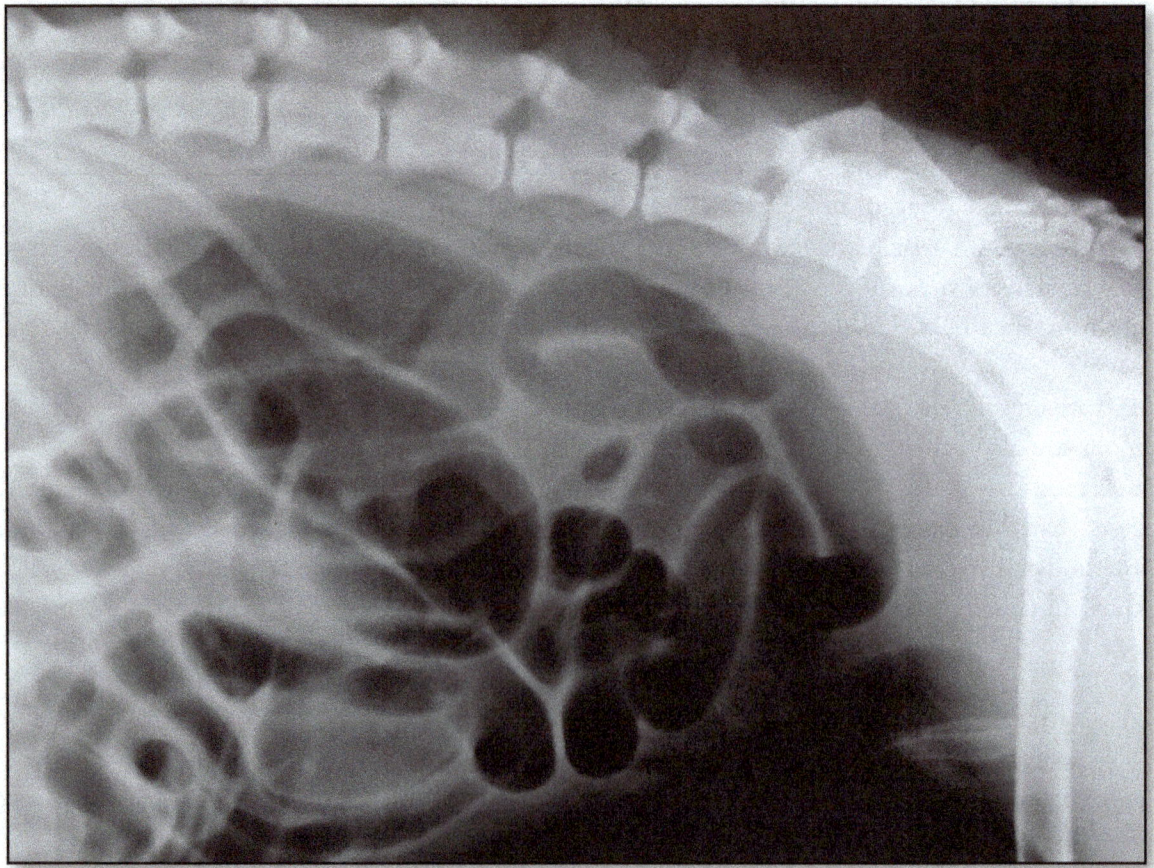

Radiograph of dog's abdomen that is dying from "Redgut"

high haematocrit (red blood cell count) of usually in excess of 65%, despite displaying very pale mucous membranes. The latter is probably mediated by haemoconcentration combined with a vast reduction in cardiac output due to endotoxic shock. Abdominosintesis (extraction of fluid from the abdomen) yields large volumes of a very putrid smelling dark red to brown fluid with large numbers of demonstrable Clostridial organisms. The combination of these findings should be considered pathognomic (confirmative) for this condition in the live dog.

The post mortem signs include: marked pallor of the mucous membranes, abdominal distention caused by loops of darkly congested and distended small intestine. The abdominal cavity is filled with 500-1500ml of foetid serosanguinous fluid. The entire small and large intestine (except the very proximal duodenal portion) is affected. There is frank haemorrhage and pooling of dark red or blackened blood within the lumen of the bowel. The mucosal surface is dark red to black (or green) in colour. The first impression upon opening the abdominal cavity is that there is intestinal strangulation instead of an extensive haemorrhagic enteritis, or severe gastro-enterorrhagia. Clinicians with no experience or knowledge of the condition may therefore not diagnose this condition and mistake it as a volvulus of the small intestine. Generalized necrosis and early rapid autolysis of the entire intestine is very apparent. Some cases show severe haemorrhage along the mesenteric edge of the intestines, while others show severe massive haemorrhage and oedema of the rectum.

There is currently no plausible explanation why only the GSD breed should be affected and if it does occur in other breeds, it is fair to assume that its incidence is very low indeed.

The aetiology (causes) and pathogenesis (circumstances that lead to the disease) are somewhat of an enigma. It has not been possible to replicate the condition in laboratory conditions. Under favourable circumstances, clostridial organisms grow profusely and produce toxins in overwhelming concentration. These toxins are thought to cause disease and subsequent death. Clostridial organisms are wide spread. A critical factor is almost certainly the presence of starch in the small intestine, providing a suitable substrate for these saccharolytic bacteria and they proliferate to immense numbers and produce correspondingly large amounts of clostridial enterotoxin. It can be speculated that this syndrome has a multifactorial origin and that nutritional factors and nutritional management may play a major pre-disposing role. Based on observations of what food affected dogs were on, it is speculated that poor digestibility and low fat percentage in dog food may predispose dogs to this condition. Another predisposing factor appears to be the sudden change from a premium diet to a very substandard or marginal diet. Such circumstances sometimes presents them self when dog owners either run out of their regular premium diet or buy a dog food of questionable quality.

Practical consideration regarding red gut (of interest to breeders)

This condition has not been diagnosed by the author in dogs fed premium diets containing a high fat % (≥ 10%) and highly digestible diets. Stricter regulations regarding quality of marginal dog food in most developed countries may provide an explanation of why this condition is not known in those parts of the world.

Preliminary trials indicate that inclusion of bacteriostatic drugs effective against clostridial organisms appear to prevent the condition. It is however important to note that the inclusion of bacteriostatic agents in dog foods has to be approved prior to its standard use.

Chapter 19 Matters and Conditions Relating to Dogs Kept in Breeding Kennels

Further research is however required including investigation into the pathogenesis and aetiology in order to explain the breed pre-disposition and its sporadic occurrence. In conclusion canine red gut is a fatal condition which affects mainly German Shepherd Dogs for which there is no treatment or vaccine. It appears that dogs fed a high quality premium diet high in fats are unlikely to suffer from red gut, in the author's experience.

19.7.9. Spirocerca lupi

Spirocerca lupi has been adequately discussed elsewhere (see 17.9) and in areas where it is present is a very common cause of sudden unexplained deaths. In some areas, the incidence of this parasite is so high that on-going preventative treatment of all dogs is indicated.

19.8. Zoonoses

A zoonosis (zoonoses = plural) is a disease that can be transmitted from animal species to humans. It is important to note that although rare, this is possible. In most cases humans acquire a zoonosis accidently. The animals they contract the disease from may or may not be symptomatic themselves. Dog owners should observe good hygienic principles and wash their hands after touching dogs and working with excreta. Because children are more investigative and likely to put anything in their mouths, it is not difficult to understand why they are at higher risk of zoonoses. As a rule, normal healthy people are at minimal risk of zoonoses with some notable exceptions.

19.8.1. Rabies

Albeit rare, rabies is a very serious zoonosis and always fatal in any mammal, including humans. Rabies is an infectious viral disease which affects the nervous system. It can only be transmitted through the saliva following a bite of rabid animals. The incubation period (interval from exposure to virus until symptoms become evident) may vary from 3-6 weeks in dogs but in exceptional circumstances may be much longer. The clinical signs in dogs are divided into separate stages (phases). The first is the prodromal stage; second the furious or excitable stage and thirdly the paralytic or dumb stage.

The prodromal phase lasts about 3 days and involves behavioural changes. Generally during this phase, not much is noticed besides friendly dogs may become more irritable and aggressive dogs more friendly. The fury phase lasts a week on average and during this phase affected dogs become irritable and aggressive. In the late stages of this phase dogs may become off-balance and seizure. During the last phase, the dog's ability to swallow becomes affected and hence the dog salivates excessively. Dogs will always die during this phase due to progressive paralysis and finally respiratory failure.

Annual vaccination of all dogs is advised in all areas where rabies is known to be endemic. In some of these areas where many clinical cases occur in dogs and exotic wildlife, it may even be prudent to have all dog handlers vaccinated against rabies as well. If one is bitten by a dog a physician should be consulted. If the animal is suspected to have rabies, your physician should immediately be informed about this as should the state veterinary authority so that they can advise on the correct course of action.

19.8.2. Bacterial infections

a) Leptospirosis

Leptospirosis is a bacterial disease spread through the urine of infected animals. Thus the main form of transmission is through contact with contaminated dog urine. Symptoms in man are mainly flu like symptoms but may progress to meningitis, jaundice and other complications. The clinical signs in the dog are fever, vomiting, diarrhoea, inappetence, anaemia and organ failure. Dogs in contact with farm animals and rodents are at increased risk. If the diagnosis is made timeously, treatment is usually very effective. Effective vaccines are available for dogs but these might not be protective against all local strains of the *Leptospira spp*.

b) Lyme disease

Lyme disease is a bacterial disease caused by *Borrelia burgdefori* which causes fever, rashes and generalised malaise. It is not a true zoonosis in the sense that one may contract the disease from the dog by direct contact but more because one may get the disease from ticks on dogs. The deer tick which lives on wildlife plays a crucial role in this disease's transmission to man.

Because it is a tick borne disease in some areas it is strongly advised that one regularly inspects oneself and the dogs following outdoor activities. It is advised that insecticidals effective against ticks are used before such excursions. Products which have a quick kill action or detaching agents are more likely to result in killing of the tick before it is able to transmit disease or to prevent it from biting humans in the first place.

c) Bacterial enteritis (Salmonellosis, *Campylobacter spp*, *Escherichia coli*)

Bacterial enteritis in dogs is very common but accurate diagnoses are seldom made. Infected dogs may be asymptomatic or show diarrhoea, abdominal pain, vomiting, shock, blood poisoning and death. Most cases will however respond well to treatment.

In humans it causes similar symptoms and the disease is usually self-limiting and resolves itself within 3-7 days. Fatal cases however have been reported in humans.

19.8.3. Endo and ectoparasites

a) Roundworms

Humans are usually incidental hosts of these worms but are not natural hosts and are rarely infected. Small children are more likely to be affected due to their habit of mouthing everything they touch. Following ingestion of the eggs or larvae, the eggs hatch and the larvae migrate through the body causing damage to the infected organs they travel through. Gardeners should be particularly vigilant.

b) Hookworms

In rare instances hookworms may harm human organs and cause disease symptoms whilst migrating through human organs and tissues. Since they can penetrate the skin of humans, they cause a condition of "sandworm infection or plumber's itch" with severe irritation and itching of the skin.

c) Tapeworms

Echinococcus and some of the other tapeworm infections in dogs pose huge potential dangers for humans. The human may act as accidental intermediate host by the inadvertent ingestion of tapeworm eggs passed by their dogs. In man the worm cysts may be located in the brain, organs, lungs, eye, muscles or connective tissues. These infections can be life threatening. This worm is present in many parts of the world.

d) Scabies

This is a disease caused by mites known as *Sarcoptes scabiei*. It causes disease in dogs and other domestic animals called mange. In humans it causes a severe itch and rash called scabies. This mange is highly contagious to other domestic animals and man. Cheyletiella mites may also cause problems but dogs are rarely affected. The latter mite has rabbits and cats as the primary host.

e) Fungal infections

Ringworm is not a worm, but it's the name given to the skin lesion caused by a fungus (mould). Ringworm causes hair loss in a circular shape with the edges showing up somewhat red. Although ringworm itself is usually not itchy, it may become infected and become itchy.

Ringworm is transmitted by the spores of the mould and direct contact with an infected animal is not always required. Dogs and cats can be carriers of the ringworm on their skin without showing any symptoms themselves. Older dogs have some immunity against ringworm infection and are less seldom affected whereas puppies are more susceptible. If there are many puppies on the premises, an outbreak of ringworm may ensue. At the earliest indication of a potential outbreak, the breeder should consult their veterinary surgeon to treat affected dogs and suggest measures to prevent further spread. Ringworm ointments, creams and shampoos are generally ineffective in treating affected dogs but may aid in decreasing the likelihood of spread by decreasing the number of infective spores released. Oral treatment using effective fungicides are indicated. During an outbreak, yet unaffected puppies may be treated using these drugs to prevent the infection from occurring in the first place and containing the outbreak.

19.8.4. Protozoal infections

a) Toxoplasmosis and pregnant women

Toxoplasmosis is strictly related to cats but it is included here as many dog owners keep cats and because it is a very important zoonosis. Toxoplasmosis poses a significant risk to women who are pregnant or plan to become pregnant. It is a rare but serious condition in both cats and dogs. The cat is the only definitive host and may act as a carrier and excretes oocysts in its faeces. Most people will during their childhood and early teens have been exposed to these oocysts and have built up immunity. This means that for those women who have already been exposed to the toxoplasma oocysts, the risk of infection is minimal and their pregnancy is not at peril as opposed to women who have never been exposed. For the latter there is a real danger that they may be infected during pregnancy, resulting in abortion or foetal defects. Pregnant women should therefore not handle the cat's litter tray. An epidemiological study showed that most people infected with toxoplasmosis got the condition from undercooked or raw meat and not from cat faeces. People that are immunocompromised (suffer from AIDS or are on immunosuppressive medication) are a lot more likely to develop clinical toxoplasmosis than others. The infection is caused by a parasite called *Toxoplasma gondi*. The clinical signs in people include fever, sore throat, muscle pain, malaise, swollen glands and vision impairment. However, most people will remain asymptomatic following infection. Also, most susceptible pregnant women will themselves not show clinical signs of disease besides very serious consequences for their pregnancy.

All animals and birds can be infected with the toxoplasmosis parasite but usually do not show any symptoms. Birds and rodents may harbour the parasite in their muscles and cats may become infected when eating their meat. Cats in turn spread the parasite in their faeces back to rodents; birds and also farm animals. Humans may then get the Toxoplasma oocysts directly from infected cat faeces or from eating infected meat from farm animals that is raw or undercooked. The critical period for infection in woman is at any stage of pregnancy. Infection of a susceptible (previously unexposed woman) may result in abortion, retarded foetal development, prematurity or stillbirth. Children from infected woman may suffer from various ailments including visual and mental disabilities, hydrocephalus (water on the brain), convulsions or death.

Treatment of an infected pregnant woman may prevent or lessen the disease in her unborn child. Treatment of an infected infant will also lessen the severity of the disease as the child grows but these options should all be discussed with an obstetrician. Affected cats usually show no symptoms. Cats are usually infective for less than a month but infected stool may remain so for up to a year.

Pregnant woman should take special precautions. First and foremost she should consult her gynaecologist, limit exposure to excreta of cats, keep cats indoors to decrease chance of them eating infected raw meat from animals, do not feed cats raw or undercooked meat and should avoid raw meat themselves. Also they should avoid stray cats.

b) Giardiasis

Giardia lamblia is a very small parasite only visible under a microscope. It can be the cause of acute or chronic diarrhoea in dogs, man and other animals. Dogs may be carriers as well. Routine hygiene and the use of disinfectants will reduce the risk of transmission. Vigilance should be increased when owners notice that their dogs are suffering from diarrhoea. Breeders suffering from chronic non responsive diarrhoea should at least mention the possibility of Giardia to their physician. Giardia is common in dog breeding colonies and is discussed in 14.4.7.

Chapter 19 Matters and Conditions Relating to Dogs Kept in Breeding Kennels

Acknowledgements

This book was created by a curious mind as a quest to serve my profession, a need to seek answers and to provide a more professional service to the needs of the dog breeder fraternity. It was completed with the support and encouragement of my lovely wife, Zelda and children, Kyle and Mira. They were victims of my frequent neglect. It is my sincere hope that this work will explain to them the many hours spent behind a computer screen and motivate my children in their own lives to distinguish themselves, ask questions and seek the answers irrespective of the efforts by others. I hope they may one-day experience gratification in both the journey and goal as I have. I thank them for the gracious response en-route.

My sincere thanks to Professor Johan Nöthling, in my eyes the giant of canine theriogenology, for his guidance and advice in matters academic in my career. He has been instrumental in laying the academic foundation for all my endeavours. Also to Professor Martin Schulman for his friendship, encouragement and assurance that I can do it.

To my partners Freek and Garreth and other colleagues and support staff at work. I thank them for their assistance and generally putting up with me. Although very many individuals have contributed in some way, several individuals need special mention. Rudi Zimmerman is singled out because he proved invaluable to improve language, logical flow and helped to make the book easier to understand by laymen. The following people also need mention and are thanked for their contributions. Drs Tania van Eeden, Freek Huberts, Vicky Reid and Mrs Sheryl Kloeck for proofreading the entire document and Drs Rachel Shuttleworth, Alan Kloeck, Sarah Miller, Louis Boag, Guy Fyvie, John Birrel and Mr. Frikkie van Kraayenburg for their proofreading of parts of the document. Shannon Mckay for her contribution on socialization. They all made valuable contributions by their constructive criticism. Dominique for the concept design of the cover and Kyle, Mira and Inge for adding conceptual ideas. Thank you all for your contributions.

Dr Sooryakanth Sasidharan is credited for his contribution to most of the genetics chapter in this book. Without his input this book would simply not be complete. I thank you very much Sasi, for your encouragement as well.

Many colleagues, fellow specialist theriogenologists and other specialists in their respective fields also need mention. Many of them have been referenced in this book and I am in awe of the great work they have published.

Collectively, the greatest contributions have been from breeders themselves. I am most appreciative of the inspiration by their passion and dedication without which this work chronicled would not exist. Thank you all, compiling this work would not have been possible without you.

About the Authors

Dr Kurt De Cramer

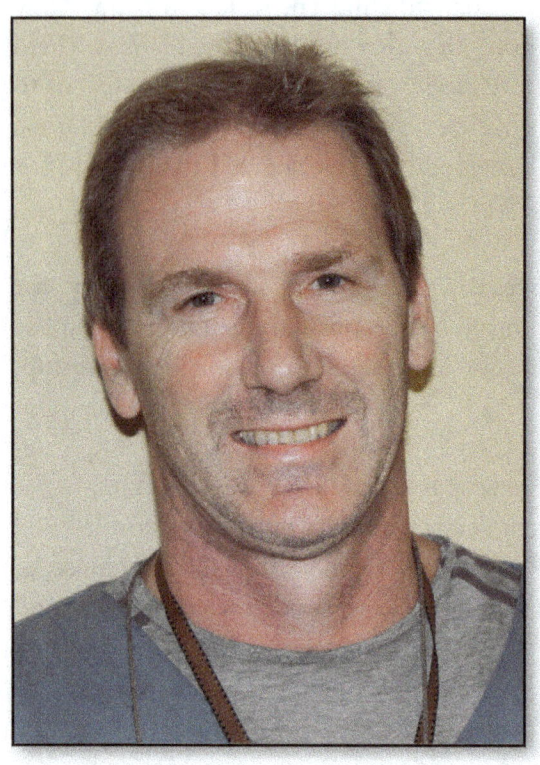

Dr Kurt De Cramer was born in Belgium in 1962, where he attended primary school. His family later immigrated to South Africa where he completed high school and qualified as a veterinary surgeon from the Faculty of Veterinary Science, Onderstepoort, University of Pretoria, in 1986. He completed his National service at the Bourke's Luck dog training unit where he was introduced to the breeding of service dogs and their health problems. He started his veterinary career at a research laboratory and entered private practice in 1992 when he co-founded the Rant-en-Dal Animal Hospital.

In furthering his studies he obtained his Master's degree MMedVet (Gyn) – Specialist theriogenologist (Animal reproduction) and PhD degree from the same university. His PhD study entailed planning elective caesarean section in high risk breeds. His thesis paved the way for planned elective caesarean sections as it is performed in women routinely and contains the discovery of the first ever confirmed monozygotic twins as well as freemartinism in dogs.

Dr De Cramer has remained in close contact with his Alma Mater through collaboration in research projects, acting as external for pre and post graduate examinations and as referee of research protocols and scientific articles. This collaboration has led to the publication of numerous articles in various international journals.

Dr De Cramer closely collaborates with dog and cat breeder associations. He has written and presented many breed specific seminars and held numerous talks on various aspects of dog and cat breeding. His habit of digitally capturing almost all cases he encounters in his practice has led to an extensive collection of digital images of veterinary interest, specifically on small animals and exotic species.

His inquisitive mind compels him to continue making a contribution to the science of dog breeding; constantly researching and solving clinical problems that breeders experience. This he manages despite time constraints placed upon him by private practice activities.

Dr De Cramer is married to Zelda and has two children, Kyle and Mira.

Dr Sooryakanth Sasidharan Priyadersini (Sasi)

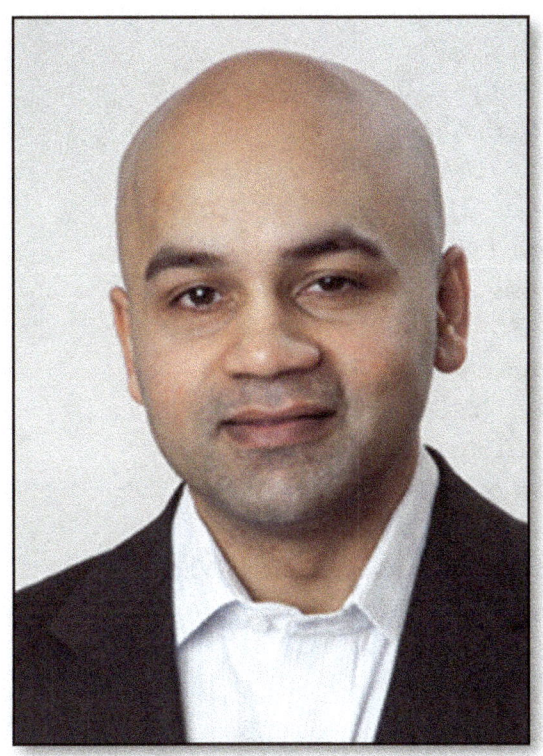

Dr Sooryakanth Sasidharan Priyadersini was born in Trivandrum, India, in 1976. He qualified as a Veterinary Surgeon from the College of Veterinary And Animal Sciences in Kerala, India in 2001 and moved to South Africa in the following year. In 2005 he obtained an MSc in Veterinary Science (Cum Laude) from the Faculty of Veterinary Science at the University of Pretoria, investigating sarcoid tumours in Cape mountain zebras. He later focused on the genetics of African cheetahs for his doctoral studies. In 2008 he moved into private practice in South Africa after passing the South African Veterinary Council Board Exam and later obtained his MRCVS from the Royal College of Veterinary Surgeons (UK) by examination in 2012. He has since been in private practice in the UK. His interests are canine and feline genomics and the evolving topics around testing for complex conditions. He firmly believes in a future where canine breeding and animal welfare is improved by genetic testing.

Keyword Index

abortion ...88
ad lib feeding ...32
agalactia ...97
aggression ...269
algae ...42
allergic dermatitis ...279
alternative healing ...261
anabolic steroid ...262
anasarca puppies see hydrops foetalis ...197
anoestrus ...55
antioxidants ...43
appetite stimulants ...37
artificial insemination ...151
artificial reproductive techniques ...151
balanoposthitis ...146
BARF diet ...23
bee sting ...283
behavioural modification ...262
benign prostatic hypertrophy ...138
biological value ...25
birth ...101
birth-mass ...187
brachycephaly ...5
breed identification ...230
breed standard ...18
breeding ...5
breeding dates ...86
breeding recommendations ...242
breeding soundness ...73
brucellosis see canine brucellosis ...165
caesarean section ...117
calcium gluconate ...116
calcium supplementation ...38
calcium: phosphorous ratio ...26
canine brucellosis ...165
canine herpesvirus ...162
canine parvovirus ...201
carbohydrates ...24
castration see neutering ...131
catflu see canine parvovirus ...201
cherry eye ...277
chilled semen ...73
chimeras ...160

chondroitin ...43
chromosomes ...217
circadian rhythm ...49
cleft lip see cleft palate ...192
cleft palate ...192
cloning ...159
coccidiosis ...205
colic ...190
colostrum ...95
congenital ...216
congenital abnormalities ...191
constipation ...35
coprophagia ...37
copulatory lock see genital lock ...60
corticosteroids ...262
cranial clefts ...191
creep feeding ...179
cruciate ligament rupture ...275
cryptorchidism ...140
cystic endometrial hyperplasia ...63
cytological dioestrus ...55
daily sperm output ...135
demodex ...256
dental care ...35
dermatophytosis see ringworm ...206
designer dogs ...221
developmental anomaly ...218
dewclaw removal ...170
deworming ...249
diabetes ...33
diarrhoea ...200
digestibility ...28
dioestrus ...55
DNA profiling ...229
Dominance ...218
dormitory effect ...56
due date see whelping date ...86
dysmaturity ...124
dystocia ...112
eclampsia see milk fever ...99
ectoparasites ...255
elbow dysplasia ...274
embryo transfer ...159

Keyword Index

encephalitozoön ...207
endoparasites ...247
enteritis ...201
ergogenic aids *see performance enhancing substances* ...44
euthanasia ...17
fading puppy ...197
false pregnancy *see pseudopregnancy* ...85
fats ...24
fecundity ...161
fertility ...71
fertilization ...79
fertilization period ...54
flat chest syndrome ...197
fleas ...257
flies ...257
foetal defects ...88
folate *see folic acid* ...41
folic acid ...41
fostering ...175
fresh semen ...151
frozen semen ...153
galactostasis ...98
gastric dilatation and volvulus ...280
gastroschisis ...194
genes ...216
genetic counselling ...242
genetic disorder ...216
genital lock ...60
genital tie *see genital lock* ...217
genomics ...216
genotype ...216
gestation length ...86
giardiasis ...206
glucosamine ...43
glucose ...199
glutamine ...42
health testing ...18
heart conditions ...281
heartworm ...251
heat cycle ...50
heat exhaustion ...282
hemiorchidectomy ...145
heritability ...219
heritability coefficient ...219
heritable ...216

heterozygous ...218
hip dysplasia ...270
homozygous ...218
hookworms ...248
hormone assays ...70
hospital-acquired disease ...205
hybridisation ...219
hydrocephalus ...195
hydrops foetalis ...197
hygiene ...259
hymen ...58
hyperfoetation ...xiv
hyperthermia *see heat exhaustion* ...282
hypertrophic osteodystrophy ...40
hypocalcaemia *see milk fever* ...99
hypoglycaemia ...199
identification of dogs ...261
inbreeding ...227
infectious juvenile pneumonia ...199
inguinal hernia ...194
inguinoscrotal hernia ...144
interoestrus interval ...49
juvenile cellulitis *see puppy strangles* ...198
kennel cough ...269
kennel management ...259
kennel vices ...268
labour induction *see parturition induction* ...93
labour *see parturition* ...101
lactation ...95
leptospirosis ...288
libido ...149
lick granuloma ...278
limb defects ...196
line breeding ...228
litter size ...84
lordosis reflex ...54
lyme disease ...289
maggots ...257
maiden bitch *see nulliparous* ...101
mammary tumours ...52
mange ...256
mastitis ...98
megaoesophagus ...278
milk fever ...99
milk replacers ...177
minute virus of canines ...165

Keyword Index

mites ...256
mixed breeds ...220
monoestrous ...50
multifactorial disease ...200
mushrooms ...44
mutation ...219
natural mating ...71
neonatal disease ...185
neonatal opthalmia ...198
neonatal septicaemia ...189
neonate ...169
neutering ...131
non-steroidal anti-inflammatory agents ...262
nosocomial disease *see hospital-acquired disease* ...205
nulliparous ...xv
Nutraceuticals ...43
Nutrition ...21
Obesity ...33
obsessive-compulsive disorder ...268
occipital hygroma ...276
oedematous puppies *see hydrops foetalis* ...197
oestrous cycle ...50
oestrus ...52
oestrus induction ...74
oestrus synchronization ...74
omega-3 and omega-6 fatty acids ...43
omphalocoel ...194
optimal breeding time ...66
optimum fertility ...71
orchitis *see testicular infection* ...142
orphan puppies ...172
osteochondritis dissicans ...26
outbreeding ...229
outcrossing *see outbreeding* ...229
outside tie *see slip mating* ...61
ovarian cysts ...64
ovariohysterectomy ...77
oxytocin ...115
panosteitis ...275
paraphimosis ...146
parentage testing ...85
parity ...52
parturition ...101
parturition date *see whelping date* ...86
parturition induction ...87

parturition management ...86
patella luxation ...275
pectus excavatum *see flat chest syndrome* ...197
penis ...145
performance enhancing substances ...44
periodontal disease ...35
persistent frenulum ...147
persistent heat ...56
pesticides ...45
phantom pregnancy *see pseudopregnancy* ...85
phimosis ...145
pica ...36
plaque ...35
poisonous plants ...44
polygenic inheritance ...221
polygynous ...81
polytocous ...50
post-whelping "blues" ...91
prebiotic ...42
predicting whelping dates ...86
pregnancy ...77
pregnancy diagnosis ...82
pregnancy length ...51
pregnancy termination ...93
prematurity ...124
prepotency ...228
priapism ...147
probiotic ...42
prolapsed gland of third eyelid *see cherry eye* ...277
prolonged pregnancy ...120
pro-oestrus ...53
prostate ...138
prostatic cancer ...139
prostatitis ...139
proteins ...25
pseudocyesis *see pseudopregnancy* ...85
pseudopregnancy ...85
puberty ...49 & 129
puerperal tetany *see milk fever* ...99
puppy temperament assessments ...266
pyometra ...65
rabies ...288 & 213
red gut ...285
reproductive cycle ...49
resorption ...80
restricted airway syndrome ...282

Keyword Index

retained deciduous teeth ...277
retained foetus ...90
retained placentas (afterbirths) ...90
rickets ...38
ringworm ...206
roundworms ...247
runts ...125
selection ...222
self-treatment ...261
semen banking ...158
semen collection ...132
semen quality ...133
sex ratios ...81
sex-linked genes ...244
sexual cycle ...49
short interoestrus intervals ...56
silent heat ...56
singleton ...119
skeletal abnormalities ...38
slip mating ...61
snake bite ...284
socialization ...263
soft pad ...276
spaying *see ovariohysterectomy* ...77
spermatogenesis ...129
spirocerca lupi ...251
split heat ...55
sterilization ...78
stillbirths ...161
stomach torsion *see gastric dilatation and volvulus* ...280
strangles ...198
stress ...267
strokes ...284
submandibular abscesses *see strangles* ...198
sudden death ...280
superfecundation ...136
superfoetation ...125
superovulation ...75
swimmer puppies ...196
tail docking ...171
tape worms ...249
taurine ...25
teeth fractures ...35
testicles ...131
testicular degeneration ...144

testicular hypoplasia ...144
testicular infection ...142
testicular neoplasia ...143
testicular torsion ...142
testicular trauma ...143
ticks ...255
tie *see genital lock* ...60
toxic milk syndrome ...191
toxins ...47 & 191
toxoplasmosis ...290
transmissible venereal tumour ...148
treats ...43
trivers-willard hypothesis ...81
twinning ...126
twisting of stomach *see gastric dilatation and volvulus* ...280
umbilical hernia ...194
urethral prolapse ...147
urine marking ...131
uterine haemorrhage ...86
uterine inertia ...112
uterine infections ...90
uterine prolapse ...92
uterine rupture ...91
uterine torsion ...89
vaccination ...210
vaginal cytology ...69
vaginal discharge ...57 & 88
vaginal fold prolapse ...57
vaginal hyperplasia *see vaginal fold prolapse* ...57
vaginal prolapse ...92
vaginitis ...62
vaginoscopy ...69
vasectomization ...130
verminosis *see worm infestation* ...247
vestibulo-vaginal strictures ...58
vitamin A ...41
vitamin B complex ...40
vitamin C ...39
vitamin D ...39
vitamin E ...42
walrus puppies *see hydrops foetalis* ...197
water ...47
water puppy *see hydrops foetalis* ...197
weaning ...180
whelping ...101

Keyword Index

whelping date ...86
whelping quarters ...105
whipworm ...249
white scours ...198
worm infestation ...247
zoonoses ...288

References

1. Abitbol,M.L., Inglis,S.R., 1997. Role of amniotic fluid in newborn acceptance and bonding in canines. Journal of Maternal-Fetal and Neonatal Medicine 6, 49-52.
2. Adesokan,H.K., Ajala,O.O., 2011. Vaginal bacterial flora and its antibiogram in bitches with vaginitis in Ibadan. Global Veterinaria 6, 316-319.
3. Ahmed,A.I.H., Versi,E., 1993. Prolonged pregnancy. Current Opinion in Obstetrics and Gynecology 5, 669-674.
4. Alan,M., Cetin,Y., Sendag,S., Eski,F., 2007. True vaginal prolapse in a bitch. Anim Reprod. Sci. 100, 411-414.
5. Al-Bassam,M.A., Thomson,R.G., O'Donnell,L., 1981. Involution abnormalities in the postpartum uterus of the bitch. Vet. Pathol. 18, 208-218.
6. Alderson, G.L.H. & Bodo I. (1992) Review of Species and Breed studies. (In Genetic conservation of domestic livestock.Vol 2. Ed. Alderson & Bodo) CABI, Wallingford.
7. Alderson,G.L.H. (1992) A system to maximise the maintenance of genetic variability in small populations. (In genetic conservation of domestic livestock. Vol 2. Ed. Alderson & Bodo) CABI, Wallingford.
8. Alexander,J.M., Wortman,A.C., 2013. Intrapartum Hemorrhage. Obstetrics and Gynecology Clinics of North America 40, 15-26.
9. Andersen A.M., Simpson M.E., 1973 The ovary and reproductive cycle of the dog (beagle). Geron-X incorporated, Los Altos California.
10. Andersen,K., 1975. Insemination with frozen dog semen based on a new insemination technique. Zuchthygiene 10, 1-4.
11. Arbeiter K 1993 Anovulatory ovarian cycles in dogs. Journal of reproduction and fertility.Supplement 47 453-456.
12. Argiolas,A., Gessa,G.L., 1991. Central functions of oxytocin. Neuroscience and Biobehavioral Reviews 15, 217-231.
13. Asher,L., Diesel,G., Summers,J.F., McGreevy,P.D., Collins,L.M., 2009. Inherited defects in pedigree dogs. Part 1: Disorders related to breed standards. The Veterinary Journal 182, 402-411.
14. Audet I, Laforest JP, Martineau GP & Matte JJ 2004 Effect of vitamin supplements on some aspects of performance, vitamin status, and semen quality in boars. Journal of animal science 82 626-633.
15. Austad,R., Lunde,A., Sjaastad,O.V., 1976. Peripheral plasma levels of oestradiol-17 beta and progesterone in the bitch during the oestrous cycle, in normal pregnancy and after dexamethasone treatment. J. Reprod. Fertil. 46, 129-136.
16. Baan,M., Taverne,M.A., de,G.J., Kooistra,H.S., Kindahl,H., Dieleman,S.J., Okkens,A.C., 2008. Hormonal changes in spontaneous and aglepristone-induced parturition in dogs. Theriogenology 69, 399-407.
17. Baan,M., Taverne,M.A., Kooistra,H.S., de,G.J., Dieleman,S.J., Okkens,A.C., 2005. Induction of parturition in the bitch with the progesterone-receptor blocker aglepristone. Theriogenology 63, 1958-1972.
18. Badinand,F., Fontbonne,A., Maurel,M.C., Siliart,B., 1993. Fertilization time in the bitch in relation to plasma concentration of oestradiol, progesterone and luteinizing hormone and vaginal smears. Journal of reproduction and fertility. Supplement 47, 63-67.
19. Bahrke,M.S., Yesalis,C.E., 2004. Abuse of anabolic androgenic steroids and related substances in sport and exercise. Current Opinion in Pharmacology 4, 614-620.
20. Bailey,R.E., 2009. Intrapartum fetal monitoring. American Family Physician 80.
21. Ball,R.L., Birchard,S.J., May,L.R., Threlfall,W.R., Young,G.S., 2010. Ovarian remnant syndrome in dogs and cats: 21 cases (2000-2007). Journal of the American Veterinary Medical Association 236, 548-553.
22. Barber,J., 2003. Parturition and dystocia. Small Animal Theriogenology 241-279.
23. Beccaglia M, Anastasi P, Grimaldi E, Rota A, Faustini M & Luvoni GC 2008 Accuracy of the prediction of parturition date through ultrasonographic measurement of fetal parameters in the queen. Veterinary Research Communications 32.
24. Beccaglia,M., Anastasi,P., Grimaldi,E., Rota,A., Faustini,M., Luvoni,G.C., 2008a. Accuracy of the prediction of parturition date through ultrasonographic measurement of fetal parameters in the queen. Veterinary Research Communications 32.
25. Beccaglia,M., Faustini,M., Luvoni,G.C., 2008b. Ultrasonographic study of deep portion of diencephalo-telencephalic vesicle for the determination of gestational age of the canine foetus. Reprod. Domest. Anim. 43, 367-370.
26. Beccaglia,M., Luvoni,G.C., 2006. Comparison of the accuracy of two ultrasonographic measurements in predicting the parturition date in the bitch. J. Small Anim Pract. 47, 670-673.
27. Beeley,L., 1986. Adverse effects of drugs in later pregnancy. Clinics in Obstetrics and Gynaecology 13, 197-214.
28. Bell,J.S., 2011. Researcher responsibilities and genetic counseling for pure-bred dog populations. Veterinary Journal 189, 234-235.
29. Bennett,D., 1974. Canine dystocia - a review of the literature. Journal of Small Animal Practice 15, 101-117.
30. Bergström,A., Fransson,B., Lagerstedt,A.S., Kindahl,H., Olsson,U., Olsson,K., 2010. Hormonal concentrations in bitches with primary uterine inertia. Theriogenology 73, 1068-1075.
31. Bergstrom,A., Fransson,B., Lagerstedt,A.S., Olsson,K., 2006. Primary uterine inertia in 27 bitches: aetiology and treatment. J. Small Anim Pract. 47, 456-460.
32. Bleicher,N., 1962. Behavior of the bitch during parturition. J. Am. Vet. Med. Assoc. 140, 1076-1082.
33. Blunden A.S. Hill CM, Brown BD & Morley CJ 1987 Lung surfactant composition in puppies dying of fading puppy complex. Research in Veterinary Science 42 113-118.
34. Böhm,A., Hoy,S., 1999. Influence of different factors on mortality in dog puppies (Beagle breed). Praktische Tierarzt 80, 856-865.
35. Boissevain,I., 2009. Galastop. Tijdschrift voor diergeneeskunde 134, 1031.
36. Bomzon,L., 1977. Rupture of the uterus following caesarean section in a bitch. Vet. Rec. 101, 38.
37. Botrü,F., Pavan,A., 2008. Enhancement Drugs and the Athlete. Neurologic Clinics 26, 149-167.
38. Bouchard,G., Plata-Madrid,H., Youngquist,R.S., Buening,G.M., Ganjam,V.K., Krause,G.F., Allen,G.K., Paine,A.L., 1992.

References

Absorption of an alternate source of immunoglobulin in puppies. American Journal of Veterinary Research 53, 230-233.

39. Bouchard,G.F., Solorzano,N., Concannon,P.W., Youngquist,R.S., Bierschwal,C.J., 1991. Determination of ovulation time in bitches based on teasing, vaginal cytology, and elisa for progesterone. Theriogenology 35, 603-611.
40. Bueno,L.M.C., Lopes,M.D., Lourenq,M.L.G., Prestes,N.C., Takahira,R.K., Derussi,A.A.P., Sudano,M.J., 2012. Lactato concentration in bitch and canine neonates born through cesarean section. Arquivo Brasileiro de Medicina Veterinaria e Zootecnia 64, 1442-1448.
41. Burke,T.M., Roberson,E.L., 1983. Fenbendazole treatment of pregnant bitches to reduce prenatal and lactogenic infections of Toxocara canis and Ancylostoma caninum in puppies. J. Am. Vet. Med. Assoc. 183, 987-990.
42. Burke,T.M., Roberson,E.L., 1985. Prenatal and lactational transmission of Toxocara canis and Ancylostoma caninum: experimental infection of the bitch at midpregnancy and at parturition. Int. J. Parasitol. 15, 485-490.
43. Burtonboy, S. Charlier P, Hertoghs J, Lobmann M, Wiseman A & Woods S 4-20-1991 Performance of high titre attenuated canine parvovirus vaccine in pups with maternally derived antibody. Vet.Rec. 128 377-381.
44. Cameron,E.Z., Linklater,W.L., 2007. Extreme sex ratio variation in relation to change in condition around conception. Biology Letters 3, 395-397.
45. Challis,J.R., 1980. Endocrinology of late pregnancy and parturition. International review of physiology 22, 277-324.
46. Challis,J.R.G., Bloomfield,F.H., Booking,A.D., Casciani,V., Chisaka,H., Connor,K., Dong,X., Gluckman,P., Harding,J.E., Johnstone,J., Li,W., Lye,S., Okamura,K., Premyslova,M., 2005. Fetal signals and parturition. Journal of Obstetrics and Gynaecology Research 31, 492-499.
47. Chan,L.Y.S., Chiu,P.Y., Siu,N.S.S., Wang,C.C., Lau,T.K., 2002. Diclofenac-induced embryotoxicity is associated with increased embryonic 8-isoprostaglandin F2+| level in rat whole embryo culture. Reproductive Toxicology 16, 841-844.
48. Chappuis, G. 1998 Neonatal immunity and immunisation in early age: lessons from veterinary medicine. Vaccine 16 1468-1472.
49. Chastant-Maillard,S., Fontbonne,A., Marseloo,N., Viaris de Lesegno,C., Thoumire,S., Reynaud,K., 2005. Assisted breeding in dogs. Point Veterinaire 36, 46-49.
50. Chatdarong,K., Tummaruk,P., Sirivaidyapong,S., Raksil,S., 2007. Seasonal and breed effects on reproductive parameters in bitches in the tropics: A retrospective study. Journal of Small Animal Practice 48, 444-448.
51. Christiansen,I.J., 1984. Dystocia, obstetric and postparturient problems. Reproduction in the Dog and Cat, 1st Edn. 197-221.
52. Concannon,P., Batista M, 1988 Canine semen freezing and artificial insemination. In: Kirk E (Ed.), Kirk E.: Current Veterinary Therapy., pp. 1247-1259.
53. Concannon,P., Hansel W., McEntee K., 1977. Changes in LH, progesterone and sexual behaviour associated with preovulatory luteinization in the bitch. Biology of Reproduction 17, 604-613.
54. Concannon,P., Rendano,V., 1983. Radiographic diagnosis of canine pregnancy: onset of fetal skeletal radiopacity in relation to times of breeding, preovulatory luteinizing hormone release, and parturition. American Journal of Veterinary Research 44, 1506-1511.
55. Concannon,P., Tsutsui,T., Shille,V., 2001. Embryo development, hormonal requirements and maternal responses during canine pregnancy. Journal of reproduction and fertility. Supplement 57, 169-179.
56. Concannon,P., Whaley,S., Lein,D., Wissler,R., 1983. Canine gestation length: variation related to time of mating and fertile life of sperm. American Journal of Veterinary Research 44, 1819-1821.
57. Concannon,P.W., 2000. Canine pregnancy: Predicting parturition and timing events of gestation. Recent Advances in Small Animal Reproduction.
58. Concannon,P.W., McCann,J.P., Temple,M., 1989. Biology and endocrinology of ovulation, pregnancy and parturition in the dog. J. Reprod. Fertil. Suppl 39, 3-25.
59. Concannon,P.W., Powers,M.E., Holder,W., Hansel,W., 1977. Pregnancy and parturition in the bitch. Biol. Reprod. 16, 517-526.
60. Crowell-Davis,S.L. 2007. Socialisation classes for puppies and kittens. CompendiumVet.com.
61. Darvelid,A.W., Linde-Forsberg C 1994 Dystocia in the bitch: A retrospective study of 182 cases. J.Small Anim.Pract. 35 402-407.
62. Daughton,C.G., Ruhoy,I.S., 2011. Green pharmacy and pharmEcovigilance: Prescribing and the planet. Expert Review of Clinical Pharmacology 4, 211-232.
63. Davidson,A.P. 2001 Uterine and fetal monitoring in the bitch. Vet.Clin.North Am.Small Anim Pract. 31 305-313.
64. Davidson,A.P., 2008. Dystocia management. Kirks' current veterinary therapy XIV 992-998.
65. Day,M.J., 2007. Immune System Development in the Dog and Cat. Journal of Comparative Pathology 137.
66. De Cramer,K.G.M., 2010. Surgical uterine drainage and lavage as treatment for canine pyometra. Journal of the South African Veterinary Association 81, 172-177.
67. De Cramer,K.G.M., van Bart. G.A., Huberts, F, 2010.Morbidity and mortality following envenomation by the common night adder (Causus rhombeatus) in three dogs. Journal of the South African Veterinary Association 83(1).
68. De Cramer,K.G.M., Stylianides,E., van Vuuren,M., Efficacy of vaccination at 4 and 6 weeks in the control of canine parvovirus. Veterinary Microbiology In Press, Accepted Manuscript.
69. de Gier,J., Kooistra,H.S., Djajadiningrat-Laanen,S.C., Dieleman,S.J., Okkens,A.C., 2006. Temporal relations between plasma concentrations of luteinizing hormone, follicle-stimulating hormone, estradiol-17+|, progesterone, prolactin, and +|-melanocyte-stimulating hormone during the follicular, ovulatory, and early luteal phase in the bitch. Theriogenology 65, 1346-1359.
70. Decaro,N., Martella,V., Buonavoglia,C., 2008. Canine Adenoviruses and Herpesvirus. Veterinary Clinics of North America - Small Animal Practice 38, 799-814.
71. Dehasse, J. 1994. Sensory, Emotional and Social Development of the Young Dog. The Bulletin for Veterinary Clinical Ethology, Vol 2, pp 6-29.
72. Derrier,M., Mercatello,A., 1997. Perioperative use of nonsteroidal antiinflammatory drugs. Clinical relevance and limites. Annales

Francaises d'Anesthesie et de Reanimation 16, 498-520.
73. Doak,R.L., Hall,A., Dale,H.E., 1967. Longevity of spermatozoa in the reproductive tract of the bitch. Journal of Reproduction and Fertility 13, 51-58.
74. Dolf,G., Gaillard,C., Schelling,C, Hofer,A., Leighton,E. (2008). Cryptorchidism and sex ratio are associated in dogs and pigs. Journal of Animal Science 86, 2480-2485.
75. Dominguez Fernandez De Tejerina,J.C., Pena Vega,F.J., 1995. Involution of placentation sites in the bitch. Medicina Veterinaria 12, 328-330+332.
76. Drobatz,K.J., Casey,K.K., 2000. Eclampsia in dogs: 31 cases (1995-1998). Journal of the American Veterinary Medical Association 217, 216-219.
77. Duffy,D.L., Serpell,J.A., 2009. Effect of early rearing environment on behavioural development of guide dogs. Journal of Veterinary Behaviour, Vol 4:6.
78. Edqvist,L.E., Johansson,E.D., Kasstrom,H., Olsson,S.E., Richkind,M., 1975. Blood plasma levels of progesterone and oestradiol in the dog during the oestrous cycle and pregnancy. Acta Endocrinol. (Copenh) 78, 554-564.
79. Eilts BE, Davidson AP, Hosgood G, Paccamonti DL & Baker DG 7-15-2005 Factors affecting gestation duration in the bitch. Theriogenology 64 242-251.
80. Ellender,L., Linder,M.M., 2005. Sports pharmacology and ergogenic aids. Primary Care - Clinics in Office Practice 32, 277-292.
81. Elwood,S., Whatling,C., 2006. Grape toxicity in dogs [5]. Veterinary Record 158, 492.
82. England,G.W.C., Concannon P W. Determination of the Optimal Breeding Time in the Bitch: Basic Considerations. Concannon P W, England G, Verstegen J, and Linde-Forsberg C. Recent Advances in Small Animal Reproduction. 2002. 6-8-2002.
83. England,G.C., 1991. ELISA determination of whole blood and plasma progestogen concentrations in bitches. Veterinary Record 129, 221-222.
84. Epe,C., Pankow,W.R., Hackbarth,H., Schnieder,T., Stoye,M., 1995. A study on the prevention of prenatal and galactogenic Toxocara canis infections in puppies by treatment of infected bitches with ivermectin or doramectin. Applied parasitology 36, 115-123.
85. Epe,C., Roesler,K., Schnieder,T., Stoye,M., 1999. Investigations into the prevention of neonatal Ancylostoma caninum infections in puppies by application of moxidectin to the bitch. Zentralbl. Veterinarmed. B 46, 361-367.
86. Evans,K.M., Adams,V.J., 2010. Proportion of litters of purebred dogs born by caesarean section. J. Small Anim Pract. 51, 113-118.
87. Fasanella,F.J., Shivley,J.M., Wardlaw,J.L., Givaruangsawat,S., 2010. Brachycephalic airway obstructive syndrome in dogs: 90 Cases (1991-2008). Journal of the American Veterinary Medical Association 237, 1048-1051.
88. Fayrer-Hosken,R., 2007. Embryo transfer in the dog and cat. Theriogenology 68, 382-385.
89. Fieni,F., Marnet,P.G., Martal J, Siliart B, Touzeau N, Bruyas JF & Tainturier D 2001 Comparison of two protocols with a progesterone antagonist aglepristone (RU534) to induce parturition in bitches. Journal of reproduction and fertility.Supplement 57 237-242.
90. Fitzgerald,K.T., Bronstein,A.C., Newquist,K.L., 2013. Marijuana Poisoning. Topics in Companion Animal Medicine 28, 8-12.
91. Fontbonne,A., Buff,S. Garnier,F., 2000. Recent data in canine reproductive physiology and hormones. Point Veterinaire 31 27-33.
92. Fontbonne,A., Badinand,F., 1993. Canine artificial insemination with frozen semen: comparison of intravaginal and intrauterine deposition of semen. Journal of reproduction and fertility. Supplement 47, 325-327.
93. Fowles,J.R., Banton,M.I., Pottenger,L.H., 2013. A toxicological review of the propylene glycols. Critical Reviews in Toxicology 43, 363-390.
94. FreedmanD., King,J.A., Elliot O. 1961. Critical period in the social development of dogs. Science, 133, pp 1016 – 1017.
95. Freshman,J.L., 2002. Semen collection and evaluation. Clin. Tech. Small Anim Pract. 17, 104-107.
96. Freshman,J.L., 2008. Pregnancy loss in the bitch. Kirks' current veterinary therapy XIV 986-989.
97. Gallant,J. 2006 Story of the African Dog.
98. Gaudet,D.A., Kitchell,B.E., 1985. Canine dystocia. Compend Contin Educ Pract Vet 7, 406-416.
99. Gendler,A., Brourman JD & Graf KE 2007 Canine dystocia: Medical and surgical management. Compendium: Continuing Education For Veterinarians 29 551-562.
100. Giesenberg,S., 2004. Pseudopregnancy in the bitch. Australian Veterinary Practitioner 34, 164-168.
101. Gillette,D.D., Filkins,M., 1966. Factors affecting antibody transfer in the newborn puppy. The American journal of physiology 210, 419-422.
102. Ginja,M.M.D., Silvestre,A.M. Gonzalo-Orden,J.M., Ferreira, A.J.A. 2010. Diagnosis, genetic control and preventive management of canine hip dysplasia: A review. The Veterinary Journal 184, 269–276.
103. Gobello,C., Corrada,Y., 2002. Noninfectious spontaneous pregnancy loss in bitches. Compendium on Continuing Education for the Practicing Veterinarian 24, 778-783.
104. Goodman,M., 2001. Ovulation timing. Concepts and controversies. Veterinary Clinics of North America - Small Animal Practice 31, 219-235, v.
105. Goodman,M., 2002. Demystifying ovulation timing. Clinical techniques in small animal practice 17, 97-103.
106. Görlinger,S., Galac,S., Kooistra,H.S., Okkens,A.C., 2005. Hypoluteoidism in a bitch. Theriogenology 64, 213-219.
107. Görlinger,S., Galac,S., Kooistra,H.S., Okkens,A.C., 2005. Hypoluteoidism in a bitch. Theriogenology 64, 213-219.
108. Gough,A., Thomas,A., 2010 Breed predispositions to disease in dogs and cats. Wiley-Blackwell, Oxford [etc.].
109. Groppetti,D., Pecile,A., Carro,A.P., Copley,K., Minero,M., Cremonesi,F., 2010. Evaluation of newborn canine viability by means of umbilical vein lactate measurement, apgar score and uterine tocodynamometry. Theriogenology.
110. Gubbels,E.J, Scholten,J, Janss,L, Rothuizen,J. (2009) Relationship of cryptorchidism with sex ratios and litter sizes in 12 dog breeds. Animal Reproduction Science 113, 187-195.

References

111. Günzel,A.R., Koivisto,P., Fougner,J.A., 1986. Electrical resistance of vaginal secretion in the bitch. Theriogenology 25, 559-570.
112. Gupta,R.C., 2012 Veterinary Toxicology.
113. Hare,E., Leighton,E.A. 2006. Estimation of Heritability of Litter Size in Labrador Retrievers and German Shepherd Dogs. Journal of Veterinary Behavior: Clinical Applications and Research 1 62-66.
114. Hedhammar,A.A., Malm,S., Bonnett,B., 2011. International and collaborative strategies to enhance genetic health in purebred dogs. The Veterinary Journal 189, 189-196.
115. Hewitt,D., England,G., 2000. Assessment of optimal mating time in the bitch. In Practice 22, 23-33.
116. Heymann,M.A., 1986. Non-narcotic analgesics. Use in pregnancy and fetal and perinatal effects. Drugs 32, 164-176.
117. Hoffmann,B., Riesenbeck,A., Klein,R., 1996. Reproductive endocrinology of bitches. Animal Reproduction Science 42, 275-288.
118. Hoffmann,B., Riesenbeck,A., Schams,D., Steinetz,B.G., 1999. Aspects on hormonal control of normal and induced parturition in the dog. Reprod. Domest. Anim. 34, 219-226.
119. Holladay,J.R. 1971 Routine use of doxapram hydrochloride in neonatal pups delivered by cesarean section. Vet.Med.Small Anim Clin. 66 28.
120. Hollinshead,F.K., Hanlon,D.W., Gilbert,R.O., Verstegen,J.P., Krekeler,N., Volkmann,D.H., 2010. Calcium, parathyroid hormone, oxytocin and pH profiles in the whelping bitch. Theriogenology 73, 1276-1283.
121. Holst,P.A.,Phemister,R.D., 1974. Onset of diestrus in the beagle bitch: definition and significance. American Journal of Veterinary Research 35 401-406.
122. Honnebier,M.B.O.M., Jenkins,S.L., Wentworth,R.A., Figueroa,J.P., Nathanielsz,P.W., 1991. Temporal structuring of delivery in the absence of a photoperiod: Preparturient myometrial activity of the rhesus monkey is related to maternal body temperature and depends on the maternal circadian system. Biology of Reproduction 45 617-625.
123. Hori,T., Tsutsui,T., Amano,Y., Concannon,P.W., 2012. Ovulation Day After Onset of Vulval Bleeding in a Beagle Colony. Reprod. Domest. Anim. 47, 47-51.
124. Hospes,R., Richter,B.R., Riesenbeck,A., Bostedt,H., 2004. Investigations on the reliability of commercial rapid blood progesterone assays in canine gynaecological diagnostics. Tierarztliche Praxis Ausgabe K: Kleintiere - Heimtiere 32, 247-251.
125. Hossein,M.S., Kim,M.K., Jang,G., Fibrianto,H.Y., Oh,H.J., Kim,H.J., Kang,S.K., Lee,B.C., 2007. Influence of season and parity on the recovery of in vivo canine oocytes by flushing fallopian tubes. Anim Reprod. Sci. 99, 330-341.
126. Humm,K.R., Adamantos,S.E., Benigni,L., Armitage-Chan,E.A., Brockman,D.J., Chan,D.L., 2010. Uterine rupture and septic peritonitis following dystocia and assisted delivery in a great dane bitch. Journal of the American Animal Hospital Association 46, 353-357.
127. Hyun,C., Filippich,L.J., 2006. Molecular genetics of sudden cardiac death in small animals : A review. The Veterinary Journal 171, 39-50.
128. Jang,G., Hong,S.G., Oh,H.J., Kim,M.K., Park,J.E., Kim,H.J., Kim,D.Y., Lee,B.C., 2008. A cloned toy poodle produced from somatic cells derived from an aged female dog. Theriogenology 69, 556-563.
129. Jeffcoate,I.A., Lindsay,F.E., 1989. Ovulation detection and timing of insemination based on hormone concentrations, vaginal cytology and the endoscopic appearance of the vagina in domestic bitches. Journal of reproduction and fertility. Supplement 39, 277-287.
130. Jöchle,W.,Andersen,A.C., 1977. The estrous cycle in the dog: A review. Theriogenology 7 113-140.
131. Johnson,C.A., 1986. Disorders of pregnancy. The Veterinary clinics of North America. Small animal practice 16, 477-482.
132. Johnson,C.A., 1991. Diagnosis and treatment of chronic vaginitis in the bitch. Veterinary Clinics of North America - Small Animal Practice 21, 523-531.
133. Johnson,C.A., 2008a. High-risk pregnancy and hypoluteoidism in the bitch. Theriogenology 70, 1424-1430.
134. Johnson,C.A., 2008b. Pregnancy management in the bitch. Theriogenology 70, 1412-1417.
135. Johnston,S.D., 1986. Parturition and dystocia in the bitch. Current Therapy in Theriogenology 500-501.
136. Johnston,S.D., Root Kustritz,M.V., Olson,P.N.S., 2001. Canine parturition - Eutocia and dystocia. Canine and Feline Theriogenology 105-128.
137. Jones,A.C.,Gosling,S.D. 2005. Temperament and personality in dogs (Canis familiaris): A review and evaluation of past research. Applied Animal Behaviour Science 95, pp 1 – 53 .
138. Kelley,R.B. (1946) Principles and methods of animal breeding. Angus & Robertson, Sydney.
139. Kelley,R., 2002. Canine reproductive management: factors affecting litter size. Proceedings of the Annual Conference of the Society for Theriogenology and American College of Theriogenology 291.
140. Kim,M.K.,Jang,G., Oh,H.J.,Yuda,F.,Kim,H.J.,Hwang,W.S.,Hossein M.S.,Kim,J.J.,Shin,N.S.,Kang,S.K.,Lee,B.C., 2007. Endangered wolves cloned from adult somatic cells. Cloning Stem Cells 9 130-137.
141. Kim,Y., Travis,A.J., Meyers-Wallen,V.N., 2007. Parturition prediction and timing of canine pregnancy. Theriogenology 68, 1177-1182.
142. King,J.W., 1978. Survival of single puppies. Veterinary Record 103, 433.
143. Kisko,C., 2011. Dog welfare: Registration of bitches undergoing repeat caesareans. Veterinary Record 168, 84.
144. Kraemer,D.C., Flow,B.L., Schriver,M.D., Kinney,G.M., Pennycook J.W., 1979. Embryo transfer in the nonhuman primate, feline and canine. Theriogenology 11 51-62.
145. Kramer,S 2007 Specifics of drug therapy during pregnancy and lactation in dogs and cats - A review. Praktische Tierarzt 88 958-967.
146. Kutzler,M.A., 2005. Induction and synchronization of estrus in dogs. Theriogenology 64, 766-775.
147. Kutzler,M.A., Mohammed,H.O., Lamb,S.V., Meyers-Wallen,V.N., 2003a. Accuracy of canine parturition date prediction from the initial rise in preovulatory progesterone concentration. Theriogenology 60, 1187-1196.
148. Kutzler,M.A., Yeager,A.E., Mohammed,H.O., Meyers-Wallen,V.N., 2003b. Accuracy of canine parturition date prediction using

fetal measurements obtained by ultrasonography. Theriogenology 60, 1309-1317.
149. Landsbergen,N., Pellicaan,C.H., Schaefers-Okkens,A.C., 2001. [The use of veterinary drugs during pregnancy of the dog]. Tijdschr. Diergeneeskd. 126, 716-722.
150. Lenard ZM, Hopper BJ, Lester NV, Richardson JL & Robertson ID 2007 Accuracy of prediction of canine litter size and gestational age with ultrasound. Australian Veterinary Journal 85 222-225.
151. Leroy,G., 2011. Genetic diversity, inbreeding and breeding practices in dogs: Results from pedigree analyses. The Veterinary Journal 189, 177-182.
152. Leroy,G., Rognon,X., 2012. Assessing the impact of breeding strategies on inherited disorders and genetic diversity in dogs. The Veterinary Journal 194, 343-348.
153. Leroyer,C., Tainturier,D., Dardenne,N., Destrumelle,S., Bencharif,D., 2002. Prediction of parturition in the bitch using measurement of plasma progesterone concentration. Revue de Medecine Veterinaire 153, 467-476.
154. Levy,X., Fontaine,E., Segalini,V., Fontbonne,A., 2009. Elective caesarean operation in the bitch using aglepristone before the pre-partum decline in peripheral progesterone concentration. Reprod. Domest. Anim 44 Suppl 2, 182-184.
155. Linde,F.C., Persson,G., 2007. A survey of dystocia in the Boxer breed. Acta Vet. Scand. 49, 8.
156. Linde-Forsberg,C., 1991. Achieving canine pregnancy by using frozen or chilled extended semen. Veterinary Clinics of North America - Small Animal Practice 21, 467-485.
157. Linde-Forsberg,C., Eneroth,A., 2000. Abnormalities in pregnancy, parturition and the periparturient period. Textbook of Veterinary Internal Medicine 1527-1539.
158. Linde-Forsberg,C., Forsberg,M., 1989. Fertility in dogs in relation to semen quality and the time and site of insemination with fresh and frozen semen. Journal of reproduction and fertility. Supplement 39, 299-310.
159. Linde-Forsberg,C., Forsberg,M., 1993. Results of 527 controlled artificial inseminations in dogs. Journal of reproduction and fertility. Supplement 47, 313-323.
160. Long,D., Mezza,R., Krakowka,S., 1978. Signs of impending parturition in the laboratory bitch. Lab Anim Sci. 28, 178-181.
161. Lopate,C. 2008 Estimation of gestational age and assessment of canine fetal maturation using radiology and ultrasonography: a review. Theriogenology 70 397-402.
162. Lush, J.L. (1945) Animal breeding plans . Iowa State College Press (3rd ed).
163. Luvoni,G.C., Beccaglia,M., 2006. The prediction of parturition date in canine pregnancy. Reprod. Domest. Anim 41, 27-32.
164. Macedo,S.P., Malm,C., Henry,M.R.J.M., Telles,L.F., Figueiredo,M.S., Fukushima,F.B., Neves,M.M., de Oliveira Cavalcanti,G.A., Chaves,M.S., Mascarenhas,R.M., de Albuquerque Lagares,M., Gheller,V.A., 2012. Endoscopic transcervical intrauterine artificial insemination in Labrador Retriever bitches. Research in Veterinary Science 92, 494-500.
165. McCarthy, J.C. & Blennerhasset, T. (1972) A preliminary estimate of the degree of inbreeding in Irish racing greyhounds. Dept Agriculture Journal 69 : 3-9.
166. Mellersh,C. DNA testing and domestic dogs. Mammalian Genome 23, 109-123. 1-2-2013.
167. Meyers-Wallen,V.N., 1995. The elective cesarian section. Current Veterinary Therapy 12 1085-1089.
168. Meyers-Wallen,V.N., 2007. Unusual and abnormal canine estrous cycles. Theriogenology 68 1205-1210.
169. Michel,E.,Reichler,I.M., 2008. Cesarean section in the dog and cat. Kleintierpraxis 53 490-498.
170. Milewski,L.M., Khan,S.A., 2006. An overview of potentially life-threatening poisonous plants in dogs and cats. Journal of Veterinary Emergency and Critical Care 16, 25-33.
171. Mir,F.,Billault,C.,Fontaine,E.,Sendra,J.,Fontbonne,A., 2011. Estimated pregnancy length from ovulation to parturition in the bitch and its influencing factors: A retrospective study in 162 pregnancies. Reproduction in Domestic Animals 46 994-998.
172. Moon-Massat,P.F.,Erb,H.N., 2002. Perioperative factors associated with puppy vigor after delivery by cesarean section. J.Am.Anim Hosp.Assoc. 38 90-96.
173. Nicholas,F.W., Crook,A., Sargan,D.R., 2011. Internet resources cataloguing inherited disorders in dogs. The Veterinary Journal 189, 132-135.
174. Nöthling,J.O. Effect of the addition of autologous prostatic fluid on the fertility of frozen-thawed dog semen after intravaginal insemination. -140pp. 1995. University of Pretoria RSAi.
175. Nöthling,J. O., Irons,P. C., Gerber, D.,Schulmann, M. L. The use of plasma progesterone concentration to predict the optimal breeding time in bitches 6 days in advance. Theriogenology 59[1], 225. 2003.
176. Nöthling,J.O., Gerber,D., Colenbrander,B., Dijkstra,M., Bakker,T., De Cramer,K., 2007. The effect of homologous prostatic fluid on motility and morphology of dog epididymal spermatozoa extended and frozen in Biladyl with Equex STM paste or Andromed. Theriogenology 67, 264-275.
177. Oh,H.J., Kim,M.K., Jang,G., Kim,H.J., Hong,S.G., Park,J.E., Park,K., Park,C., Sohn,S.H., Kim,D.Y., Shin,N.S., Lee,B.C., 2008. Cloning endangered gray wolves (Canis lupus) from somatic cells collected postmortem. Theriogenology 70, 638-647.
178. Okkens AC, Hekerman TW, de Vogel JW & van HB 1993 Influence of litter size and breed on variation in length of gestation in the dog. Vet.Q. 15 160-161.
179. Olson P.N., Thrail M.A., Wykes P.M., Husted P.W., Nett T.M., Sawyer H.R., 1984. Vaginal cytology. Part I. A useful tool for staging the canine oestrous cycle. The compendium of continuing education 6, 288-297.
180. Olson,P.N., Johnston,S.D., Root,M.V., Hegstad,R.L., 1992. Terminating pregnancy in dogs and cats. Animal Reproduction Science 28, 399-406.
181. Olson,P.N., Wrigley,R.H., Husted,P.W., Bowen,R.A., Nett,T.M., 1989. Persistent estrus in the bitch. Textbook of Veterinary Internal Medicine 1792-1796.
182. Onclin,K.,Verstegen,J.P.,1999. Comparisons of different combinations of analogues of PGF2 alpha and dopamine agonists for the termination of pregnancy in dogs. Vet.Rec. 144 416-419.

References

183. Ostrander,E.A., 2012 Genetics of the Dog. CAB International.
184. Pearson,H., 1973. The complications of ovariohysterectomy in the bitch. Journal of Small Animal Practice 14, 257-266.
185. Pfaffenberger,C.J. (1963) The new knowledge of dog behavior . Howell, New York.
186. Phemister RD, Holst PA, Spano JS & Hopwood ML 1973 Time of ovulation in the beagle bitch. Biol.Reprod. 8 74-82.
187. Poffenbarger,E.M.,Olson,P.N.,Chandler,M.L.,Seim,H.B.,Varman,M. 1991. Use of adult dog serum as a substitute for colostrum in the neonatal dog. American Journal of Veterinary Research 52 1221-1224.
188. Poppenga,R.H., 2010. Poisonous plants. EXS 100, 123-175.
189. Poppenga,R.H., Oehme,F.W., 2010 Pesticide Use and Associated Morbidity and Mortality in Veterinary Medicine., pp. 285-301.
190. Pretzer,S.D., 2008. Bacterial and protozoal causes of pregnancy loss in the bitch and queen. Theriogenology 70 320-326.
191. Pretzer,S.D., 2008. Medical management of canine and feline dystocia. Theriogenology 70 332-336.
192. Puschner,B., Wegenast,C., 2012. Mushroom Poisoning Cases in Dogs and Cats: Diagnosis and Treatment of Hepatotoxic, Neurotoxic, Gastroenterotoxic, Nephrotoxic, and Muscarinic Mushrooms. Veterinary Clinics of North America - Small Animal Practice 42, 375-387.
193. Rehfeld, C.E. (1970). Definition of relationships in a closed beagle colony. Am.J.Vet.Res . 31 : 723-32.
194. Robinson,R., 1973. Relationship between litter size and weight of dam in the dog. Veterinary Record 92, 221-223.
195. Ronsse,V., Verstegen,J., Thiry,E., Onclin,K., Aeberl+¬,C., Brunet,S., Poulet,H., 2005. Canine herpesvirus-1 (CHV-1): Clinical, serological and virological patterns in breeding colonies. Theriogenology 64, 61-74.
196. Root Kustritz,M.V., 2007. The value of canine semen evaluation for practitioners. Theriogenology 68, 329-337.
197. Sampson,J., 2011. How the Kennel Club is tackling inherited disorders in the United Kingdom. The Veterinary Journal 189, 136-140.
198. Schlafer,D.H., 2012. Diseases of the canine uterus. Reprod. Domest. Anim. 47, 318-322.
199. Schroeder,M., Munnich,A., Falkenberg,U., Heuwieser,W., 2006. Tocodynomometry as a non-invasive method for monitoring labour patterns, delivery and dystocia in the dog to reduce neonatal mortality. Reprod Domest Anim 4131.
200. Schutte AP 1967 Canine vaginal cytology. 3. Compilation and evaluation of cellular indices. Journal of Small Animal Practice 8 313-317.
201. Scott, J.P., Fuller, J.L. 1965. Dog Behaviour, the Genetic Basis. Univ. of Chicago Press, Chicago.
202. Seefeldt,A., Schöne,J., Brussow,N., Bunck,C., Hoppen,H.O., Beyerbach,M., Gunzel-Apel,A.R., 2007. Relevance and accuracy of ovulation timing with regard to prediction of parturition in the dog. Tierarztliche Praxis Ausgabe K: Kleintiere - Heimtiere 35, 188-192.
203. Slutsky,J., Raj,K., Yuhnke,S., Bell,J., Fretwell,N., Hedhammar,A., Wade,C., Giger,U., 2013. A web resource on DNA tests for canine and feline hereditary diseases. The Veterinary Journal.
204. Smith,F.O., 1986. Postpartum diseases. Vet. Clin. North Am. Small Anim Pract. 16, 521-524.
205. Smith,F.O., 2007. Challenges in small animal parturition--timing elective and emergency cesarian sections. Theriogenology 68, 348-353.
206. Soderberg,S.F., 1986. Canine breeding management. The Veterinary clinics of North America. Small animal practice 16, 419-433.
207. Spady,T.C., Ostrander,E.A., 2008. Canine Behavioral Genetics: Pointing Out the Phenotypes and Herding up the Genes. The American Journal of Human Genetics 82, 10-18.
208. Stolla,R., Dusi-F+ñrber,B., Stengel,B., Schmid,G., Braun,J., 1999. Dystocia in the bitch: A retrospective study. Wiener Tierarztliche Monatsschrift 86, 145-149.
209. Summers,J.F., Diesel,G., Asher,L., McGreevy,P.D., Collins,L.M., 2010. Inherited defects in pedigree dogs. Part 2: Disorders that are not related to breed standards. The Veterinary Journal 183, 39-45.
210. Tamler,R., Mechanick,J.I., 2007. Dietary Supplements and Nutraceuticals in the Management of Andrologic Disorders. Endocrinology and Metabolism Clinics of North America 36, 533-552.
211. Taverne MA, Okkens AC & van Oord R 1985 Pregnancy diagnosis in the dog: a comparison between abdominal palpation and linear-array real-time echography. Veterinary Quarterly 7 249-255.
212. Toaff,M.E., Hezroni,J., Toaff,R., 1977. Effect of diazepam on uterine activity during labor. Israel Journal of Medical Sciences 13, 1007-1012.
213. Traas,A.M., 2008. Resuscitation of canine and feline neonates. Theriogenology 70, 343-348.
214. Traas,A.M., Casal,M., Haskins,M., Henthorn,P., 2006. Genetic counseling in the era of molecular diagnostics. Theriogenology 66, 599-605.
215. Trivers,R.L., Willard,D.E., 1973. Natural selection of parental ability to vary the sex ratio of offspring. Science 179, 90-92.
216. Tsutsui,T., 1989. Gamete physiology and timing of ovulation and fertilization in dogs. Journal of reproduction and fertility. Supplement 39, 269-275.
217. Tsutsui,T., Hori,T., Kawakami,E., 2001. Intratubal transplantation of early canine embryos. J. Reprod. Fertil. Suppl 57, 309-314.
218. Tsutsui,T., Hori,T., Kirihara,N., Kawakami,E., Concannon,P.W., 2006. Relation between mating or ovulation and the duration of gestation in dogs. Theriogenology 66, 1706-1708.
219. Tsutsui,T., Murata,Y., 1982. Variations in body temperature in the late stage of pregnancy and parturition in bitches. Nippon juigaku zasshi. The Japanese journal of veterinary science 44, 571-576.
220. Tsutsui,T., Shimizu,T., Ohara,N., Shiba,Y., Hironaka,T., Orima,H., Ogasa,A., 1989. Relationship between the number of sperms and the rate of implantation in bitches inseminated into unilateral uterine horn. Nippon juigaku zasshi. The Japanese journal of veterinary science 51, 257-263.
221. Tsutsui,T., Takahashi,F., Hori,T., Kawakami,E., Concannon,P.W., 2009. Prolonged duration of fertility of dog ova. Reprod. Domest. Anim. 44, 230-233.

222. Ubbink, G.J., Knol, B.W. & Bouw, J. (1992) The relationship between homozygosity and the occurrence of specific diseases in Bouvier Belge des Flandres dogs in the Netherlands. Vet. Quart . 14: 137-40.
223. Urfer,S.R., 2009. Inbreeding and fertility in Irish Wolfhounds in Sweden: 1976 to 2007. Acta Veterinaria Scandinavica 51.
224. van Arendonk,J.A.M., Liinamo,A.E., 2005. Animal breeding and genomics: Perspectives for dog breeding. The Veterinary Journal 170, 3-5.
225. Van Duijkeren,E., 1992. Significance of the vaginal bacterial flora in the bitch: A review. Veterinary Record 131, 367-369.
226. Van Hooft,P., Prins,H.H., Getz,W.M., Jolles,A.E., Van Wieren,S.E., Greyling,B.J., Van Helden,P.D., Bastos,A.D., 2010. Rainfall-driven sex-ratio genes in African buffalo suggested by correlations between Y-chromosomal haplotype frequencies and foetal sex ratio. BMC Evolutionary Biology 10.
227. Veronesi,M.C.,Panzani,S.,Faustini,M.,Rota,A., 2009. An Apgar scoring system for routine assessment of newborn puppy viability and short-term survival prognosis. Theriogenology 72 401-407.
228. Veronesi,M.C., Battocchio,M., Marinelli,L., Faustini,M., Kindahl,H., Cairoli,F., 2002. Correlations among body temperature, plasma progesterone, cortisol and prostaglandin F2alpha of the periparturient bitch. J. Vet. Med. A Physiol Pathol. Clin. Med. 49, 264-268.
229. Verstegen,J., Dhaliwal,G., Verstegen-Onclin,K., 2008a. Canine and feline pregnancy loss due to viral and non-infectious causes: A review. Theriogenology 70, 304-319.
230. Verstegen,J., Dhaliwal,G., Verstegen-Onclin,K., 2008b. Mucometra, cystic endometrial hyperplasia, and pyometra in the bitch: Advances in treatment and assessment of future reproductive success. Theriogenology 70, 364-374.
231. Verstegen-Onclin,K., Verstegen,J., 2008. Endocrinology of pregnancy in the dog: a review. Theriogenology 70, 291-299.
232. Vilà,C.,Maldonado,J.E.,Wayne,R.K.,1999. Phylogenetic relationships, evolution, and genetic diversity of the domestic dog. Journal of Heredity 90, 71–77.
233. Volkmann,D.H., Kutzler,M.A., Wheeler,R., Krekeler,N., 2006. The use of deslorelin implants for the synchronization of estrous in diestrous bitches. Theriogenology 66, 1497-1501.
234. Von Heimendahl A & Cariou M 2009 Normal parturition and management of dystocia in dogs and cats. In Practice 31 254-261.
235. Wahl,J.M., Herbst,S.M., Clark,L.A., Tsai,K.L., Murphy,K.E., 2008. A review of hereditary diseases of the German shepherd dog. Journal of Veterinary Behavior: Clinical Applications and Research 3, 255-265.
236. Warren,J.B.,Anderson,J.M.,2010. Newborn respiratory disorders. Pediatrics in review 31 (12),487-496.
237. Willis, M.B. (1989) Genetics of the Dog. Witherbys, London.
238. Wilson,B.J., Wade,C.M., 2012. Empowering international canine inherited disorder management. Mammalian Genome 23, 195-202.
239. Wilson,M.S., 1993. Non-surgical intrauterine artificial insemination in bitches using frozen semen. Journal of reproduction and fertility. Supplement 47, 307-311.
240. Wood, J.L.N., Lakhani, K.H., Henley, W.E., 2004. An epidemiological approach to prevention and control of three common heritable diseases in canine pedigree breeds in the United Kingdom. The Veterinary Journal 168 14–27.
241. Zonturlu,A.K., Aksoy,O.A., Kacar,C., 2008. Gestation duration and rectal temperature changes during peripartum period in dogs. Journal of Applied Animal Research 33, 199-200.

www.ingramcontent.com/pod-product-compliance
Lightning Source LLC
Chambersburg PA
CBHW080902010526
44118CB00016B/2238